Novel Pharmacological Interventions for Alcoholism

Claudio A. Naranjo Edward M. Sellers
Editors

Novel Pharmacological Interventions for Alcoholism

With 51 Illustrations

Springer-Verlag
New York Berlin Heidelberg London Paris
Tokyo Hong Kong Barcelona Budapest

Claudio A. Naranjo
Addiction Research Foundation
Toronto, Ontario M5S 2S1
Canada

Edward M. Sellers
Addiction Research Foundation
Toronto, Ontario M5S 2S1
Canada

Library of Congress Cataloging-in-Publication Data
International Society for Biomedical Research on Alcoholism. Congress (5th : 1990 : Toronto, Ont.)
Novel pharmacological interventions for alcoholism : proceedings of the satellite symposium to the Fifth Congress of the International Society for Biomedical Research on Alcoholism, Toronto, Canada, 16–17, June 1990 / editors, C.A. Naranjo, Edward M. Sellers.
p. cm.
Includes bibliographical references and index.
ISBN 0-387-97741-4
1. Alcoholism—Chemotherapy—Congresses. 2. Alcoholism—Research--Methodology—Congresses. 3. Alcoholism—Animal models—Congresses. I. Naranjo, C. A. II. Sellers, E. M. (Edward M.) III. Title.
RC565.I546 1990
616.86′1061—dc20 91-37646

Printed on acid-free paper.

Production managed by Henry Krell; manufacturing supervised by Jacqui Ashri.
Camera-ready copy prepared by the editors.
Printed and bound by BookCrafters Inc., Chelsea, MI.
Printed in the United States of America.

9 8 7 6 5 4 3 2 1

ISBN 0-387-97741-4 Springer-Verlag New York Berlin Heidelberg
ISBN 3-540-97741-4 Springer-Verlag Berlin Heidelberg New York

Acknowledgments

This book is derived from the Satellite Symposium to the Fifth Congress of the International Society for Biomedical Research on Alcoholism (ISBRA-90) entitled "Novel Pharmacological Interventions for Alcoholism," which was held on June 16 and 17, 1990, at the Addiction Research Foundation in Toronto, Canada. Financial support for the meeting was generously provided by several institutions listed below. Their generous contributions made this symposium possible.

We would like to acknowledge the help of all the contributors to this book. They promptly and efficiently attended to our several requests. It has been a pleasure to work with them. The Ewing Marion Kauffman Foundation (U.S.A.) deserves special mention for providing generous financial support. We would also like to thank the staff of the Clinical Pharmacology Program, Addiction Research Foundation, for their many contributions to the symposium and to the book. Mrs. Linda Neuman helped with the preparation of several manuscripts. Also, Dr. Usoa Busto and Ms. Karen Bremner helped with the organization and implementation of the symposium as well as the editing of the book.

We would also like to thank the other members of the Program Committee, Drs. R. Deitrich, L. Grupp, and L. Reid, for helping us to organize this Conference.

We would like to gratefully acknowledge the following institutions which helped to defray part of the costs of the symposium:

Abbott Laboratories (U.S.A.)
Addiction Research Foundation (Canada)
Ciba-Geigy (U.S.A.)
Eli Lilly Canada
Ewing Marion Kauffman Foundation (U.S.A.)
Hoffman-La Roche, Inc. (U.S.A.)
Lilly Research Laboratories (U.S.A.)
Novopharm (Canada)
Rhone-Poulenc Pharma, Inc. (Canada)
Roche Pharmaceuticals (U.S.A.)
Squibb Canada, Inc.

Contents

Part III. Opioids and Alcohol Consumption

Part IV. The Role of Other Neurotransmitters in Regulating Alcohol Intake

Poster Papers

General Methodologic Issues

Serotonin and Alcohol Consumption

Opioids and Alcohol Consumption

The Role of Other Neurotransmitters in Regulating Alcohol Intake

Contributors

Manuella S. Adrian Statistical Research, Addiction Research Foundation, Toronto, Ontario M5S 2S1, Canada

Zalman Amit Center for Research on Drug Dependency, Concordia University, Sir George Williams Campus, Montreal, Quebec, Canada

Bruce Berg University of Pennsylvania, School of Medicine, Addiction Research Center, Philadelphia, PA 19104, USA

Edward J. Bilsky Addictions Research Laboratory, Rensselaer Polytechnical Institute, Troy, NY 12180-3590, USA

Bruna Brands Clinical Pharmacology Program, Addiction Research Foundation, Toronto, Ontario, M5S 2S1, Canada

Che-Ping Cheng Section on Cardiology, Bowman Gray School of Medicine, Winston-Salem, NC 27103, USA

Jonathan Chick Royal Edinburgh Hospital, Edinburgh EH10 5DF Scotland

Richard A. Deitrich University of Colorado, Dept. of Pharmacology, Denver, CO 80262, USA

John Delconte Addictions Research Laboratory, Rensselaer Polytechnical Institute, Troy, NY 12180-3590, USA

Jorgan A. Engel Department of Pharmacology, University of Goteborg, 33 Goteborg, Sweden

Morris D. Faiman The University of Kansas, School of Pharmacy, Department of Pharmacology & Toxicology, Lawrence, KS 66045-2500, USA

Janice C. Froehlich Indiana University, School of Medicine, Emerson Hall 421, Indianapolis, IN 46223, USA

David V. Gauvin University of Oklahoma, Department Psychiatry & Behavioral Sciences, Research Bldg, Oklahoma City, OK 73190, USA

Larry A. Grupp Department of Pharmacology, University of Toronto, Toronto, Ontario M5S 1A8, Canada

Guy Higgins Psychopharmacological Research, Addiction Research Foundation, Toronto, Ontario M5S 2S1, Canada

Christopher Hubbell Addictions Research Laboratory, Rensselaer Polytechnical Institute, Troy, NY 12180-3590, USA

Adam Jaffe Yale University, School of Medicine, New Haven, CT 06511, USA

Henry R. Kranzler Department of Psychiatry, The University of Connecticut, Health Center, School of Medicine, Farmington, CT 06032, USA

Collins E. Lewis Department of Psychiatry, Jewish Hospital, St. Louis, MO 63110, USA

Markku Linnoila Lab. of Clinical Studies, NIH Clinical Centre, Bethesda, MD 20892, USA

John Littleton Department of Biochemistry, Kings College, Strand, London WC2R 2LS, UK

Jorge Mardones Department of Pharmacology, Faculty of Medicine, University of Chile, Santiago, Chile

William J. McBride Indiana University School of Medicine, Department of Psychiatry, Indianapolis, IN 46223, USA

Roger E. Meyer Department of Psychiatry, University of Connecticut Health Center, Farmington, CT 06032, USA

H.T. Nagasawa Medical Research Laboratories, VA Medical Center, Minneapolis, MN 55417, USA

Claudio A. Naranjo Departments of Pharmacology and Medicine, University of Toronto and Clinical Pharmacology Program, Addiction Research Foundation, Toronto, Ontario M5S 2S1, Canada

Michael Nichols Addictions Research Laboratory, Rensselaer Polytechnical Institute, Troy, NY 12180-3590, USA

Stephanie O'Malley Yale University School of Medicine, New Haven, CT 06511, USA

Isidore Pelc Department of Psychiatry and Medical Psychology, Free University of Brussells, Brugman Campus, 4-1020 Brussells, Belgium

Michael Phillips New York Medical College, St. Vincents Medical Center, Staten Island, NY 10310, USA

Larry D. Reid Department of Psychology and Neuroscience, Rensselaer Polytechnical Institute, Department of Psychology, Troy, NY 12180-3590, USA

Edward M. Sellers Departments of Pharmacology, Medicine and Psychiatry, University of Toronto and Psychopharmacology Research, Addiction Research Foundation, Toronto, Ontario M5S 2S1, Canada

William Shoemaker University of Connecticut Health Center, School of Medicine, Farmington, CT 06032, USA

John D. Sinclair Research Labs, Alko Ltd., POB 350 SF-00101, Helsinki, Finland

Tony Toneatto Behavioral Treatment Research, Addiction Research Foundation, Toronto, Ontario M5S-2S1, Canada

E. Vavrousek-Jacuba University of Connecticut Health Center, School of Medicine, Farmington, CT 06032, USA

J.R. Volpicelli University of Pennsylvania, School of Medicine, Addiction Research Center, Philadelphia, PA 19104, USA

Walter Zieglgänsberger Clinical Neuropharmacology, Max Planck Institut für Psychiatrie, Kraepelinstr. 2, D-8000 München 40, Germany

Part I
General Methodologic Issues

1
Animal Models for Testing Drug Effects on Alcohol Consumption

R.A. Deitrich

Introduction:

Perhaps there is no area of alcohol related research so diverse in the methods used than the area of preference testing. The number and variety of paradigms for testing an animal's preference or rejection of alcohol solutions seeming is limited only by the number of investigators in the field. This has led to an amazing variety of paradigms and interpretations. While there are now a number of accepted findings, the path to these findings would have been greatly accelerated if a standardized testing paradigm had been employed by investigators in order to make comparisons between laboratories easier. Many studies are internally consistent but the effects observed may be peculiar to the paradigm used and not generally applicable.

An example from another field may illustrate the situation. Many years ago, testing for analgesic effects of opiate like drugs was an important topic for animal research. A simple procedure was developed which consisted of placing a rat's tail over a photoelectric cell and a heat lamp was positioned such that the rat flicked its tail away in a few seconds. The lengthening of this time was a measure of the effectiveness of the analgesic. This became known as the tail-flick test and was the standard test for many years. Later it was used to validate newer techniques, making a stable base for comparison between laboratories (D'Amour and Smith, 1941). Had a similar standardized procedure for alcohol preference testing been instituted 20 years ago, much time and effort might have been saved. In any case, it is the thesis of this paper that such a standardized procedure should be instituted even now so that comparisons between laboratories can be more easily made. Exactly what this procedure should be is open to debate, but assuming that it is desirable, if not necessary, a suggested paradigm will be presented. Such a paradigm would be used either as the method of testing or as a check on whatever procedure is used. There are a number of areas that need attention. Some of these are:

A. What animal model should be used?

If the goal of a study is to measure the effectiveness of some drug to reduce alcohol intake, then obviously one must have some intake to begin with. A great majority of the studies have been carried out with rats, for a variety of reasons such as size and expense. As a result of these considerations, a vast literature has been developed using rats as a model. Other studies have been done with dogs, pigs, and primates, but the expense and relatively small data base make these animals less desirable. The use of primates has the advantage that they are much closer to humans phylogenetically. The disadvantage, besides expense, however is that they are often used over and over in experiment after experiment with unknown consequences to the most recent protocol.

There are a variety of techniques used to obtain sufficient intake of ethanol in rodents to be able to measure a decrease. One may use an inbred strain with significant intake, for example the M520/N or MR/N rats (Li and Lumeng, 1984). Another procedure often employed is to screen a large group of randomally bred animals and use the high drinkers, or sometimes both the high and low drinkers (Gill et al, 1984). In effect, this is the technique used for the base generation for a selective breeding program. A more advantageous procedure is to actually use animals that have been selectively bred for ethanol preference from a genetically defined base population. While there are four rat lines currently bred for ethanol preference, the UChA and UChB (Mardones and Segovia-Riquelme, 1983), the AA and ANA rats (Eriksson and Rusi 1981) the P and NP (Li et al 1981) and SP and SNP lines (Fadda, 1990), none of them were bred from a genetically defined, reproducible, heterogeneous stock. Currently a well-designed breeding project to do this is underway with the high (HAD) and low (LAD) alcohol drinking rats (Froehlich et al, 1990) using the N/Nih heterogeneous stock of rats as a base. These rats, although in short supply, are the best compromise at the moment. It should be pointed out, that while the selection

Another issue that has not usually been approached is the issue of single caging of animals. It has been known for many years that single caging animals is a stress condition (Conger et al 1951). Yet nearly all preference studies are done on singly caged animals because it is impossible to determine which animal is drinking without direct observation, or by video taping. However, if a laboratory is set up to automatically record alcohol intake (Lawrin et al, 1986; Gill et al, 1989a), then, by the use of microchip identification bars implanted in each animal, it is possible to determine which animal is responsible for a given bout of drinking.

A "naturalistic" environment for rats has been studied by Ellison (1981). In this situation rats are allowed to roam freely in a large enclosure and then drinking habits can be assessed, provided that the animals are individually identified. If direct observation is required it is very labor intensive.

B. How should the ethanol be presented?

Again a variety of techniques have been employed. Often animals are pre-exposed to ethanol, whether to select high drinkers or to initiate their drinking in a no-choice situation. Clearly pre-exposure increases subsequent preference for ethanol (Li et al, 1981). Other methods are used to increase drinking such as sweetening the solutions (Reid et al - this conference, York 1981, Gilbert 1978) with saccharine or sucrose.

The sweetening agent is either left in the solution or faded out (Samson et al, 1989) after the animals are "hooked". The problems which can arise are in the interactions between the sweetening agent and the drug which is used. A separate demonstration that the drug does not change the selection of the sweetened solution vs water is an important, if seldom used control. A novel and useful, if somewhat labor intensive technique is to use the flavor pairing technique (Deutsche and Eisner, 1977; Waller et al, 1984). In this technique the ethanol is directly self-administered into the stomach through an indwelling catheter, depending upon which flavored solution the rat chooses. This requires much more equipment and surgery but has the advantage that it largely bypasses taste. It is probably too expensive and cumbersome for routine testing.

Another technique is to fluid deprive the animals for a varying period of time and then measure the ethanol intake in a short period. This is termed acceptance and differs from preference, which is measured over a longer time period. The advantages of the acceptance technique are clear for studies of short half-life drugs. In the usual 24 hour paradigm, ethanol drinking may take place over several hours, whereas a drug's effect may be evident only for a small fraction of that time. By using fluid deprived animals, the time of measurement can more closely approximate the duration of drug effect. The disadvantage to the technique is that there is almost never any demonstration that preference correlates with acceptance. In one attempt at this in mice, the correlation between preference and acceptance was only 0.247 although this was significant ($p<0.05$ $n = 110$) (Anderson and McClearn, 1981).

A varient of the acceptance paradigm is the limited access procedure (Linseman, 1987). Animals are given access to a choice of ethanol and water only for a brief period during the day. Water is freely available at other times. It has been possible to obtain sustained alcohol consumption in this way. It offers a number of advantages over the fluid deprivation model in that thirst is not a motivation and yet short half-life drugs can be studied. It is still important to ascertain the correlation of alcohol intake with the classical preference paradigm, however.

Neither the acceptance nor limited access procedures are useful if the goal is to achieve tolerance and dependence since the alcohol intake is transient.

How long should the data be collected? Of course the longer that this is done, the more likely the data will be valid. In any case, a two week period would seem to be the minimum.

C. How should the data be presented?

For the use of non-automated systems, data collection at least once a day is essential and needs to be reported in both preference ratio (ml of ethanol/ ml total fluid), total fluid and gm/kg/day ethanol consumed. If blood ethanol levels can be obtained with a minimum of disturbance by breath or eyeball vapor techniques during the drinking period as well as during the non-drinking period, this is valuable information. Several automated procedures for recording data on a minute by minute basis are available (Beardsley and Meisch, 1981; Lawrin et al, 1986; Gill et al 1989a). The advantages of these systems is that a much finer determination of the drinking habits of the animals can be ascertained. They are particularly useful for studies of unrestricted drinking but they probably are not necessary for the fluid deprived (acceptance) or the limited access paradigms since all drinking takes place in a short time span.

D. How should drug interaction be measured?

This is the meat of studies to alter an animal's preference for ethanol. Regardless of the theoretical basis on which a particular drug is tried, certain principles should apply. First, there should be a consistent dose-response relationship in the effects of the drug. This is one reason that it is necessary to have animals that consume considerable amounts of ethanol, otherwise there will be no room to demonstrate a significant dose-related decrease. Often, to improve the comparisons, an animal is used as its own control. This adds complicating factors unless it is done carefully. First, the delivery of the drug or vehicle should be alternated so that every animal does not experience ethanol first with vehicle and then with the active compound. Ideally, enough animals would be used to make it unnecessary to use an animal more than once. The use of inbred strains or selectively bred lines should decrease the variance so that using animals as their own controls would not be necessary. If pre-exposure is used, each animal is used as its own control, and at least three doses of the drug are used, the animal will have been through the testing procedure at least five times. Randomization of the exposures to active drug and placebo in a balanced design is critical if this paradigm is followed.

Proper pharmacological evidence should be obtained. For example if a serotonin receptor agonist decreases drinking, a serotonin receptor antagonist might be expected to increase drinking, or at least block the decrease by the agonist. Specificity of the compound for ethanol vs. other fluid intake should be investigated. This is not to suggest that a drug might not be useful even if it also decreases intake of food, water or other pharmacologically active agents, just that the interpretation of the data may be somewhat different in such a situation.

E. Should non-drinking animals be studied?

Much greater use could be made of the animals that do not drink (Samson et al, 1989). After all, the goal of therapy or prevention of alcoholism is to decrease alcohol intake. We should understand why animals or people do not drink excessively. Perhaps we could apply that knowledge to prevent alcohol intake.

F. Basal comparison protocol:

1. Animal model: Selectively bred animals (e.g. HAD and LAD rats) or heterogeneous stock (N/Nih rats or HS mice).

2. Ethanol presentation: At least two weeks of preference testing at 10% w/v ethanol vs. water or ethanol in sweetened solution vs. sweetened solution.

3. Data collection: Preference ratio, grams/kg/day, fluid intake, blood ethanol levels at peak ethanol intake.

4. Drug interactions. Dose response relationships. Randomized presentation if each animal is its own control. Investigation of the specificity of any action on ethanol preference. Controls for interactions with flavoring or sweetening agents. Changes in total food or fluid intake.

REFERENCES

Anderson, S.M., and McClearn, G.E., 1981. Ethanol consumption: Selective breeding in mice. Behavior Genetics 11, 291-301.

Beardsley, P.M., and Meisch, R.A., 1981. A precision drinking device for rats tested with water, etionitazene, and ethanol. Pharm. Biochem. Behav. 14, 871-876.

Conger, J.J., Sawrey, W.L., and Turrell, E.S., 1958. The role of social experience in the production of gastric ulcers in hooded rats placed in a conflict situation. J. Soc. Psych. 57, 214-220.

D'Amour, F., and Smith, D.L., 1941. A method for testing loss of pain sensation. J. Pharmacol. Exptl. Therap. 72, 74-79.

Deutsch, J.A., Eisner, A., 1977. Ethanol self-administration in the rat induced by forced drinking of ethanol. Behav. Biol. 20, 81-90.

Ellison, G.D., 1981. A novel animal model of alcohol consumption based on the development of extremes of ethanol preference in colony-housed but not isolated rats. Behav. Neurol. Biol. 31, 324-330.

Eriksson, K., and Russi, M., 1981. Finnish selection studies on alcohol related behaviors: General outline, in McClearn, G.E., Deitrich, R.A. and Erwin, V.G., eds., Development of Animal Models as Pharmacogenetic Tools. Res. Monograph No. 6, National Institute on Alcohol Abuse and Alcoholism, Washington, D.C. pp. 87-117.

Fadda, F., Mosca, E., Colombo, G., and Gessa, G.L., 1990. Alcohol-preferring rats: Genetic sensitivity to alcohol-induced stimulation of dopamine metabolism. Physiol. Behav. 47, 727-729.

Froehlich, J.C., Harts, J., Lumeng, L., and Li, T.-K., 1990. Naloxone attenuates voluntary ethanol intake in rats selectively bred for high ethanol preference. Pharm. Biochem. Behav. 35, 385-390.

Gilbert, R.M., 1978. Schedule induction and sweetness as factors in ethanol consumption and preference by rats. Pharm. Biochem. Behav. 8, 739-741.

Gill, K., Amit, Z., and Ogren, S.O., 1984. Selective depletion of norepinephrine in brain by N-2-chloroethyl-n-ethyl-2-bromobenzylamine fails to alter the voluntary consumption of ethanol in rats. Neuropharmacology 23, 1379-1383.

Gill, K., Mundl, W.J., Cabilio, S., and Amit, Z., 1989. A microprocessor controlled data acquisition system for research on feeding and drinking behavior in rats. Physiol. Behav. 45, 741-746.

Gill, T.J., III, Smith, G.J., Wissler, R.W., and Kunz, H.W., 1989. The rat as an experimental animal. Science 245, 269-275.

Lawrin, M.O., Naranjo, C.A., and Sellers, E.M., 1986. Identification of new drugs for modulating ethanol consumption. Psychopharm. Bull 22, 1020-1025.

Li, T.-K., and Lumeng, L., 1984. Alcohol preference and voluntary alcohol intakes of inbred rat strains and the National Institutes of Health heterogeneous stock of rats. Alc.: Clin. Exp. Res. 8, 485-486.

Li, T.-K., Lumeng, L., McBride, W.J., and Waller, M.B., 1981. Indiana selection studies on alcohol related behaviors, in McClearn, G.E.,

Deitrich, R.A. and Erwin, V.G., eds., Development of Animal Models as Pharmacogenetic Tools. Res. Monograph No. 6, National Institute on Alcohol Abuse and Alcoholism, Washington, D.C. pp. 171-191..

Linseman, M.A., 1987. Alcohol consumption is free-feeding rats: Procedural, genetic and pharmacokinetic factors. Psychopharmacology 92, 254-261.

Mardones, J., and Segovia-Riquelme, N., 1983. Thrity-two years of selection of rats by ethanol preference: UChA and UChB strains. Neurobehav. Toxicol. Teratol. 5, 171-178.

Pickett, R.A., III, and Collins, A.C., 1975. Use of genetic analysis to test the potential role of serotonin in alcohol preference. Life Sci. 17, 1291-1296.

Privette, T.H., Hornsby, R.L., and Myers, R.D., 1988. Buspirone alters alcohol drinking induced in rats by tetrahydropapaveroline injected into brain monoaminergic pathways. Alcohol 5, 147-152.

Samson, H.H., Tolliver, G.A., Lumeng, L., and Li, T.-K., 1989. Ethanol reinforcement in the alcohol nonpreferring rat: Initiation using behavioral techniques without food restriction. Alc.: Clin. Exp. Res. 13, 378-384.

Waller, M.B., McBride, W.J., Gatto, G.J., Lumeng, L., and Li, T.-K., 1984. Intragastric self-infusion of ethanol by ethanol-preferring and non-preferring lines of rats. Science 225, 78-80.

York, J.L., 1981. Consumption of intoxicating beverages by rats and mice exhibiting high and low preferences for ethanol. Pharm. Biochem. Behav. 15, 207-214.

2
Animal Models for Screening Drugs to Decrease Alcohol Consumption

J.D. Sinclair

Abstract

Improved methods for treating alcoholism are greatly needed, and the use of pharmacological agents holds great promise. Development was previously hindered by the lack of an accepted animal model. Great emphasis has been placed upon designated criteria for an animal model of alcoholism, but such face validity is unimportant for finding better treatments. What really is needed is predictive validity -- the ability to predict which drugs will reduce alcohol drinking in alcoholics. The simple model of rats voluntarily selecting unflavored ethanol has been shown to possess good predictive validity (Sinclair, 1987) and is currently being used for screening drugs for potential usefulness in alcoholism treatment.

The next step should be development of special animal models for screening drugs that act on specific components of alcohol drinking: e.g., blocking the deprivation-induced increase in craving or the accompanying arousal, correcting underlying disorders promoting drinking in some individuals, suppressing stimuli triggering drinking (e.g., withdrawal sensations or stimuli arising from the first drink after abstinence), satisfying the alcohol craving or blocking tolerance to satiety signals from alcohol. Particularly promising are drugs that block alcohol reinforcement and thus could be used to extinguish the alcohol-drinking response.

There is increasing evidence that pharmacological agents alter alcohol drinking in laboratory animals and in humans, and that pharmacological suppression of alcohol intake represents a feasible approach for improved treatment of alcoholism (Sinclair, 1987). The search for drugs that are useful against alcoholism must eventually proceed to clinical trials. Before that, however, a method is needed for screening the vast multitude of possibly beneficial drugs. This screening, by necessity, requires a good animal model.

Face validity vs. predictive validity

Much effort has been devoted to developing and testing various animal models to see if they have face validity for alcoholism, i.e., whether the animals display various designated characteristics seen in human alcoholics. Face validity, however, is not relevant for screening potential alcoholism-treatment drugs. What really is needed is predictive validity (Sinclair, 1980): a model that will accurately predict which drugs will suppress alcohol drinking by alcoholics. Face validity often is correlated with predictive validity, and it is initially the only guide for what may be useful models. But the two do not necessarily go together.

Establishing the predictive validity of an animal model requires extensive data on the effects of the drug in the model and clinical data with which to compare it. Sufficient data has been accumulated for the two-bottle self-selection animal model in which rats have access to an unflavored alcohol solution, water, and food. As reviewed elsewhere (Sinclair, 1987), the results with this model match rather closely the available findings with humans and more specifically the clinical findings with alcoholics. One can, of course, find fault with many of the clinical studies -- and also with some of the laboratory experiments. Nevertheless, I believe the results as a whole indicate that this model possesses good predictive validity.

The self-selection model is currently being used as a general screening procedure for drugs that suppress alcohol drinking in alcoholics, and it probably will continue to serve this purpose well in the near future.

Now, however, I believe we should turn our attention to the development of animal models for more specific components of alcohol drinking and abuse.

Components of alcohol drinking and alcoholism

In general we have been working on alcohol drinking as if it were a monolithic behavior. It is clear, however, that alcohol drinking is composed of a variety of separate components in any one individual and that different factors may involved in different alcoholics. Some likely components can be illustrated with the following working working hypothesis about alcoholism.

Alcohol drinking is seen as a learned response, reinforced largely by specific effects of ethanol in the central nervous system. Some people, as a result of genetics, environment, or a combination, have their alcohol-drinking response reinforced so strongly and so often that eventually it comes to dominate their behavior, preventing them from leading a healthy, productive life; and society classifies them as alcoholics.

The probability of the alcohol-drinking response being emitted is, of course, not constant. It varies according to what stimuli are present, the state of the individual, and the immediate drinking history.

The probability of making most responses (e.g., socializing, sexual behaviors, eating, drinking, consuming specific flavors, bar pressing, exercising) is increased after a period in which the response cannot be emitted (see Sinclair & Bender, 1978). In the case of the alcohol-drinking response, this is seen in rats (Sinclair, 1972, 1979; Sinclair & Senter, 1967, 1968) and monkeys (Sinclair, 1971; Kornet et al., 1990) as the alcohol-deprivation effect -- a strong, temporary rise in alcohol consumption accompanied by arousal when alcohol is first returned. In alcoholics it is seen as a progressive increase in craving for alcohol during abstinence (Voltaire et al., 1989). In normal rat strains the increase develops slowly over days of deprivation (Sinclair et al., 1973b), but in the heavy-drinking AA and P rat lines (Sinclair & Li, 1989) and also human alcoholics (Rankin et al., 1979) an increase develops during only a few hours of deprivation.

The alcohol-drinking response is learned to various stimuli, some external and some internal. One class of stimuli to which alcohol drinking may be learned by many alcoholics consists of the sensations occurring at the beginning of withdrawal, and these sensations may become conditioned to and then elicited by other stimuli. Another class of stimuli always present when alcohol is drunk are those from the alcohol itself: the sight, smell, and taste of the beverage, and the initial feelings produced by the alcohol. These sensations may help to produce a priming effect in an alcoholic from the first drink after being abstinent; central effects, perhaps related to the stimulation of appetite and the loss of behavioral inhibitions may also contribute.

Deficiencies in the satiety mechanism which terminates imbibing after a certain amount of alcohol has been consumed may also contribute to the over-indulgence. The satiety process with alcohol is poorly understood, but one factor which could affect it is the rapid development of tolerance (Sinclair et al., 1989) to the satiety-mediating effects of ethanol.

Drugs for affecting specific components

From the preceding description, one can postulate various classes of drugs, acting on separate components of alcohol drinking, which could be useful in the treatment of alcoholism.

-- Drugs which block positive reinforcement from alcohol

If alcohol drinking is a learned response, it could be extinguished by emitting it repeatedly while reinforcement is blocked by a drug. Such drugs might also be useful in conjunction with other drugs that produce adverse effects if ethanol is consumed. Although punishing a response that still produces positive reinforcement is ineffective (Sinclair & Thomas, this volume), punishing alcohol drinking while the positive reinforcement is blocked might be more beneficial.

-- Drugs that correct underlying disorders

If alcohol drinking in some individuals is only a symptom of one of various underlying, perhaps inherent, disorders, their alcoholism could be treated with drugs that corrected the disorder. This explanation of drinking, however, seems unlikely because it does not account for the gradual development of alcoholism. It seems more likely that a disorder might only contribute to the development, e.g., by increasing the amount of reinforcement from alcohol. In this case, drugs counteracting the disorder could be used as a preventative against the development of alcoholism, as a factor to help prevent relearning of the alcohol-drinking response after extinction, or as a means for removing stimuli (e.g., depressive feelings) to which alcohol drinking has been learned.

-- Drugs which block the alcohol-deprivation effect

The increase in craving produced by abstinence is probably a major factor in the resumption of drinking by binge-style alcoholics and in relapse after forced abstinence. Alcohol itself, of course, prevents the increase (Sinclair et al., 1973b) and morphine, apparently acting as substitution drug, also does (Sinclair et al., 1973a). A drug with this ability but without addictive potential should be very useful. Even drugs which blocked the accompanying arousal might be beneficial.

-- Drugs promoting cue exposure

The ability of stimuli to trigger the alcohol-drinking response might be lessened by cue exposure (Litt et al., 1990): another form of extinction in which the patient goes through all the motions of alcohol drinking under normal drinking conditions but does not take alcohol. It might be possible to find a drug that improved this procedure. In addition, a drug that blocked the positive reinforcement from alcohol could be given as a security measure in case the person proceeded to drink alcohol, in which case there would be an extinction trial.

-- Stimulus-attenuating drugs

The triggering of alcohol drinking by withdrawal-like sensations might be eliminated by drugs that counteracted or blocked such sensations. The supposed first-drink priming effect might be suppressed by drugs that blocked reception of stimuli from alcohol itself.

-- Drugs enhancing satiety

Substitution drugs with some effects similar to alcohol might satisfy the desire for alcohol and help prevent or terminate drinking. This seems the most likely explanation for the prolonged specific suppression of alcohol drinking by morphine and other opiate agonists (Critcher et al., 1983: Ho, 1980, Ho, 1982; Sinclair et al., 1973a), but again it is necessary to find a drug with this ability and without addictive potential. Drugs which enhanced the satiety effects from alcohol itself or prevented the development of tolerance to the satiety effects could help limit alcohol drinking.

Specific animal models

Screening drugs for the ability to affect these separate components will require specific animal models. Some procedures currently available -- mainly ones used in our laboratory -- are outlined below.

The ability of naloxone to block positive reinforcement from alcohol was suspected initially because it blocks the stimulatory effect of alcohol on locomotor activity in mice or improved tilting plane performance in rats (Sinclair et al., 1982). The increase in head-poking by rats after ingestion of small amounts of ethanol (Gill, 1989) might provide a similar test. Screening with these models is limited to the degree that the stimulatory effect is actually correlated with reinforcement.

The ability of naloxone and other opiate antagonists to promote extinction of the alcohol-drinking response was suggested by several findings. Monkeys working for alcohol infusions showed an extinction burst -- a temporary increase in responding -- when an antagonist was first administered (Altshuler & Shippenberg, 1982). In rats, the first injection of an antagonist before a 1 hour alcohol-drinking session produced little suppression, but subsequent injections produced progressively less drinking, in a manner resembling the classical extinction curves (Sinclair, 1990). The suppression persisted long after the antagonist should have been removed from the body. The subsequent increase appeared to be reacquisition because it occurred more rapidly in AA rats which receive more reinforce from alcohol and acquire ethanol-reinforced responses more rapidly (Hyytiä & Sinclair, 1989).

Identifying procedures that weaken the alcohol-drinking response or otherwise decrease the motivation for alcohol could also be done with operant responding. Increasing the effort or the number of responses required for each ethanol reinforcement lowers the total daily amount of alcohol obtained (Sinclair, 1974; Hyytiä & Sinclair, 1990). Under such conditions motivation-reducing procedures should suppress responding but ones that merely limit the maximal amount of alcohol that can be consumed should be ineffective. Rats working for intracranial infusions of ethanol (Li, 1990) also provides an excellent procedure for making such distinctions and also for eliminating taste factors.

Animal models used for screening drugs used against disorders (e.g., depression) that might underlie alcohol drinking are beyond the present scope. In another direction, however, it has been found (Kampov-Polevoy et al., 1990) that rats inherently differ along a "personality" dimension similar to that distinguishing Cloninger's (1989) Type 1 and Type 2 alcoholics. Consequently, it was suggested that the heaviest alcohol drinking rats at the two extremes of this dimension might be developed into specific animal models for the two types of alcoholics.

Screening drugs for their ability to counteract the alcohol-deprivation effect is done simply by administering the drug during a week when alcohol-experienced rats are deprived but terminating the administration early enough for all of the drug to be eliminated before alcohol is returned. In this way it was discovered that morphine (Sinclair et al, 1973a) but not cyanamide (Sinclair & Gribble, 1985) blocks the alcohol-deprivation effect. Drugs with suspected arousal-suppressing capability can be administered just before alcohol is returned to deprived rats to see if they block deprivation-induced drinking.

Finding drugs to block withdrawal-like symptoms that may trigger drinking could be done with various animal models involving chronic ethanol administration (Freund, 1980). A simpler procedure, however, might be provided with our proposed hangover model, measuring hyperthermia, increase wheel running, and other aftereffects of a single ethanol injection (Sinclair & Gustafsson, 1987; Sinclair & Taira, 1988). Development of an animal model for the suspected first-drink priming effect will, however, first require a demonstration that such an effect occurs in animals.

Computer-monitored drinkometers (Gill, 1989) or operant chambers (Hyytiä & Sinclair, 1989) could be used for testing drugs for their ability to increase alcohol satiety. Such drugs would be expected to decrease the duration of individual bouts but not the initial rate of consumption after deprivation. Screening could also be done by seeing if the drugs specifically enhanced the suppressive effect of intubated ethanol on voluntary alcohol drinking (Sinclair et al., 1973b)

Application

If there is ever to be practical benefit, the drugs found to be effective with such animal models must next be tested with an increasingly expensive series of clinical trials. The entire process seems to require a tripartite collaboration, involving (1) a laboratory conducting the basic research and screening with animal models, (2) a clinical center organized for conducting the trials scientifically, and (3) some agency to cover the expenses. Furthermore, there must be understanding and good communication between the three parties, which can be difficult because of the different backgrounds of the people involved. Establishment of such collaboration, however, is probably the most important step for obtaining improved alcoholism treatments.

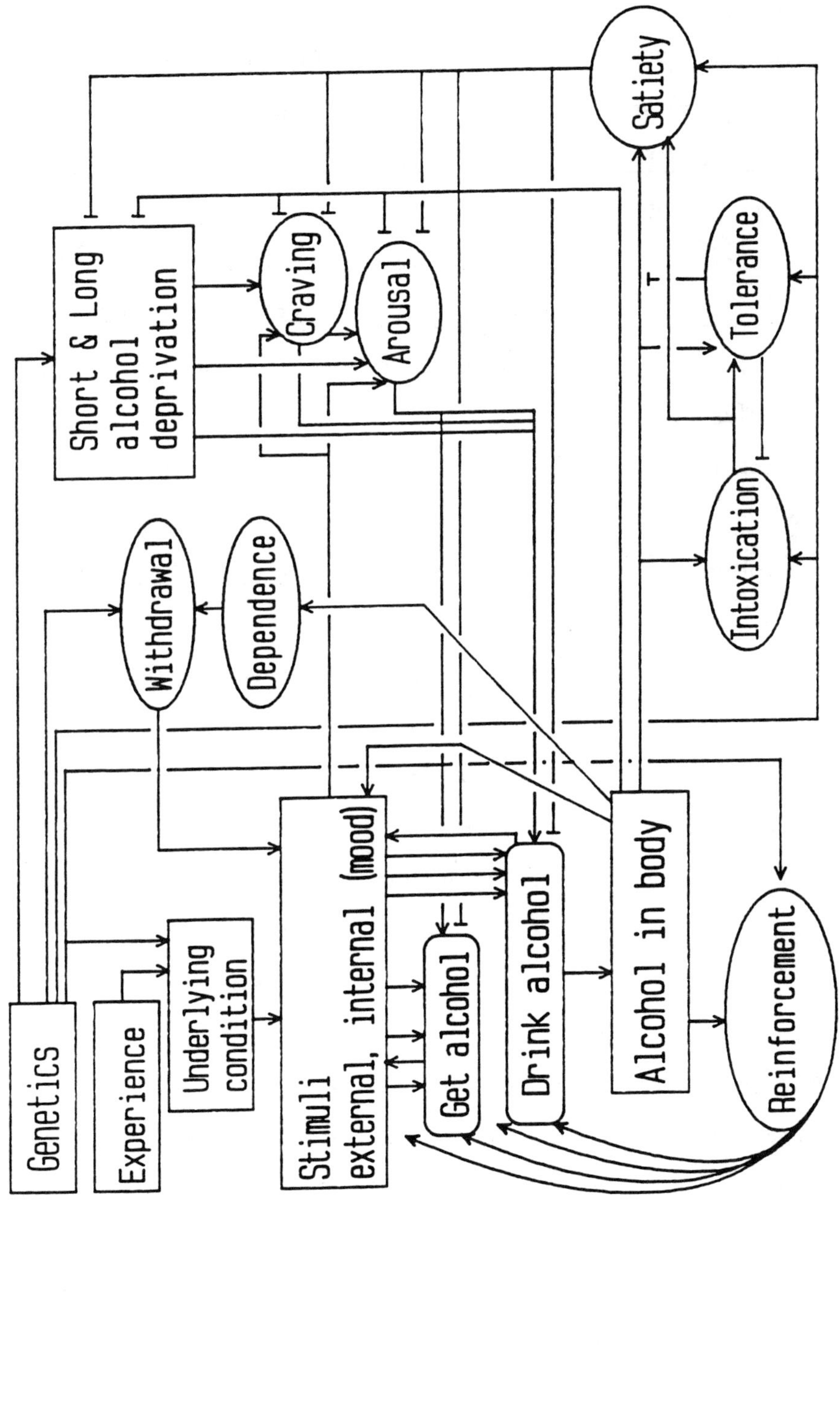

Genetics
Experience
Underlying condition
Stimuli external, internal (mood)
Get alcohol
Drink alcohol
Alcohol in body
Reinforcement
Withdrawal
Dependence
Short & Long alcohol deprivation
Craving
Arousal
Intoxication
Tolerance
Satiety

References

Altshuler, H.L and T.S.Shippenberg. Tetrahydroisoquinoline and opioid substrates of alcohol actions. Beta-Carbolines and Tetrahydroisoquinolines, Progress in Clinical Biological Research, 90: 329-344, 1982.

Cloninger, C.R. Clinical heterogeneity in families of alcoholics. In: Genetic Aspects of Alcoholism K. Kiianmaa, B. Tabakoff and T. Saito (eds.), Helsinki: The Finnish Foundation for Alcohol Studies, pp. 55-65, 1989.

Critcher, E.C., C.I. Lin, J. Patel and R.D. Myers. Attenuation of alcohol drinking in tetrahydroisoguinoline-treated rats by morphine and naltrexone. Pharmacol Biochem Behav 18: 225-229, 1983.

Fruend, G. Comparison of alcohol dependence, withdrawal and hangover in humans and animals. In: Animal Models in Alcohol Research K.Eriksson, J.D.Sinclair, K.Kiianmaa (eds.) London: Academic, pp. 293-308, 1980.

Gill, K. J. A critical evaluation of the use of animal models in alcohol research: An examination of voluntary alcohol consumption in rodents. Doctor Thesis, Dept Psychology, Concordia University, 1989.

Ho, A.K.S. Ethanol preference, withdrawal and toxicities: modification by pharmacological agents. In K. Eriksson, J.D.Sinclair, & K.Kiianmaa (Eds.) Animal Models in Alcohol Research, London: Academic Press, pp. 173-178, 1980.

Ho, A.K.S. Suppression of ethanol consumption by MET-enkephalin in rats. Journal of Pharmacy and Pharmacology 34: 118-119,

1982.

Hyytiä, P. and J. D. Sinclair. Demonstration of lever pressing for oral ethanol by rats with no prior training or ethanol experience. Alcohol 6: 161-164, 1989.

Hyytiä, P., and J. D. Sinclair. Differential reinforcement and diurnal rhythms of lever pressing for ethanol in AA and Wistar rats. Alcoholism: Clinical and Experimental Research (in press, 1990).

Kampov-Polevoy, A. B., O. P. Kasheffskaya and J. D. Sinclair. Initial acceptance of ethanol: Gustatory factors and patterns of alcohol drinking. Alcohol 7: 83-85, 1990.

Li, T.-K. Genetic and neurobiological substrates of alcohol-seeking behavior & alcoholism. Presented at the 20th Nordic Meeting on Biological Alcohol Research, Espoo, Finland, May 13-15, 1990 (Second plenary abstract in proceedings).

Litt, M.D., N.L. Cooney, R.M. Kadden and L. Gaupp L. Reactivity to alcohol cues and induced moods in alcoholics. Addictive Behaviors 15: 137-146, 1990.

Kornet, M., C. Goosen and J.M.Van Ree. The effect of naltrexone on alcohol consumption after alcohol deprivation in rhesus monkeys. Presented at the 20th Nordic Meeting on Biological Alcohol Research, Espoo, Finland, May 13-15, 1990 (Abstract 20 in proceedings).

Rankin, H., R. Hodgson and T.Stockwell. The concept of craving and its measurement. Behaviour, Research and Therapy 17: 389-396, 1979.

Sinclair, J. D. The alcohol-deprivation effect in monkeys. Psychonomic Science 25: 21-22, 1971.

Sinclair, J.D. The alcohol-deprivation effect: Influence of various factors. Quarterly Journal of Studies on Alcohol 33: 769-782, 1972.

Sinclair, J.D. Rats learning to work for alcohol. Nature 249: 590-592, 1974.

Sinclair, J.D. Alcohol-deprivation effect in rats genetically selected for their ethanol preference. Pharmacology, Biochemistry & Behavior 10: 597-602, 1979.

Sinclair, J.D. Comparison of the factors which influence voluntary drinking in humans and animals. In: Animal Models in Alcohol Research K.Eriksson, J.D.Sinclair, K.Kiianmaa (eds.) London: Academic, pp. 119-137, 1980.

Sinclair, J.D. The feasibility of effective psycho-pharmacological treatments for alcoholism. British Journal of Addiction 82, 1213-1223, 1987.

Sinclair, J.D. Drugs to decrease alcohol drinking. Annals of Medicine In press, 1990.

Sinclair, J.D., J.Adkins, and S.Walker. Morphine-induced suppression of voluntary alcohol drinking in rats. Nature 246: 425-427, 1973a.

Sinclair, J.D. and D.O.Bender. Compensatory behaviors: Suggestion for a common basis from deficits in hamsters. Life Sciences 22: 1407-1412, 1978.

Sinclair, J.D. and P.A.Gribble. Cyanamide injections during alcohol deprivation increase alcohol drinking. Alcohol 2: 627-630, 1985.

Sinclair, J.D. and K. Gustafsson. Behavioral changes in rats on the day after acute ethanol intoxication. Alcohol 4: 503-507, 1987.

Sinclair, J.D., A.D.Lê, and K.Kiianmaa. The AA and ANA rat lines selected for differences in voluntary alcohol consumption. Experientia 45: 798-805, 1989.

Sinclair, J.D. and T.-K.Li. Long and short alcohol deprivation: Effects on AA and P rats. Alcohol 6: 505-509, 1989.

Sinclair, J.D., M.Rusi, M.M.Airaksinen, and H.L.Altshuler. Relating TIQ's, opiates, and ethanol. Beta-Carbolines and Tetrahydroisoquinolines, Progress in Clinical Biological Research, 90: 365-376, 1982.

Sinclair, J.D. and R.J.Senter. Increased preference for ethanol in rats following alcohol deprivation. Psychonomic Science 8: 11-12, 1967.

Sinclair, J.D. and R.J.Senter. Development of an alcohol-deprivation effect in rats. Quarterly Journal of Studies on Alcohol 29: 863-867, 1968.

Sinclair, J.D and T.Taira. Hangover hyperthermia in rats: relation to tolerance and external stimuli. Psychopharmacology 94, 161-166, 1988.

Sinclair, J.D., S.Walker, and W.Jordan. Alcohol intubation and its effect on voluntary consumption. Quarterly Journal of Studies on Alcohol 34: 726-743, 1973b.

Sinclair, J.D., S.Walker, and W.Jordan. Behavioral and physiological changes associated with various durations of alcohol deprivation. Quarterly Journal of Studies on Alcohol 34: 744-757, 1973c.

Voltaire, A. O.Beck, S. Borg and H. Stibler. Clinical and biochemical features of relapse in alcohol dependent patients during longterm abstinence. Presented at the 19th Annual Nordic Meeting on Biological Alcohol Research, Varberg, Sweden, April 9-12, 1989 (Abstract 20 in proceedings).

3
Medications for Alcohol Abuse and Dependence: Methodology for Clinical Studies

E.M. Sellers and M.B. Sobell *

The ideal initial requirement for any clinical studies with medications to modify alcohol consumption is that there is extensive pre-clinical pharmacology with the compounds. At a minimum there should be sufficient evidence to suggest that the medication modifies ethanol self-administration, discriminative stimulus properties, place preference, development of tolerance or alcohol withdrawal or withdrawal behaviours (Bozarth, 1987). Despite the existence of reliable methods for conducting such studies, there are no current medications under study where there has been more than fragmentary pre-clinical information.

Even in the presence of such evidence, there will be a number of medications for which no pre-clinical study would anticipate efficacy in decreasing alcohol consumption; for example, drugs which modify mood (e.g. anxiety, depression), or drugs which produce conditioned aversive responses. Table 1 summarizes mechanisms whereby medications could have therapeutic utility in the treatment of alcohol abuse or dependence.

DEFINING THE DEPENDENT VARIABLES

Alcohol Consumption

The primary dependent variable which medications should be expected to modify is alcohol consumption. However, alcohol drinking patterns vary considerably among individuals irrespective of mean daily consumption. In addition, mean level of consumption is independent of the within-subject variations suggesting that variation per se is a feature of drinking pattern which should be given equal attention to average daily consumption (Sellers et al, 1990).

From a public health perspective, peak drinking may be important because of its association with accidents, violence and possibly certain organic complications such as brain damage. On the other hand it is clearly established that average consumption of between 3 and 4 standard drinks per day over long periods of time are associated with a significant increase risk of alcohol liver disease (Seventh Special Report, 1990).

---

*The views expressed in this manuscript are those of the authors and do not necessarily reflect those of the Addiction Research Foundation.

Table 1: Medication Development to Reduce Alcohol Consumption

---

I. INITIAL STUDIES POSSIBLE IN LABORATORY ANIMALS

A. Directed at Modifying Alcohol Reinforcing Properties
   1. Antagonize the reinforcing effects
      a) direct
      b) indirect
   2. Substitute for the reinforcing effects
      a) direct
      b) indirect
   3. Provoke an unconditioned aversive or dysphoric reaction
   4. Modify ethanol biodisposition

B. Directed at Modifying Mood, Motivation or Cognition
   1. Treat primary or secondary mental disorders
   2. Suppress target symptoms that may prompt or sustain use or that may prevent the reduction, cessation or resumption of use
   3. Facilitate the learning or retention of a new behaviour

II. INITIAL STUDIES POSSIBLE IN HUMANS ONLY

A. Human
   1. Non-specific substitute for the reinforcing effects
   2. Induce dysphoric symptoms which produce mild malaise
   3. Augment self-efficacy by providing cues that active medication is part of treatment
   4. Provoke a conditioned aversive or dysphoric physiologic reaction
   5. Decrease the desire to drink

Craving

In common use, craving is a "strong desire or intense longing". However, the concept of craving in the alcohol field has a number of shortcomings (Kozlowski and Wilkinson, 1987a,b). For example, the word promises more than it can deliver since conceptually components of craving are multiple (Kozlowski and Wilkinson, 1987a,b). In addition, popular and technical meanings of this word are not similar and researchers who use this term cannot agree among themselves as to what it means or how to measure it. Not only do researchers not agree on what the term means, but patients as well are unable to give reliable reports as to what they understand craving to mean

(Kozlowski et al, 1989). Importantly, the term can deceptively simplify the behavioural etiology of a complex addictive disorder.

Despite these shortcomings, the notion has figured prominently in the field. Certainly with respect to the behaviour of interest, namely heavy alcohol use, there are a number of features of that behaviour which are of interest and might serve as secondary dependent variables. For example an individual's: desire to use; intention to use; probability of actual use; desire to change or enhance mood; desire to change internal state and the strength of that desire. Each of these in turn is affected by a number of contextual features, many of which are observable or reportable upon by the individual (e.g. setting, time of day, actual opportunity to drink, avoidance behaviours instead of drinking, actual use and the overall time frame).

Such concurrent measures help to operationalize "craving". Craving alone as a term should probably be reserved as a quantitative descriptor of strong desires to take alcohol and not used as a dependent variable in its own right.

FEATURES OF CLINICAL TRIALS

Design

Clinical efficacy trials for the development of medications in this field should generally be: randomized, double-blind, placebo-controlled; parallel group; and include two or more drug dose levels in addition to the placebo condition. However, the trial can be "dose-controlled" (i.e. dose constant), "concentration-controlled" (i.e. dose titrated to achieve a particular concentration or concentration range, e.g. high, low), or "response-controlled" (i.e. dose titrated to achieve a particular response, e.g. success in the absence of important toxicity). In this regard it cannot be assumed that drugs developed for other indications will have the same dose response curve or concentration effect relationship, hence particular consideration should be given to "response-controlled" studies.

Patient selection and entry into studies can occur in one of three ways: abstinent individuals entering after a period of post-detoxication; individuals entering after a self-achieved period of abstinence or non-hazardous drinking; reduction in drinking per se is a goal of the medication treatment and occurs at the beginning of treatment. Medications focussed on relapse prevention might use the second option while drugs modify ethanol reinforcement or directed at the interaction of ethanol consumption behaviour the other two.

Duration

Four published clinical trials with serotonin uptake inhibitors demonstrate onset of an effect quite rapidly (Naranjo et al, 1984,1987,1989,1990a). A recent study with citalopram has confirmed that short-term studies of a week or less can given an indication whether the drug is going to be effective (Naranjo et al,

1990b). For initial efficacy studies of a medication's ability to initiate a decrease in alcohol consumption trials should probably be 4-8 weeks in duration. However, studies of long-term medication use or relapse prevention will normally be conducted over a period of 24-52 weeks. In addition, long-term follow-up of patients for a 1-2 year period would be required in relapse prevention and multi-centre efficacy trials.

Patient Population for Initial Clinical Trials

In general, the goal of medication development in this area would be to develop medications for individuals in whom non-hazardous drinking or abstinence is the goal. Minimum characteristics of individuals to enter such studies would be individuals abusing or dependent on alcohol who are consuming more than 4 standard drinks per day (3 for women) on average or consuming greater than 6-8 standard drinks on any one day on more than one occasion per week. Initial clinical trials should study individuals who are not severely dependent (DSM-IIIr), without cirrhosis or progressive alcoholic hepatitis or other irreversible organic complications of alcohol abuse and without severe impairment of psychosocial functioning. Risk factors should be controlled in order to have a group of individuals with a favourable probability of response (i.e. < 2 previous serious formal treatment attempts and have not been unemployed for more than 3 months). In addition, the study should be directed in individuals who do not have any other DSM-IIIr axis I diagnosis requiring treatment and do not currently meet DSM-IIIr criteria for abuse or dependence on any other drug excepting tobacco.

Primary Outcome Variables

The key primary outcome variables are: a reduction in alcohol consumption to non-hazardous levels both with respect to a decrease in average consumption (< 4 standard drinks) and an abolition of peak drinking days (≥ 8 standard drinks/day); a significant improvement in biochemical and other indicators of organic function if abnormal initially; in longer term trials (> 6 months), a significant improvement in patient specific psychosocial function.

Measurement of Alcohol Consumption

The different approaches that can be incorporated into clinical trials to monitor alcohol consumption include: self-reports; daily monitoring booklets; daily urine alcohol; breath alcohol; liver function tests and corroboration by collaterals. In contrast to popular opinion, self-reports and daily monitoring booklets are extremely reliable. Correlations of urine alcohols with daily monitoring booklets are acceptably high (range of 0.5-0.7) (Naranjo et al, 1984,1987,1989,1990a).

Compliance

Compliance is known to be importantly confounded with outcome in many areas of drug treatment. However, compliance should not be used as a dependent variable. In order to sort compliant and non-compliant individuals with respect to adherence to study protocols it is important to include detailed procedural compliance measures for both the study procedures and medication use. Procedural compliance measures include records of appointments kept, monitoring booklets returned, daily urine samples submitted, pill count, homework assignments and participation in various parts of the study. Monitoring of medication compliance can be achieved through measurement of drug concentrations in plasma or urine, the use of inert markers in the medication (e.g. riboflavin), measures of biological activity (e.g. blockade of serotonin uptake by platelets into platelets by serotonin uptake inhibitors) or the use of newer medication event monitoring systems that can record the opening and closing of medication vials (Naranjo et al, 1984,1987,1989,1990a).

Other Variables

Theoretic considerations suggest that self-efficacy, reasons and situations for drinking, situational confidence, mood and health beliefs may interact importantly and specifically with medications.

For example, it seems possible that emergent somatic symptoms secondary to a drug during a clinical trial might provide cues to individuals and persuade them that they were receiving a drug which might be helpful. Such factors introduce potential potent pharmacologic and sociobehavioural interactions into clinical trials. Greater care is needed to anticipate them and to understand and separate them from selective drug effects.

Integration with Psychosocial Treatment

In general, medications are likely to serve as important adjuncts to other treatment interventions. For example, the efficacy of serotonin uptake inhibitors suggests they may be useful in the initiation of a reduction in consumption. For maintenance of this decrease a sustained behavioural change is needed. The role of medications for such change at this point is unclear.

In parallel and conjunction with medication development, motivationally focussed psychosocial interventions for use in combined pharmacological-psychological treatment should be developed. An important feature of psychosocial treatments is that they could explicitly interlock with the specific mechanism of action of the drug. For example, a drug that works as a cognitive enhancer should be combined with a non-pharmacologic strategy that enhances the patient's perception of self-efficacy or provide a new skill to learn. Alternately, the psychosocial intervention component should enhance a health belief that medications are effective and how they can be effective (e.g. in reduction of anxiety).

CONCLUSIONS

Over the past five years progress has been made in finding medications which may have clinical utility. The strategies for initial drug development are now established and should now be applied. Medications with larger effects, trial designs which enhance drug effects and psychosocial interventions that complement pharmacologic treatments should have top future priority.

ACKNOWLEDGEMENTS

We thank our colleagues, Dr. C.A. Naranjo, Dr. L.C. Sobell, Dr. T. Toneatto who have through ongoing colleagueship undoubtedly planted unbeknownst to us the seeds of ideas in this manuscript.

REFERENCES

Bozarth MA (ed.). Methods of Assessing the Reinforcing Properties of Abused Drugs. Springer-Verlag, New York, 1987.

Kozlowski LT, Wilkinson DA. Use and misuse of the concept of craving by alcohol, tobacco, and drug researchers. Br J Addict 1987a; 82: 31-36.

Kozlowski LT, Wilkinson DA. Comments on Kozlowski & Wilkinson's "Use and misuse of the concept of craving by alcohol, tobacco and drug researchers": A reply from the authors. Br J Addict 1987b; 82: 489-492.

Kozlowski LT, Mann RE, Wilkinson DA, Poulos CX. "Cravings" are amibiguous: Ask about urges or desires. Addict Behav 1989; 14: 443-445.

Naranjo CA, Sellers EM, Roach CA, Woodley DV, Sanchez-Craig M, Sykora K. Zimelidine-induced variations in alcohol intake in nondepressed heavy drinkers. Clin Pharmacol Ther 1984; 35(3): 374-381.

Naranjo CA, Sellers EM, Sullivan JT, Woodley DV, Kadlec K, Sykora K. The serotonin uptake inhibitor citalopram attenuates ethanol intake. Clin Pharmacol Ther 1987; 41(3): 266-274.

Naranjo CA, Sullivan JT, Kadlec KE, Woodley-Remus DV, Kennedy G, Sellers EM. Differential effects of viqualine on alcohol intake and other consummatory behaviors. Clin Pharmacol Ther 1989; 46(3): 301-309.

Naranjo CA, Kadlec KE, Sanhueza P, Woodley-Remus D, Sellers EM. Fluoxetine differentially alters alcohol intake and other consummatory behaviors in problem drinkers. Clin Pharmacol Ther 1990a; 47(4): 490-498.

Naranjo CA, Sellers EM, Kadlec KE, Poulos CX. Citalopram decreases the desire for alcohol. Abstracts of Satellite Symposium "Novel

Pharmacological Interventions for Alcoholism", 5th ISBRA Conference (Toronto, Ontario), 1990b.

Sellers EM. Models of human alcohol abuse and dependence. Abstracts of British Association for Psychopharmacology Meeting (Cambridge, England) 1990: 7.

Seventh Special Report to the U.S. Congress on Alcohol and Health. Chapter V. Medical consequences. Editorial Experts, Inc., Virginia, 1990. pp. 107-138.

4
Some Issues in the Evaluation of a Pharmacotherapy of Alcoholism

R.E. Meyer

Disulfiram has been used as an adjunct in alcohol rehabilitation in the United States for approximately 50 years. Evidence of clinical efficacy, based on a double blind and placebo controlled trial, was examined only recently by Fuller et al. in a large collaborative study supported by the United States Department of Veterans Affairs (1). That study failed to find significant differences in treated vs. control subjects relative to percentage of subjects remaining abstinent, or the length of time to the first drink. Among subjects who drank, subjects on usual clinical doses of disulfiram (250 mg. per day) had fewer drinking days. In addition to conclusions on efficacy, the study by Fuller et al. broke important methodological ground that should inform subsequent pharmacotherapy trials in the alcohol field. The study drew attention to the need for a larger patient pool from which to admit subjects. Medical contraindications (usually secondary to the alcoholism) prevent the inclusion of a substantial percentage of alcoholic patients in drug treatment trials. In addition, many patients refuse to volunteer for a treatment that might result in toxic side effects either alone, or in combination with accidental or intentional alcohol consumption.

In this study, compliance with prescribed medication (or placebo) appeared to represent an important patient characteristic that was more predictive of treatment outcome than the treatment itself. The use of a riboflavin marker with the medication (or placebo) served as a useful measure of compliance. By employing a pharmacologically inactive dose of disulfiram (1 mg.), as well as a separate placebo condition (i.e., 2 placebo conditions), the investigators could differentiate the effects of expectancy from true pharmacological efficacy. The active treatment group received 250 mg. of disulfiram per day. Finally, in addition to self-reports of alcohol use, symptoms of alcohol dependence and alcohol-related problems, the authors used objective biological markers (blood and urine measures of ethanol) to determine the recurrence of alcohol use.

In a number of ways, studies of pharmacological treatments for chronic alcoholism are more complex than other areas of treatment research (including other clinical psychopharmacology). In addition to the problems of recruiting and retaining a sufficiently large sample for the study, there is a need to be certain that subjects from the treatment and control groups have equal access to (and make comparable use of) nonpharmacological modes of treatment. If assignment to treatment is truly random, then one must presume that important patient characteristics should be distributed equally across groups. Finally, there is a need to define specific measures of treatment efficacy that are both reliable and valid. For example, will the treatment improve the rate of abstinence among patients? Will it improve the duration of abstinence? Will it facilitate a moderate drinking outcome, or will it modify the potency of alcohol as a reinforcer? If the target is a moderate drinking outcome, Fuller et al. reported that self-report measures may not be valid enough to confirm such an outcome (1). A number of biological measures (2-7) have been suggested as a means of validating data from patients and collateral informants. For some drugs, it will be important to monitor blood levels because of altered pharmacokinetics in alcoholic patients (8).

Recently, there has been renewed interest in pharmacotherapies for alcoholism and other addictive disorders that has been fueled by reports of successful pharmacotherapies for opiate addiction (9,10) and other addictive disorders (11-13), as well as by the pace of scientific discovery in the neurosciences. There is a developing body of knowledge that suggests possible mechanisms for alcohol intoxication, reinforcement, anxiolysis, and tolerance (14). An understanding of the biological basis of these effects may provide pharmacological tools to modify the course of alcoholism. Progress in characterizing patient samples to include prognostic criteria such as severity of alcohol dependence (15), co-morbid psychopathology (16), and other characteristics (17) are important methodological developments over the past decade. The application of more rigorous statistical methodologies (such as survival analysis to deal with the problem of patient dropout) have increased confidence in the scientific rigor of treatment research in this field.

In a recent review, this author described the prospects for a rational pharmacotherapy in the rehabilitation of alcohol-dependent patients (18). The review identified six areas of opportunity for new pharmacotherapy initiatives:

1. Drugs that may reverse or ameliorate the central nervous system signs and symptoms of protracted abstinence.

2. Drugs that may have a primary effect on the desire to consume alcohol as part of a general effect on consummatory behavior.

3. Drugs that may improve the cognitive capacity of patients with alcohol-induced impairments.

4. Drugs that appear to block the reinforcing effects of alcohol.

5. Other types or forms of antidipsotropic agents which may be less problematic than the present formulation of disulfiram.

6. Specific nonaddicting psychotropic drugs for co-morbid psychiatric disorders administered in conjunction with alcohol treatment.

While these six areas reflect the apparent range of potential pharmacotherapy, those drugs which appear to diminish alcohol consumption on the basis of a general effect on consummatory behavior (e.g., serotonin uptake inhibitors) have been the most extensively studied over the past decade (19-21). Naltrexone, a narcotic antagonist, has also been studied in the treatment of obesity and, recently, in alcoholic patients (22). At this juncture, it is unclear whether these drugs (serotonin uptake inhibitors and/or naltrexone) reduce the intensity of desire (appetite) for alcohol, or reduce its reinforcing potency; or whether they facilitate a sense of satiation that would lead to a moderation of intake. In general, outcome has been reported as a modest decrease in alcohol consumption among heavy drinkers.

For the most part, the serotonin uptake inhibitors have not been studied in individuals who fulfill the DSM-III-R diagnosis of alcohol dependence. Kranzler and Orrok have suggested that serotonin uptake inhibitors could be combined in a program of aftercare involving a cognitive behavioral approach to relapse prevention which is designed to teach alcohol-dependent patients how to cope with high risk situations in which drinking is likely to occur (23). There is at least one clinical trial currently underway comparing fluoxetine and placebo in alcohol-dependent individuals who also receive relapse prevention training (Kranzler, personal communication).

To date, pharmacotherapy of other addictive disorders has been most successful when focused on the treatment of the symptoms and signs of the residual (dysphoric) state following acute withdrawal. Labelled as "protracted abstinence" in studies of opiate addicts at the Addiction Research Center at Lexington, Kentucky (24), it was characterized by altered responsivity to opiate drugs, as well as other evidence of altered physiology. Dole (25) postulated that chronic exposure to heroin caused persistent residual changes in cellular function that obliged addicts to resume opiate self-administration (after detoxification) in order to maintain normal function. He conceived of methadone maintenance as a treatment for heroin addiction which would reduce drug hunger and reduce the likelihood of intravenous heroin use. Methadone maintenance represents one example of same-class drug substitution to alter addictive behavior. It is the single most effective example of this approach. Nicotine chewing gum appears to reduce some of the protracted withdrawal symptoms associated with cigarette smoking, while improving the early rate of recovery (26). One of the problems with same class drug substitution, however, is that these drugs have the same discriminative stimulus properties as the original drug of abuse. Animal experiments suggest that low doses of such drugs serve as powerful cues for drug self-administration (27). Hence, this type of approach could increase the desire to use certain drugs and make relapse more likely. In the early phase of the present cocaine epidemic, methylphenidate was proposed as a treatment for cocaine addicts (28). Unfortunately, clinical experience has not borne out the early enthusiasm for this approach. Similarly, chlordiazepoxide appears to mimic the discriminative and reinforcing stimulus properties of ethanol. Early enthusiasm for chronic chlordiazepoxide treatment of protracted abstinence symptoms in alcoholics (29) was not borne out by clinical experience which demonstrated the high likelihood of patterns of cross-dependence associated with this treatment (30). Most clinicians would agree that chlordiazepoxide and other benzodiazepines do not appear to have a place in the treatment of alcoholism, apart from the treatment of acute alcohol withdrawal.

With regard to alcoholism, there are no current candidates for the pharmacotherapy of the symptoms and signs of protracted withdrawal. These include persistent anxiety and depressive symptoms (in the absence of a coexisting anxiety or mood disorder); abnormalities of sleep architecture and subjective complaints of insomnia; neuroendocrine abnormalities such as nonsuppression in the dexamethasone suppression test; persistent alterations in the gating of auditory evoked potentials; and neuropsychological deficits (18). As is true of other addictive disorders, there is increased risk of relapse in the first three to six months after withdrawal--suggesting that the symptoms of protracted abstinence may increase the probability of relapse. It is tempting to consider drug treatments for some of the symptoms and signs of protracted abstinence. Unfortunately, there are no present candidate drugs. Potential targets include central nervous system hyperexcitability, anxiety and depressive symptoms, altered circadian rhythm, cognitive impairment, and insomnia. Research related to other addictive disorders suggests that it may be possible to reverse some of the signs and symptoms of protracted abstinence associated with some drugs of abuse by using medications with a different drug stimulus profile than the original drug of abuse. These drugs would not be associated with increased risk of cross dependence. Gawin and Kleber (11) employed desipramine to reverse the theoretical dopamine depletion following chronic cocaine administration. Others have employed imipramine (31) or bromocripitine (12) for this function. Halikas and associates used carbamazepine in an open trial theoretically to suppress limbic kindling, which has been associated with chronic cocaine administration (13). As research advances our understanding of the reversible residual CNS effects of chronic ethanol administration, it may be possible to identify non-addicting drugs to advance the recovery process, or to reverse the signs and symptoms of protracted abstinence.

One of the problems in assessing the efficacy of pharmacotherapy in the treatment of alcoholism has been the high prevalence of co-morbid psychiatric disorders in alcoholic patients. Antisocial personality disorder, which is quite prevalent in male alcoholics (32,33), is associated with poor prognosis in alcohol treatment (34), and is not treatable with known pharmacotherapies. In general, the presence of co-morbid psychopathology in an alcohol-dependent male patient is a poor prognostic sign; while female alcoholics with major depression appear to have a better outcome than other female alcoholic patients (including those without any other psychiatric disorder) (34,35). Alcoholic patients with co-morbid psychopathology would appear to be ideal for studies in which psychotropic medication is used in conjunction with standard alcoholism treatment in a treatment/matching design. In addition to issues of gender and severity of alcohol dependence, a number of issues need to be addressed in such studies:

1. Many of the symptoms of anxiety and depression present during the early phases of recovery disappear over the first two to four weeks after acute withdrawal. Formal psychiatric diagnoses should be made after this initial period.

2. Research studies should employ diagnostic interview schedules to reduce some of the error variance associated with differences between raters, as well as errors of omission and commission that lead to unacceptable levels of criterion variance. While there is good reliability for Axis I DSM-III-R (36) criteria, diagnoses of personality disorders (Axis II) are quite unreliable (apart from the diagnosis of antisocial personality disorder). Additional interview schedules might be used to improve the reliability of Axis II diagnoses.

3. Clinical judgement is critical in choosing the proper pharmacological and nonpharmacological treatments.

4. Outcome assessments must separately evaluate the psychiatric disorder and the problem of alcohol use. Psychotropic drugs may be effective in treating the co-morbid psychiatric problem, but may be able of little use in controlling the alcoholism.

The Problem of Craving

DSM-III-R criteria for alcohol dependence disorder emphasize alcohol consummatory behavior (rather than tolerance and physical dependence), its primacy in relationship to other behavioral options, and impaired control over drinking behavior (36). Efforts to operationalize criteria for treatment efficacy have focused on abstinence or moderation of drinking (as measured by self- or significant other-report, and/or biological markers associated with drinking). Many investigators have asked subjects to record their desire to drink on a visual analogue scale of "craving." Some studies ask subjects to record their level of "craving" retrospectively (last week; last month), while other studies ask subjects to record "craving" on the day of examination, or daily while in treatment. The validity of the visual analogue scale (relative to the probability of alcohol consumption) has not been systematically examined in each of these contexts (i.e., retrospective, daily, or on the day of examination). Thus, by itself, "craving" is not a useful measure of treatment outcome.

Questions have also been raised about the usefulness of the construct itself (37,38). Mello (39) argued against the position that the subjective awareness of "craving" should serve as an explanation for relapse or "loss of control." She regarded the term as a mentalist construct which was unnecessary, if one viewed alcohol consumption like any other operant (i.e., a behavior whose frequency was controlled by its consequences). In contrast to Mello's Skinnerian perspective, a number of investigators have attempted to identify a specific psychophysiological state associated with "craving" in alcoholic subjects (40-45).

At least two distinct constructs must be differentiated: "craving" or "drug hunger" associated with protracted abstinence, and "craving" associated with previous episodes of alcohol consumption. The latter, theoretically, can occur at any point in recovery. Some of the issues associated with protracted abstinence have been described above. Issues related to stimulus specific "craving" will be discussed here.

Wikler proposed the use of narcotic antagonists for the treatment of the stimulus specific "craving" of heroin addicts (46). He postulated that heroin addicts experience a strong desire for heroin in "street" settings in which they had previously experienced true pharmacological withdrawal (47). The withdrawal symptoms had been paired to these settings by Pavlovian conditioning. He was able to demonstrate "conditioned abstinence" in heroin addicts (48) and in addicted rats (49). Wikler also postulated that drug self-administration results in "counter adaptive" conditioning. Over time, the <u>anticipation</u> of a heroin injection becomes associated with physiological effects which counter the pharmacological effects of the injected heroin. Siegel has theorized that this conditioning of drug opposing effects ("opponent process conditioning") may explain the development of tolerance to heroin and alcohol (50). Stewart et al. have postulated that environmental stimuli associated with previous drug (or alcohol) administration elicit drug-like <u>reinforcing</u> effects which could account for conditioned place preference in animals (51), as well as the tendency of alcoholics (and addicts) to return to their old drinking (or drug-using) environments. They argue that while opponent process conditioning and conditioning of drug effects may be occurring concurrently, the latter is responsible for increased risk of relapse ("craving"), while the former may account for "learned tolerance." At this juncture, this hypothesis has not been systematically tested, although Meyer and Dolinsky (52) have suggested that neuroendocrine parameters may provide a more useful indicator of conditioned "craving" than traditional psychophysiologic measures of autonomic arousal. The latter do not clearly differentiate conditioned withdrawal from conditioned alcohol-like effects.

What are the implications of these Pavlovian conditioning theories of relapse for a pharmacotherapy of alcoholism? As described above, Wikler proposed using a narcotic antagonist to block the effects of injected heroin in addicts encouraged to self-administer their drug. He theorized that this would lead to extinction of conditioned Pavlovian responses (withdrawal symptoms and/or "counter adaptive" responses) and operant responding for heroin. Meyer and Mirin (53) observed that addicts on naltrexone dramatically reduced their self-administration of heroin. This was associated with a decline in self-reported "craving" for heroin which appeared to be related to the realization that they could not get "high" while on the narcotic blocking drug. The results of this study suggested that "craving" was associated with a mental set in which subjects felt that heroin was "available." Consumption of the narcotic antagonist made heroin "unavailable," with a consequent decline in "craving" for the narcotic. Follow-up of subjects in the community indicated that the greatest challenge facing the clinician would be to develop techniques to enhance compliance with the prescribed treatment. The laboratory data did not support the feasibility of systematic extinction of heroin-related responses in subjects on naltrexone.

In general, alcoholic subjects experience some increase in self-reported "craving" or "desire to drink" when they hold, sniff, or consume an alcoholic beverage (or a placebo which they believe contains ethanol) in the laboratory (40-41,43-44). For alcoholics, but not controls, the increase in "craving" is associated with some measure of autonomic arousal (increased skin conductance or heart rate). All alcoholics do not show this response. It appears to be more likely in more seriously alcohol-dependent subjects who drink the beverage in the laboratory than in subjects who merely hold and sniff the alcoholic beverage (but are not allowed to drink it). It is unclear whether self reports of "craving" in the laboratory conform to the experience in the community where other cues (e.g., negative mood states, familiar drinking environment) may be more relevant. It is also unclear whether the laboratory paradigm for craving in alcoholics would be a useful test for the efficacy of a medication designed to modify stimulus specific "craving" responses. Kranzler and Bauer (54) are using this type of cue exposure paradigm to assess potential pharmacotherapies for cocaine "craving."

Are there possible pharmacotherapies for stimulus specific "craving" in alcoholics? At this writing, there is no pharmacological antagonist for alcohol intoxication, anxiolysis, or reinforcement. Peachey and Annis have utilized calcium carbimide as part of a relapse prevention program, where patients are instructed to use this reversible aldehyde dehydrogenase inhibitor when they expect to be in "high risk" situations (55). By consuming calcium carbimide, the patient is creating an "alcohol unavailable" condition analogous to the "heroin unavailable" condition created by naltrexone consumption. Essentially, the pharmacotherapy becomes a behavioral tool to modify the stimulus conditions that would otherwise signal "alcohol availability" and associated "craving." In the absence of a known biological substrate for stimulus specific "craving," it is impossible to speculate on other potential pharmacotherapies for the modification of this subjective state.

In summary, if the investigator chooses to assess the effect of pharmacotherapy on subjective "craving" or "desire to drink" in the alcoholic, it is important to keep the following points in mind. Is the drug designed to affect "craving" associated with "protracted abstinence," or specific stimulus conditions? If the former, it will be important to secure other measures of protracted abstinence. If the latter, it will be important to secure a full stimulus history, along with the subjective measure. During treatment, does the patient fail to experience the usual "craving" in familiar drinking settings, or in association with specific negative mood states? Does the patient find it easier to avoid "high risk" situations? Craving, by itself, does not fully characterize disposition to drink. The patient may experience a strong subjective desire to drink and concomitantly a strong wish to avoid drinking which he/she may act on by consuming a drug like calcium carbimide, going to an AA meeting, or practicing coping skills learned in treatment. "Craving" is a continuous measure which, by itself, is not a sufficient outcome measure. In association with other drinking-related outcome assessments, it may be informative.

We are at a very early stage in developing new pharmacotherapies (and tools for their assessment) for the treatment of alcoholic patients. Optimally, we will see the development of specific treatments for specific aspects of the disorder. One can imagine the integration of pharmacotherapy with other treatment modalities, as in the work of Peachey and Annis (55). It is possible that research in the neurosciences will generate treatments for protracted abstinence and cognitive impairment in the alcoholic in the early stages of recovery. This might be followed by a broadly based rehabilitation program that includes an aldehyde dehydrogenase inhibitor or an ethanol antagonist to assist the individual to cope with stimulus specific "craving," and/or a psychotropic drug for the treatment of co-morbid psychopathology. It will be a challenge for clinicians and clinical investigators to collaborate in the development of clinically and theoretically sound assessments, and in the integration of new knowledge into practice.

This paper was supported by grant 5 P50 AA03510 from the National Institute on Alcohol Abuse and Alcoholism.

References

1. Fuller, R.K., Branchey, L., Brightwell, D.R., et al. Disulfiram treatment of Alcoholism: A Veterans Administration cooperative study. JAMA 256:1449-1455, 1986.
2. Chick, J., Kreitman, N., Plant, M. Mean cell volume and gamma-glutamyl-transpeptidase as markers of drinkers in working men. Lancet 1:1249-1251, 1981.
3. Reyes, E., Miller, W.R., Serum gamma-glutamyl-transpeptidase as a diagnostic aid in problem drinkers. Addict Behav 5:59-65, 1980.
4. Irwin, M., Baird, S., Smith, T., et al. The use of laboratory tests to monitor heaving drinking. Am J Psychiatry 145:595-599, 1988.
5. Behrans, U.J., Worner, T.M., Braly, L.F., et al. Carbohydrate-deficient transferrin, a marker for chronic alcohol consumption in different ethnic populations. Alcohol Clin Expres 12:427-432, 1988.
6. Israel, Y., Orrego, H., Niemalla, O. Immune responses to alcohol metabolites: Pathogenic and diagnostic implications. Semin Liver Dis 8:81-90, 1988.
7. Voltaire, A., Beck, O., Borg, S., et al. Clinical and biochemical characteristics during long-term abstinence in relation to relapses. Results from a longitudinal study of alcohol dependent male patients. Paper presented at the Research Society on Alcoholism, Toronto, Canada, June 1990.

8. Ciraulo, D.A., Alderson, L.M., Chapron, D.J., et al. Imipramine disposition in alcoholics. J Clin Psychopharmacol 2:2-7, 1982.
9. Dole, V.P., Nyswander, M.E. A medical treatment for diacetyl morphine (heroin) addiction. JAMA 193:646-650, 1965.
10. Kleber, H. Clinical experience with narcotic antagonists. In S. Fisher & A.M. Freedman (eds.), Opiate Addiction: Origins and Treatment. Washington, DC: 1974, 211- 222.
11. Gawin, F.H., Kleber, H.D., Byck, R. et al. Desipramine facilitation of initial cocaine abstinence. Arch Gen Psychiatry 46:117- 121, 1989.
12. Dackis, C., Gold, M.S., Sweeney, D. et al. Single dose bromocriptine reverses cocaine craving. Psychiatry Res 20:261-264, 1987.
13. Halikas, J., Kemp, K., Kuhn, K. et al. Carbamazepine for cocaine addiction? Lancet 1:623-624, 1989.
14. Seventh Special Report to the U.S. Congress on Alcohol and Health from the Secretary of Health and Human Services. Neuroscience, Chapter 4, pp. 69-105, 1990, U.S. Department of Health and Human Services.
15. Babor, T.F., Cooney, N.L., Lauerman, R.J. The dependent syndrome concept as a psychological theory of relapsed behavior: An empirical evaluation of alcoholic and opiate addicts. Br J Addict 82:393-405, 1987.
16. Meyer, R.E. How to understand the relationship between psychopathology and addictive disorders: Another example of the chicken and the egg. In R.E. Meyer (ed.), Psychopathology and Addictive Disorders. New York: Guilford Press, 1986, 3-16.
17. Finney, J.W., Moos, R.H. Matching patients with treatments: Conceptual and methodological issues. J Stud Alcohol 47:122-134, 1986.
18. Meyer, R.E. Prospects for a rational pharmacotherapy of alcoholism. J Clin Psychiatry 50:403-412, 1989.
19. Naranjo, C.A., Sellers, E.M., Roach, C.A., et al. Zimelidine-induced variations in alcohol intake by nondepressed heavy drinkers. Clin Pharmacol Ther 35:374-381, 1984.

20. Amit, Z., Brown, Z., Sutherland, A., et al. Reduction in alcohol intake in humans as a function of treatment with zimelidine: Implications for treatment. In C.A. Naranjo & E.M. Sellers (eds.), Research Advances in New Psychopharmacological Treatments for Alcoholism. Amsterdam: Elsevier, 1985, 189-198.
21. Naranjo, C.A., Sellers, E.M., Sullivan, J.T., et al. The serotonin uptake inhibitor citalopram attenuates ethanol intake. Clin Pharmacol Ther 41:266-274, 1987.
22. Volpicelli, J.R., Alterman, A., Hayashida, M. et al. Naltrexone in the treatment of alcohol dependence: Initial findings. In L.B. Reid (ed.), Opioids, Bulimia, Alcohol Abuse, and Alcoholism. New York: Springer Verlag, 1989.
23. Kranzler, H.R., Orrok, B. The pharmacotherapy of alcoholism. In A. Tasman, R.E. Hales, & A.J. Frances (eds.), Annual Review of Psychiatry, Vol. 8. Washington, DC: American Psychiatric Association Press, 1989, 359-379.
24. Martin, J.R., Jasinski, D.R. Physiological parameters of morphine dependence in man--Tolerance, early abstinence, protracted abstinence. J Psychiatr Res 7:9-17, 1969.
25. Dole, V.P. Narcotic addiction, physical dependence and relapse. N Eng J Med 286:988-992, 1972.
26. Hughes, J.R., Miller, S. Nicotine gum to help stop smoking. JAMA 252:2855-2858, 1984.
27. DeWit, H., Stewart, J. Drug reinstatement of heroin reinforced responding in the rat. Psychopharmacol 79:28-31, 1983.
28. Khantzian, E.J. Cocaine dependence: An extreme case and marked improvement with methylphenidate treatment. Am J Psychiatry 140:784-785, 1983.
29. Kissin, B. The use of psychoactive drugs in the long-term treatment of chronic alcoholics. Ann NY Acad Sci 252:385-395, 1975. 30.
30. Meyer, R.E. Anxiolytics and the alcoholic patient. J Stud Alcohol 47:269-273, 1986.
31. Rosecan, J. The treatment of cocaine abuse with imipramine, l-tyrosine, and l-tryptophan. Presented at the 7th World Congress of Psychiatry, Vienna, Austria, July 14-19, 1983.

32. Hesselbrock, M.N., Meyer, R.E., Keener, J.J. Psychopathology in hospitalized alcoholics. Arch Gen Psychiat 42:1050- 1055, 1985.
33. Schuckit, M.A. The clinical implications of primary diagnostic groups among alcoholics. Arch Gen Psychiatry 42:1043- 1049, 1985.
34. Rounsaville, B.J., Dolinsky, Z.S., Babor, T.F., et al. Psychopathology as a predictor of treatment outcome in alcoholics. Arch Gen Psychiatry 44:505- 513, 1987.
35. Schuckit, M.A., Winokur, G. A short-term follow-up of women alcoholics. Dis Nerv Syst 33:672-678, 1978.
36. American Psychiatric Association: Diagnostic and Statistical Manual of Mental Disorders (DSM-III-R), 3rd edition rev., Washington DC, APA 1987.
37. Drummond, D.C., Cooper, T., Glautier, S.P. Conditional learning in alcohol dependence: Implications for cue exposure treatment. Brit J Addict 85:725-743, 1990.
38. Newlin, D.B., Hotchkiss, B., Cox, W.M., et al. Autonomic and subjective responses to alcohol stimuli with appropriate control stimuli. Addict Behav 14:625-630, 1989.
39. Mello, N.K. A semantic aspect of alcoholism. In H.D. Cappell & A.E. LeBlanc (eds.), Biological and Behavioral Approaches to Drug Dependents. Toronto: Addiction Research Foundation, 1978, 73-85.
40. Ludwig, A.M., Wikler, A., Stark, L.H. The first drink: Psychobiological aspects of craving. Arch Gen Psychiatry 30:539-548, 1974.
41. Kaplan, R.F., Meyer, R.E., Stroebel, C.F. Alcohol dependence and responsivity to an ethanol stimulus as predictors of alcohol consumption. Br J Addict 78:259-267, 1983.
42. Dolinsky, C.S., Morse, D.E., Kaplan, R.F., et al. Neuroendocrine, psychophysiological, and subjective reactivity to an alcohol placebo in male alcoholic patients. Alcoholism: Clin Exper Res 11:296-300, 1987.
43. Hodgson, R., Rankin, H., Stockwell, T. Alcohol dependence and the priming effect. Behav Res Ther 17:379-387, 1979.

44. Laberg, J.C., Ellertsen, B. Psychophysiological indications of craving in alcoholics: The effects of cue exposure. Br J Addict 82:1341-1348, 1987.
45. Monti, P.M., Binkoff, J.A., Abrams, D.B. et al. Reactivity of alcoholics and nonalcoholics to drinking cues. J Abnorm Psychol 96:122-126, 1987.
46. Wikler, A. Requirements for extinction of relapse-facilitating variables and for rehabilitation in a narcotic antagonist treatment program. In M.C. Braude, L.S. Harris, J.P. Smith, E.A. May, J.E. Villareal (eds.), Narcotic Antagonists. New York: Raven Press, 1971, 399-414.
47. Wikler, A. Dynamics of drug dependence: Implications of a conditioning theory for research and treatment. In S. Fisher & A.M. Freedman (eds.), Opiate Addiction: Origins and Treatment. Washington, DC: Winston Press, 1974, 7-22.
48. Wikler, A. Conditioning factors in opiate addiction and relapse. In D.M. Wilmer & G.G. Kassebaum (eds.), Narcotics. New York: McGraw-Hill, 1965, 85-100.
49. Wikler, A., Pescor, F.T. Classical conditioning of morphine abstinence: Reinforcement of opioid-drinking behavior and relapse in morphine-addicted rats. Psychopharmacologia 10:255-284, 1967.
50. Siegel, S. Morphine tolerance acquisition as an associative process. J Exp Psychol [Anim Behav] 3:1-13, 1977.
51. Stewart, J., DeWit, H., Eikelboom, R. Role of unconditioned and conditioned drug effects in the self-administration of opiates and stimulants. Psychol Rev 91: 251-268, 1984.
52. Meyer, R.E., Dolinsky, Z.S. Ethanol beverage anticipation: Effects on plasma testosterone and luteinizing hormone levels--A pilot study. J Stud Alcohol 51:350-355, 1990.
53. Meyer, R.E., Mirin, S.M. The Heroin Stimulus: Implications for a Theory of Addiction. New York: Plenum Press, 1979.

54. Kranzler, H.R., Bauer, L.O. Effects of bromocriptine on subjective and autonomic responses to cocaine-associated stimuli. In L.S. Harris (ed.), Problems of Drug Dependence 1990. Proceedings of the 52nd Annual Scientific Meeting, The Committee on Problems of Drug Dependence, Inc., in press.

55. Peachey, J.E., Annis, H.M. New strategies reusing the alcohol-sensitizing drugs. In C.A. Naranjo & E.M. Sellers (eds.), Research Advances in New Psychopharmacological Treatments for Alcoholism. Amsterdam: Excerpta Medica, 1985, 199-216.

Part II
Serotonin and Alcohol Consumption

5
Serotonin and Alcohol Consumption

W.J. McBride, W.J. Murphy, L. Lumeng, and T.-K. Li

1.1 ABSTRACT

The involvement of serotonin (5-HT) in alcohol consumption was studied in lines of rats selectively bred for disparate alcohol drinking behavior. Neurochemical data indicated that the alcohol-preferring (P) line and the high alcohol-drinking (HAD) line had lower CNS levels of 5-HT and/or 5-hydroxyindoleacetic acid compared with their respective counterparts, the alcohol-nonpreferring (NP) and low alcohol-drinking (LAD) rats. In addition, higher densities of cortical 5-HT_{1A} receptors were found in the P compared with the NP rats. Pharmacological studies indicated that agents which increase the actions of 5-HT or mimic its effects at 5-HT_1 or 5-HT_2 receptors can decrease the alcohol intake of P and HAD rats. Overall, the data suggest that (a) innate abnormalities exist in 5-HT systems in the CNS of P and HAD rats which may be associated with their high alcohol intake and (b) multiple 5-HT receptor subtypes might be involved in regulating alcohol consumption.

1.2 INTRODUCTION

The involvement of serotonin (5-HT) in alcohol consumption was studied in two pairs of lines of rats selectively bred for disparate alcohol drinking. One pair is the alcohol-preferring (P) line and the alcohol-nonpreferring (NP) line, derived from a stock of Wistar rats [6]. The second pair is the high alcohol-drinking (HAD) line and the low alcohol-drinking (LAD) line derived from the N/Nih heterogeneous stock rats [5]. The P and HAD lines will generally consume, under free-choice conditions, greater than 5g ethanol/kg body wt/day while the NP and LAD rats drink less than 1g ethanol/kg body wt/day. The P line of rats will orally self-administer ethanol under operant-responding conditions [10, 17] and will drink sufficient amounts to elevate blood alcohol to pharmacologically relevant levels [11]. The P rat appears to consume alcohol for its CNS positive-reinforcing actions and not solely for its caloric value, taste or smell [19]. Although the HAD line has not been as well studied as the P rats, there is evidence that the HAD animals also find alcohol rewarding and will orally self-administer ethanol under operant conditions [4]. The objective of this article is to present neurochemical and neuropharmacological data implicating the involvement of CNS 5-HT systems in regulating alcohol consumption of P and HAD rats.

1.3 INNATE NEUROCHEMICAL DIFFERENCES AND EFFECTS OF ALCOHOL

Several neurochemical studies were undertaken to determine if there were any innate differences in the CNS 5-HT system between the high alcohol-consuming lines and their respective low-alcohol drinking line, and if acute and/or chronic alcohol altered the neuronal activity of CNS 5-HT pathways.

1.3.1 CNS Levels of 5-HT and Alcohol Drinking

The levels of 5-HT and/or its major metabolite 5-hydroxyindoleacetic acid (5-HIAA) were 12-26% lower ($P < 0.05$) in the nucleus accumbens (Acb), frontal cortex, cerebral cortex, hippocampus, striatum, thalamus and hypothalamus of the P compared with the NP rats [13, 14]. Moreover, similar differences for 5-HT and/or 5-HIAA levels have been found in most of the same CNS regions of the HAD line compared with the LAD rats, most notably in the Acb, frontal cortex, hippocampus and hypothalamus [2]. Since the low alcohol intake of the NP and LAD lines resembles that of a general population of rats whereas the alcohol consumption of P and HAD rats is unusually high, the results suggest that lower CNS contents of 5-HT and/or 5-HIAA are associated with high alcohol-seeking characteristics.

1.3.2 Effects of Ethanol on 5-HT Systems

The i.p. administration of 2.5g ethanol/kg increased the levels of 5-HIAA approximately 20% ($P < 0.05$) in the Acb, frontal cortex and anterior striatum of P rats [12], which is interpreted to indicate enhanced activity of 5-HT neurons projecting to these 3 regions. Furthermore, it appears that the 5-HT projection to the Acb from the dorsal raphe nucleus (DR) develops tolerance with chronic consumption of alcohol by the P rat, since the increase in 5-HIAA following the challenge dose of ethanol is blunted in alcohol-tolerant P rats compared with nontolerant P rats [12]. Thus, alcohol increases the activity of the DR 5-HT pathway to the Acb and chronic free-choice alcohol drinking desensitizes this response.

1.3.3 Densities of 5-HT Receptors and Alcohol Drinking

The densities of 5-HT receptors were examined in alcohol-naive P and NP rats using standard membrane binding assays (with cortical and hippocampal preparations) and, as well, with quantitative autoradiography. Using membrane preparations, the densities of 5-HT_{1A} sites, labelled with [^{3}H] 8-OH DPAT [21], were higher in the cerebral cortical and hippocampal membranes from the P than from the NP line. On the other hand, the densities of 5-HT_2 sites, labelled with [^{3}H] ketanserin, were not different in membranes of the posterior cortex for the P and NP lines [20]. Quantitative autoradiography of the anterior portion of the cerebral cortex and of the hippocampus using [^{3}H] 8-OH DPAT, demonstrated higher densities of 5-HT_{1A} sites in the cingulate cortex, all layers of the frontal cortex, and the ventral portion of the hippocampus [7].

Overall, the neurochemical data suggest an up-regulation of 5-HT_{1A} receptors in the CNS of P rats. This up-regulation may be caused by decreased innervation or functioning of the 5-HT systems projecting to these regions. Such a decreased innervation or functioning is suggested by the lower contents of 5-HT/5-HIAA observed in the CNS regions of the P compared with the NP rats [13, 14]. In addition, recent immunocytochemical data also suggest lower 5-HT innervations in certain CNS regions of the P compared with the NP rats [22].

1.4 NEUROCHEMICAL ALTERATIONS OF ALCOHOL INTAKE

If the lower contents of 5-HT/5-HIAA observed in several CNS regions of the P and HAD lines are associated with their high alcohol-seeking characteristics and indicate reduced innervation and/or functioning of these systems, then enhancing the physiologically effective pool of 5-HT or mimicking the actions of 5-HT in these animals might decrease alcohol drinking.

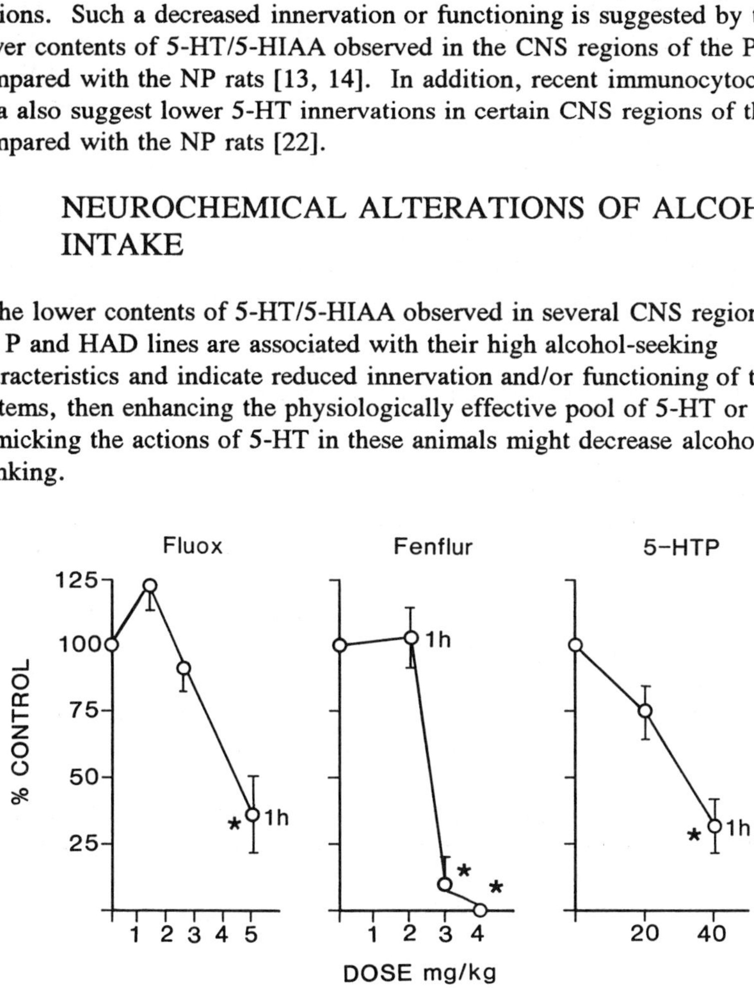

Figure 1. Effects of i.p. administration of fluoxetine (Fluox), fenfluramine (Fenflur) and D,L-5-hydroxytryptophan (5-HTP) on the intake of 10% (v/v) ethanol after the first hour (1 h) by female P rats during a 4-hour period of alcohol availability. Food and water were available ad libitum. Control intakes were 0.9 $\pm$ 0.1 g/kg (3.3 $\pm$ 0.1 ml) after 1 hour and 2.8 $\pm$ 0.2 g/kg (10.0 $\pm$ 0.4 ml) after 4 hours. *$P < 0.05$ vs. control for first hour with ANOVA and post-hoc Dunnett test.

1.4.1 Effects of Agents Which Enhance 5-HT Actions

A very elegant study demonstrated that the intragastric (i.g.) administration of 10 mg/kg fluoxetine, a selective 5-HT uptake inhibitor, once a day for 7 days markedly reduced the i.g. self-administration of 20% ethanol by P rats while the i.g. self-administration of H_2O increased [15]. Fluoxetine also reduced the oral intake of alcohol by P (Fig. 1) as well as by HAD rats (data not shown). These findings are consistent with several reports that 5-HT uptake inhibitors effectively reduce alcohol drinking in rats not selectively bred for alcohol drinking [8]. In addition, other agents which enhance the actions of 5-HT by increasing its extracellular levels, such as fenfluramine (a releaser) and D,L-5-hydroxytryptophan (a precursor), can reduce oral alcohol consumption of the P rat (Fig. 1). These pharmacological data are consistent with the hypothesis that lower functioning of certain 5-HT systems is associated with high alcohol drinking. However, these studies do not indicate which 5-HT receptor or receptors might be involved in mediating alcohol intake. Therefore, studies were undertaken with more selective agents to determine the possible involvement of 5-HT_{1A}, 5-HT_{1B} and 5-HT_2 receptors in alcohol consumption.

1.4.2 Effects of 5-HT Agonists on Alcohol Consumption

In general, 5-HT agonists acting at different subtypes of 5-HT receptors all significantly reduced alcohol drinking of P and HAD rats (Table 1). The 5-HT_{1A} agonist 8-OH DPAT [1, 3] effectively reduced alcohol consumption of P and HAD rats (Table 1). TFMPP, which behaves like a 5-HT_{1B} agonist under certain experimental conditions [18] but also has high affinity for other 5-HT sites [3], was very effective at reducing ethanol intake in both P and HAD animals (Table 1). The 5-HT_2 agonist DOI [1] reduced alcohol drinking of the P rat but had a biphasic effect on ethanol intake of the HAD line (Table 1). Low doses of DOI significantly increased alcohol intake of HAD rats while higher doses markedly decreased consumption.

Overall, the pharmacological studies suggest the involvement of 5-HT_{1A}, 5-HT_{1B} and 5-HT_2 receptors in mediating alcohol drinking. Although the nature of this involvement is not clear, the results indicate that activating 5-HT receptors generally produces decreased alcohol consumption by the P and HAD rats.

1.4.3 Effects of 5-HT Antagonists on Alcohol Drinking

If 5-HT agonists generally reduce alcohol intake of P and HAD rats, then antagonists might be expected to produce the converse effect. Therefore, studies were undertaken to examine the effects of 5-HT_{1A} and 5-HT_2 antagonists on alcohol drinking (Fig. 2).

Table 1. Effects of I.P. Administration of 5-HT Agonists on 10% Ethanol Intake of P and HAD Rats During Scheduled Availability of Alcohol

Agent	Receptor	Line	mg/kg[a]	Intake[b]
8-OH DPAT	5-HT_{1A}	P	1	75% lower
		HAD	0.3	85% lower
TFMPP	5-HT_{1B}	P	1	100% lower
		HAD	0.3	70% lower
DOI	5-HT_2	P	1[c]	50% lower
		HAD	0.5[d]	65% higher
		HAD	4[d]	75% lower

[a]ED_{50} value (1st hour) unless otherwise noted. [b]Maximal effect that was observed during the first hour. Lower or higher values were statistically different from control intakes (ANOVA, post-hoc Dunnett test). [c]Highest dose used. [d]Biphasic effect.

Spiroxatrine, a possible 5-HT_{1A} antagonist [16], did not alter alcohol consumption of HAD (Fig. 2) or P [9] rats when administered by itself. Similarly, pindolol another 5-HT_{1A} antagonist [1], had no effect on alcohol consumption (Fig. 2). However, when spiroxatrine was given with either fluoxetine or 8-OH DPAT, it markedly augmented the actions of both 5-HT agents in reducing alcohol intake of P rats [9]. These studies indicate that spiroxatrine is not functioning as an antagonist but appears to be acting as a partial agonist and/or modulator at 5-HT_{1A} receptors. These results further support the idea that activating 5-HT_{1A} receptors reduces alcohol intake.

The i.p. administration of LY53857, a 5-HT_2 antagonist [1], significantly reduced alcohol consumption of the HAD rats (Fig. 2). The findings that a 5-HT_2 antagonist decreases ethanol intake while a 5-HT_2 agonist, DOI, has a biphasic action (Table 1) could indicate that 5-HT_2 receptors might be involved in CNS circuitry promoting alcohol consumption of HAD rats. The 5-HT_2 antagonist blocks the 5-HT systems normally activated by ethanol, thereby inhibiting the positive reinforcing actions of alcohol and decreasing its consumption. Low dose DOI acts as a "primer" for the 5-HT systems and potentiates the reinforcing properties of alcohol. However, high doses of DOI maximally activate the 5-HT_2 systems such that alcohol has little positive

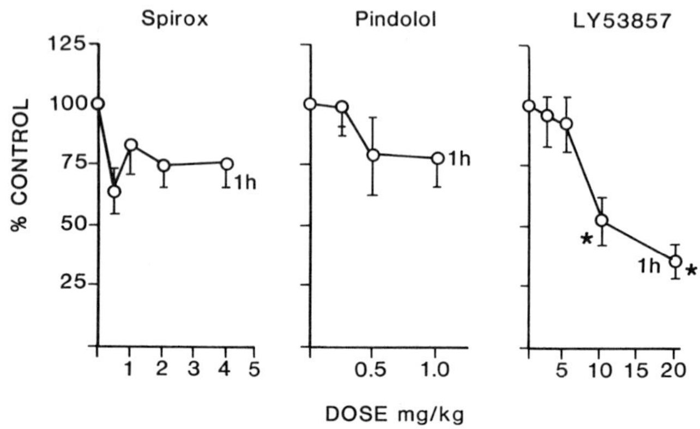

Figure 2. Effects of i.p. administration of spiroxatrine (Spirox), Pindolol and LY 53857 on the intake of 10% (v/v) ethanol after the first hour (1 h) by male HAD rats during a 4-hour period of alcohol availability. Food and water were available ad libitum. Control intakes were 0.81 $\pm$ 0.06 g/kg (5.0 $\pm$ 0.1 ml) for the first hour and 1.6 $\pm$ 0.1 g/kg (10 $\pm$ 1 ml) for the 4 hours. *$P < 0.05$ vs. control for first hour with ANOVA and post-hoc Dunnett test.

effect and, as a consequence, alcohol intake decreases.

1.5 CONCLUSIONS

The neurochemical data for 5-HT and/or5-HIAA content in the CNS of the P and HAD lines are consistent with the hypothesis that high alcohol-seeking characteristics are associated with lower innervation and/or functioning of certain 5-HT pathways (e.g., DR projections to the Acb and frontal cortical areas). The higher densities of CNS 5-HT_{1A} receptors in the P compared with NP rats suggests that up-regulation of this receptor might also be associated with high ethanol intake. The pharmacological data suggest that 5-HT_{1A}, 5-HT_{1B} and 5-HT_2 receptors might all play a role in regulating alcohol consumption of P and HAD rats. Obviously, any interpretations of the pharmacological data must take into consideration possible peripheral actions of the agent, the possibility of the drug acting at multiple receptor types, and the possibility that the 5-HT agent may have effects on several neuronal systems some of which are involved in mediating general appetitive, motivational and/or other behaviors. Despite these reservations, the present findings indicate that future studies exploring the involvement of 5-HT_{1A}, 5-

HT_{1B} and $5\text{-}HT_2$ receptors in the mediation of alcohol drinking would be fruitful and could lead to the development of pharmacological interventions for alcoholism.

1.6 ACKNOWLEDGEMENTS

The skillful technical assistance of Suzann Geisler, Steve Cunningham, Simon Katner, Eyassu Chernet and Florianne Franada and the secretarial support of Jeanne Wilson are deeply appreciated. Studies reported in this article were supported by AA 03243, AA 07462 and AA 07611. LY 53857 and fluoxetine were gifts from Eli Lilly and Co.

1.7 REFERENCES

1. Glennon, R.A. Serotonin receptors: clinical implications. Neurosci. Biobehav. Rev. 14: 35-47, 1990.

2. Gongwer, M.A., Murphy, J.M., McBride, W.J., Lumeng, L., Li, T.-K. Regional brain contents of serotonin, dopamine and their metabolites in the selectively bred high- and low-alcohol drinking lines of rats. Alcohol 6: 317-320, 1989.

3. Hoyer, D. J. Functional correlates of serotonin $5\text{-}HT_1$ recognition sites. Receptor Res. 8: 59-81, 1988.

4. Levy, A.D., McBride, W.J., Murphy, J.M., Lumeng, L., Li, T.-K. Genetically selected lines of high- and low-alcohol drinking rats: operant studies. Soc. Neurosci. Abstr. 14: 41, 1988.

5. Li, T.-K., Lumeng, L., Dolittle, D.P., McBride, W.J., Murphy, J.M., Froehlich, J.C., Morzorati, S. Behavioral and neurochemical associations of alcohol-seeking behavior. In: Biomedical and social aspects of alcohol and alcoholism. (Kuriyama, K., Takada, A., Ishii, H., eds.) Amsterdam, Elsevier, 1988, pp. 435-438.

6. Lumeng, L., Hawkins, T.D., Li, T.-K. New strains of rats with alcohol preference and nonpreference. In: Alcohol and aldehyde metabolizing systems. Vol 3 (Thurman, R.G., Williamson, J.R., Drott, H., Chance, B., eds.) New York, Academic Press, 1977, pp. 537-544.

7. McBride, W.J., Guan, X.-M., Chernet, E., Lumeng, L., Li, T.-K. Regional differences in the densities of serotonin-1A receptors between P and NP rats. Alcoholism: Clin. Exp. Res. 14: 316, 1990.

8. McBride, W.J., Murphy, J.M., Lumeng, L., Li, T.-K. Serotonin and ethanol preference. In: Recent Developments in Alcoholism, Vol.. 7 (Galanter, M. ed.) New York, Plenum, 1989, pp. 187-209.

9. McBride, W.J., Murphy, J.M., Lumeng, L., Li, T.-K. Spiroxatrine augments fluoxetine-induced reduction of ethanol intake by the P line of rats. Pharmacol. Biochem. Behav. 34: 381-386, 1989.

10. Murphy, J.M., Gatto, G.J., McBride, W.J., Lumeng, L., Li, T.-K. Operant responding for oral ethanol in the alcohol-preferring P and alcohol-nonpreferring NP lines of rats. Alcohol 6: 127-131, 1989.

11. Murphy, J.M., Gatto, G.J., Waller, M.B., McBride, W.J., Lumeng, L., Li, T.-K. Effects of scheduled access on ethanol intke by the alcohol-preferring (P) line of rats. Alcohol 3: 331-336, 1986.

12. Murphy, J.M., McBride, W.J., Gatto, G.J., Lumeng, L., Li, T.-K. Effects of acute ethanol administration on monoamine and metabolite content in forebrain regions of ethanol-tolerant and -nontolerant alcohol-preferring (P) rats. Pharmacol. Biochem. Behav. 29: 169-174, 1988.

13. Murphy, J.M., McBride, W.J., Lumeng, L., Li, T.-K. Regional brain levels of monoamines in alcohol-preferring and -nonpreferring lines of rats. Pharmacol. Biochem. Behav. 16: 145-149, 1982.

14. Murphy, J.M., McBride, W.J., Lumeng, L., Li, T.-K. Contents of monoamines in forebrain regions of alcohol-preferring (P) and -nonpreferring (NP) lines of rats. Pharmacol. Biochem. Behav. 26: 389-392, 1987.

15. Murphy, J.M., Waller, M.B., Gatto, G.J., McBride, W.J., Lumeng, L., Li, T.-K. Effects of fluoxetine on the intragastric self-administration of ethanol in the alcohol preferring P line of rats. Alcohol 5: 283-286, 1988.

16. Nelson, D.L., Taylor, E.W. Spiroxatrine: a selective serotonin-1A receptor antagonist. Eur. J. Pharmacol. 124: 207-208, 1986.

17. Penn, P.E., McBride, W.J., Lumeng, L., Gaff, T.M., Li, T.-K. Neurochemical and operant behavioral studies of a strain of alcohol-preferring rats. Pharmacol. Biochem. Behav. 8: 475-481, 1978.

18. Schechter, M.D. Use of TFMPPP stimulus properties as a model of 5-HT_{1B} receptor activation. Pharmacol. Biochem. Behav. 31: 53-57, 1988.

19. Waller, M.B., McBride, W.J., Gatto, G.J., Lumeng, L., Li, T.-K. Intragastric self-infusion of ethanol by ethanol-preferring and -nonpreferring lines of rats. Science 225: 78-80, 1984.

20. Wong, D.T., Lumeng, L., Threlkeld, P.G., Reid, L.R., Li, T.-K. Serotonergic and adrenergic receptors in alcohol-preferring and -nonpreferring rats. J. Neural Transm. 71: 207-218, 1988.

21. Wong, D.T., Threlkel, P.G., Lumeng, L., Li, T.-K. Higher density of serotonin-1A receptors in the hippocampus and cerebral cortex of alcohol-preferring P rats. Life Sci. 46: 231-235, 1990.

22. Zhou, F.C., Bledsoe, S., Lumeng, L., Li, T.-K. Serotonergic immunostained terminal fibers are decreased in selected brain areas of alcohol-preferring P rats. Alcoholism Clin. Exp. Res. 14: 355, 1990.

6

Serotonergic and Dopaminergic Involvement in Ethanol Intake

J.A. Engel, C. Enerback, C. Fahlke, P. Hulthe, E. Hard, K. Johannessen, L. Svensson, and B. Soderpalm

Ethanol, being a simple molecule, is known to influence the activity of a number of biological systems and therefore it is not suprising that ethanol has a very complex psychopharmacodynamic profile. The understanding of the neurochemical basis of these various pharmacological effects is of course imperative for the development of new pharmacological treatment strategies for decreasing alcohol consumption in man. All the diverse effects of ethanol can in all probability not be related to one single neurotransmitter system. In fact, as indicated by data from our research group as well as from others, we have to consider that different neurotransmitters and perhaps also hormones are involved in the mediation of the pharmacological effects of ethanol (fig. 1). To what degree they participate in the regulation of ethanol consumption is one of many challenges we have to face in ethanol research. One way to view this is that multiple neurotransmitters and hormones collectively orchestrate the reward profile of ethanol, ethanol being the conductor and every instrument/transmitter being able to play the reward tune to some degree, but not until all instruments are playing together the full reward symphony will be experienced. Furthermore, adding to the complexity, we also have to take into account that the various biological systems may be differentially sensitive to ethanol i.e. they display different dose-response ranges (cf. Engel and Liljequist, 1983).

Needless to say the final behavioral outcome will be determined by factors related to the individual and it should be emphasized that these are not only genetic but may also be state dependent including hormonal state and the age of the individual (cf.Engel 1985).

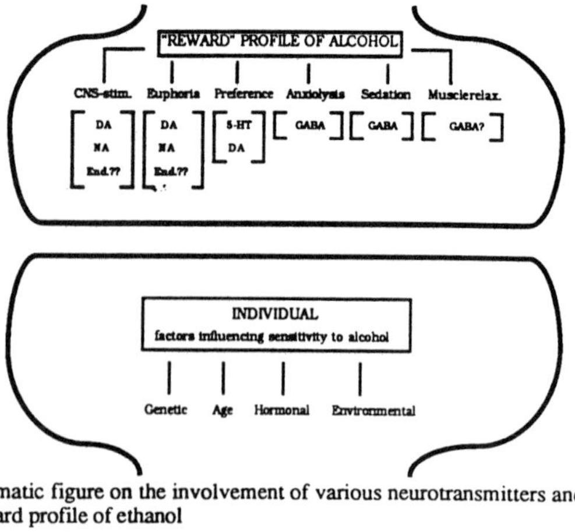

FIGURE 1. Schematic figure on the involvement of various neurotransmitters and individuallly related factors in the reward profile of ethanol

CATECHOLAMINES

Ample evidence has accumulated over the past decade indicating that the catecholamines (CA) are implicated in the brain reward systems and that the CA are directly or indirectly involved in the stimulatory and euphoric effects of ethanol in experimental animals as well as in man (Engel 1977, 1985). The first, indirect pharmacological evidence for a causal relationship between ethanol induced stimulation of behavior and of cateholaminergic activity was provided by data showing that the CA-synthesis inhibitor α-methyltyrosine antagonized the ethanol-induced locomotor-stimulation in rodents and the euphoria and stimulation in man (see Engel 1977).

We have recently obtained direct, biochemical support for the notion that ethanol can activate central dopaminergic systems by means of a new technique, in vivo voltammetry. With this method it is possible to monitor rapid changes in extracellular concentrations of dopamine (DA) and 3,4-dihydroxyphenylacetic acid (DOPAC) in discrete brain areas in real time and in awake, freely moving animals.

Square wave voltammetry was used to produce the voltammograms and Tacussel carbon fibre electrodes (diameter 8 μm) were utilized as working electrodes. The electrodes were electrochemically pretreated according to Gonon and co-workers (1981) before they were used. This electrode will generate distinct peaks for ascorbic acid and DA+DOPAC (cf. Engel et al. 1988).

Male rats from an unselected stock of the Wistar strain were used. They were presented with a free choice between water and increasing concentrations of 2-6% ethanol for a 3 week habituation period, during which time the amounts of ethanol and water consumed were measured. Rats drinking more than 75% of their daily liquid intake in the form of ethanol solution were defined as high preferring rats (HP) and those drinking less than 25% ethanol solution were defined as low preferring rats (LP). Oral daily intake of ethanol in our HP rats was about 5g/kg/24hr and that of the LP less than 1g/kg/24hr. The rats were alcohol free for at least 4 weeks prior to the voltammetry experiment.

When the electrode was placed in the caudate nucleus a 15-20% increase in the DA+DOPAC peak was observed in both the LP and HP rats with no significant

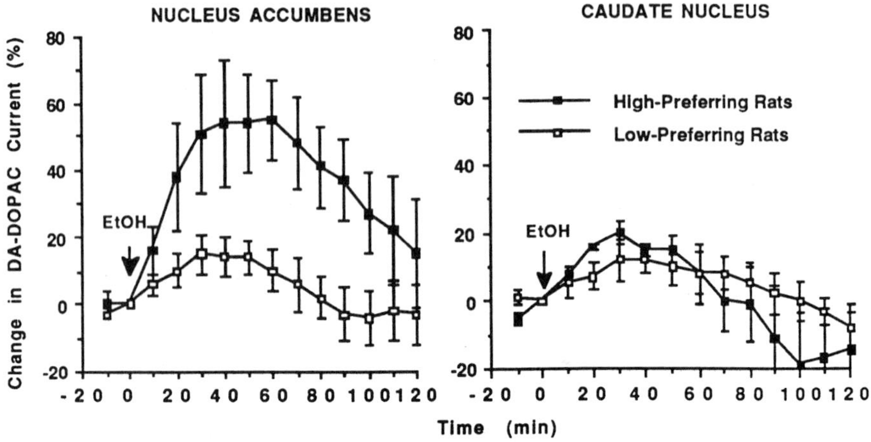

FIGURE 2. Electrochemical detection of DA+DOPAC by means of square wave voltammetry at an electrochemically pretreated carbon fibre electrode. Ethanol (EtOH) administered i.p. 1.25 g/kg to awake freely moving rats. Shown are the means ± SEM of 4-6 rats. Maximum current increase in nucleus accumbens: HP rats: 55±12% (n=5, $p<0.01$), LP rats: 15±6% (n=6, $p<0.05$). Caudate nucleus: HP rats: 20±3% (n=4, $p<0.01$), LP rats: 12±4% (n=4, $p<0.05$).

difference between the two groups (fig. 2). However, when the carbon-fibre electrode was placed in the nucleus accumbens, the enhancing effect of ethanol on DA metbolism was much more marked in the HP than in the LP rats (HP: 55%, LP: 15%, $p<0.05$), indicating that the mesolimbic DA system is more sensitive to ethanol in the HP than in the LP rats. In preliminary experiments, using a new carbon-fibre electrode (Textron, diameter 30 μm) that was electrochemically pretreated and nafion coated making it selectively sensitive for DA, we found that the ethanol-induced DA release in nucleus accumbens was more marked in the HP than in the LP rats. Furthermore, by means of microdialysis in awake animals Imperato and Di Chiara (1986) recently reported that ethanol produced an increased DA release, that was more marked in the nucleus accumbens than in the striatum. Taken together these data implicate the mesolimbic DA system in the rewarding effects of ethanol and provide further support for the notion that the mesolimbic DA system is a constituent of the brain reward circuitry (see Wise and Bozarth 1984, Engel et al. 1985). However, using ex vivo biochemistry Fadda et al. (1990) recently found in their inbred strains of high and low preferring rats a differential sensitivity to ethanol induced stimulation of DA metabolism not only in tuberculum olfactorium and prefrontal cortex but, in contrast to our findings, also in the caudate nucleus. Whether factors related to genetic breeding are responsible for this discrepancy remains to be elucidated.

Considering the importance of the catecholamines for some of the reinforcing pharmacological effects of ethanol, it would be of interest to study the effect of drugs, that reduce the influence of these neurotransmitters, on the behavioral effects induced by ethanol. Recently it has been reported that the calcium channel antagonists of the dihydropyridine class reduce both the synthesis and release of DA in the mouse and the rat brain (Pileblad and Carlsson 1986, 1987). Thus the dihydropyridines may represent a new class of drugs that under certain circumstances can reduce the influence of catecholamines. Consequently we investigated how the L-type calcium channel antagonist, nifedipine, affected some of the biochemical and behavioral effects of ethanol.

Nifedipine in a dose that had no effect per se, completely antagonized the locomotor stimulatory effect of a low dose of ethanol in mice (fig. 3). Furthermore, in a two bottle

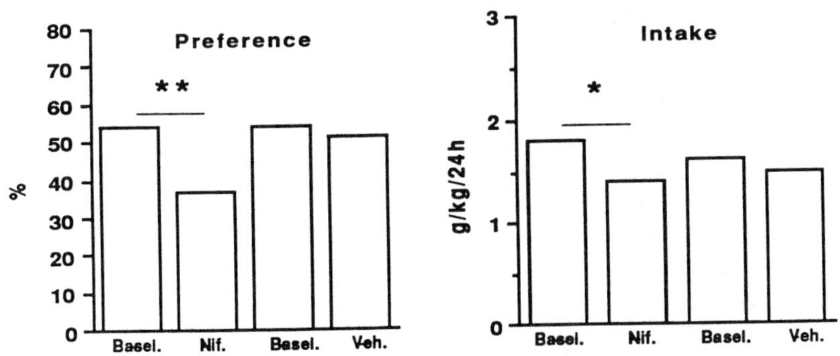

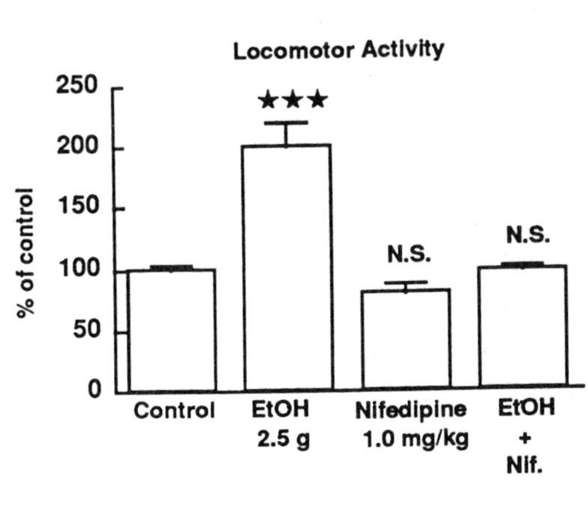

FIGURE 3. The effects of nifedipine on ethanol preference and intake (upper panels). Ethanol consumption in a free choice situation was recorded during a 3 day period in rats treated 2 times daily with nifedipine (Nif, 5 mg/kg p.o.) or vehicle (Veh) and compared with a 3 weeks baseline period (Basel). * $p<0.05$, ** $p<0.02$. The lower panel shows the effects of nifedipine on ethanol induced locomotor stimulation in mice. Nifedipine was administered p.o. 20 minutes and ethanol i.p. 5 minutes before the start of locomotor activity recording. Comparisons with control . *** $p<0.001$. (Data from Engel et al. 1988)

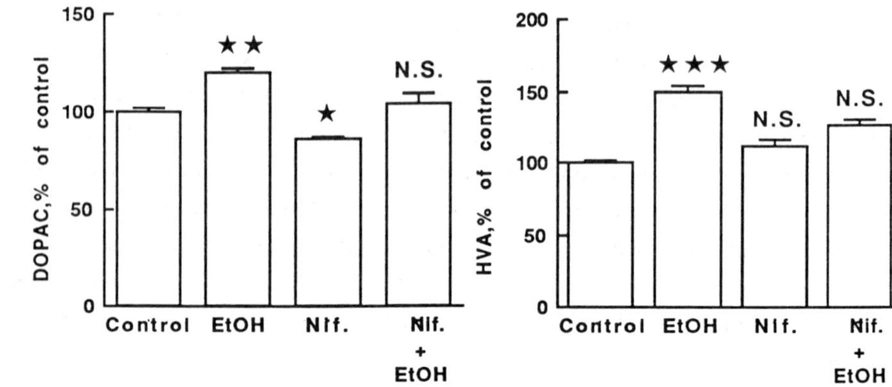

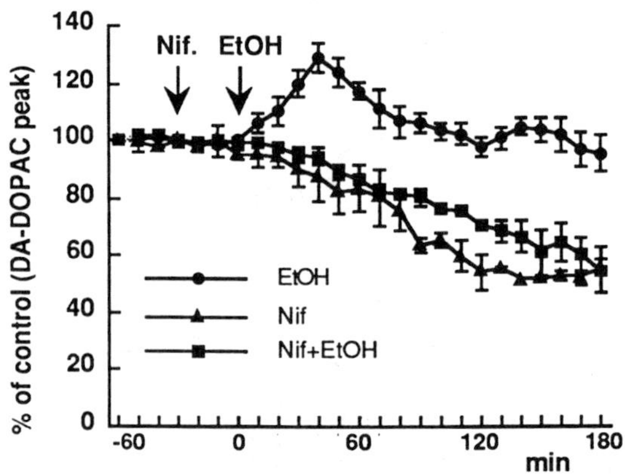

FIGURE 4. Ex vivo biochemical evidence for an inhibitory effect of nifedipine on ethanol induced changes in dopamine metabolism (upper panels). Nifedipine (Nif, 5 mg/kg p.o.) was administered 70 minutes and ethanol (EtOH, 2.5 g/kg) 40 minutes before decapitation. DOPAC and HVA were measured by means of HPLC with electrochemical detection. Shown are the means +/- SEM of 4 mice. Comparisons with control. * $p<0.05$, ** $p<0.01$, *** $p<0.001$. The lower panel shows in vivo voltammetric evidence for an inhibitory effect of nifedipine on ethanol induced changes in dopamine metabolism in nucleus accumbens. Each datum point represents the mean of 3-5 rats +/- SEM. (Data from Engel et al. 1988)

choice situation between water and 6% ethanol both intake of and preference for ethanol was significantly reduced by nifedipine in an unselected strain of Wistar rats (fig. 3). No effect on water intake was observed indicating a selective effect on ethanol intake.

Biochemical correlates to the behavioral findings are shown in figure 4. In one study using conventional postmortem analyses of DA metabolites by means of HPLC with electrochemical detection we found that locomotor stimulatory doses of ethanol increased DA-metabolism in both striatum and the DA-rich limbic region in mice and that this effect was significantly reduced by nifedipine. Using the in vivo voltammetry method in anaesthetized rats we obtained additional biochemical data indicating that the L-type calcium channel antagonist nifedipine could reduce the ethanol induced increase in DA-metabolism (fig. 4). Since blood alcohol levels were not changed by nifedipine it seems unlikely that the behavioral and biochemical results could be explained by interference with ethanol metabolism.

Taken together these results show that a calcium channel blocker of the dihydropyridine type can antagonize some of the behavioral (locomotor stimulatory and preference for ethanol) and biochemical (stimulation of DA metabolism) effects of ethanol. The theoretical implication from these studies is that some of the behavioral and biochemical effects of ethanol may involve alterations in the calcium movements even though the nature of this effect remains to be clarified. It should, however, be emphasized that nifedipine, in addition to blocking Ca^{2+} channels, has been shown to be able to i.a. potentiate adenosine and interact with the peripheral benzodiazepine receptor ligands and also to block flurazepam induced sleep (cf. Swanson and Green 1986).

The clinical implication is that these drugs may provide an alternative pharmacological treatment approach for moderating ethanol intake in problem drinkers. This suggestion is based on the fact that the alcohol preference model has been shown to be a useful animal model for preclinical screening of drugs that reduce alcohol consumption in man (see Naranjo et al. 1987, Naranjo and Sellers 1989). Needless to say clinical studies have to be undertaken to test this hypothesis.

SEROTONIN

Already two decades ago Myers and Veale (1968) presented data implicating brain serotonin (5-HT) in the regulation of preference for ethanol. Since then, a large amount of animal studies has shown that various pharmacological manipulations of central 5-HT neurotransmission alter ethanol consumption and preference (see table 1; McBride 1989, Zabik 1989). Thus it has been shown that manipulations leading to a decrease in 5-HT function has usually, but not always, been shown to increase ethanol intake. The findings are consistent when serotonin neurons have been destructed anatomically or by neurotoxins such as 5,6-dihydroxytryptamine (5,6-DHT) or 5,7-DHT. The reported results appear to be less consistent when the 5-HT synthesis inhibitor *para*-chlorophenylalanine (PCPA) has been used as the pharmacological tool. This is possibly due to the fact that PCPA is a less specific 5-HT tool and also interferes with other neurotransmitter systems such as the catecholamines.

Conversely, it has been shown that ethanol intake decreases after manipulations that enhance 5-HT function. The administration of 5-HT precursors such as tryptophan and

	Ethanol intake/preference
Anatomical lesions of 5-HT systems	↑
Neurotoxins (5,6-DHT, 5,7-DHT)	↑
PCPA	(↑)
Tryptophan	(↓)
L-5-HTP	↓
5-HT (icv)	↓
Fenfluramine (5-HT-releaser)	↓
5-HT-uptake inhibitors zimelidine citalopram alaproclate fluoxetine fluvoxamine indalpine viqualine	↓
Quipazine (unselective 5-HT receptor agonist)	↓
TFMPP (unselective 5-HT_1 receptor agonist)	↓
8-OH-DPAT (5-HT_{1A} receptor agonist)	↓
Ipsapirone (5-HT_{1A} receptor agonist)	↓
Buspirone (5-HT_{1A} agonist / DA antagonist)	↓
Ondansetron (5-HT_3 receptor antagonist)	0
Granisetron (5-HT_3 receptor antagonist)	0
LY 53857 (5-HT_2 receptor antagonist)	0
D-5-HTP	0

TABLE 1. The role of serotonin for the regulation of intake and preference of ethanol.

L-5-hydroxytryptophan (L-5-HTP), but not D-5-HTP, intracerebral administration of 5-HT and postsynaptic unselective 5-HT agonists such as quipazine and *meta*-trifluoromethylphenylpiperazine (TFMPP) have all been reported to decrease ethanol intake and preference.

Furthermore all selective 5-HT uptake inhibitors tested including zimelidine, citalopram, alaproclate, fluoxetine, fluvoxamine, indalpine and viqualine consistently and repeatedly have been shown to diminish ethanol intake in laboratory rats when offered as a free-choice with water.

Thus the serotonin systems appear to be involved in ethanol intake and preference. On the basis of these animal data the 5-HT uptake inhibitors zimelidine, citalopram and fluoxetine have been tested in non-depressed, high alcohol consumers by Naranjo et al.

(1989). These studies demonstrate that both zimelidine and citalopram do attenuate ethanol intake in this group of subjects and provide strong support for a role of 5-HT in regulating ethanol intake also in humans. In addition these clinical findings cross validate the results obtained in experimental animals.

The existence of multiple 5-HT receptor subtypes has been demonstrated and at present it is believed that 5-HT_{1A}, $_{1B}$, $_{1C}$, $_{1D}$, 5-HT_2 and 5-HT_3 sites are present in the rat brain. So far very little work has been performed to identify the 5-HT receptor subtypes responsible for the mediation of ethanol preference or intake except for the findings by Murphy et al. (1985) who reported that the 5-HT_2 receptor antagonist LY 53857 appears to be without effect on ethanol intake by the alcohol preferring (P) line rats. Using the 5-HT_2 recptor antagonist, ritanserin, we found in preliminary experiments that this drug had no effect on ethanol intake or preference in an unselected strain of Wistar rats. Furthermore buspirone has been shown to attenuate volitional alcohol intake in monkeys (Collins and Myers 1987). However, buspirone is not selective for the 5-HT_{1A} receptor but has also potent antidopaminergic properties (Hjorth and Carlsson 1982). This additional effect could, however, be advantageous in the treatment of problem drinkers considering the complex psychopharmacological profile of ethanol (see Introduction).

To further elucidate the involvement of the 5-HT receptor subtypes we investigated the effect of the specific 5-HT_{1A} agonists, 8-OH-DPAT (8-hydroxy-2-(di-n-propylamino) tetralin) and ipsapirone, on ethanol intake and preference in the rat using the free choice paradigm. Male rats from an unselected stock of Wistar rats were used. They were presented with a free choice between water and gradually increasing ethanol concentrations from 2-6% ethanol for a 3 week habituation period during which time the amounts of ethanol and water consumed was measured. In these studies, rats drinking more than 60% of their daily fluid intake in the form of ethanol solution were defined as HP rats and those drinking less than 30% ethanol solution were defined as LP rats.

8-OH-DPAT, 0.125 mg/kg s.c. twice daily for three days, caused a significant reduction of ethanol intake and ethanol preference in the high preference group but interestingly not in the low preference group (fig. 5). Water intake was unaffected. Thus the effect of the 5-HT_{1A} agonist is restricted to the high preference group. Assuming that increased ethanol consumption in the preference situation reflects positive reinforcing actions, these findings support the hypothesis that interference with

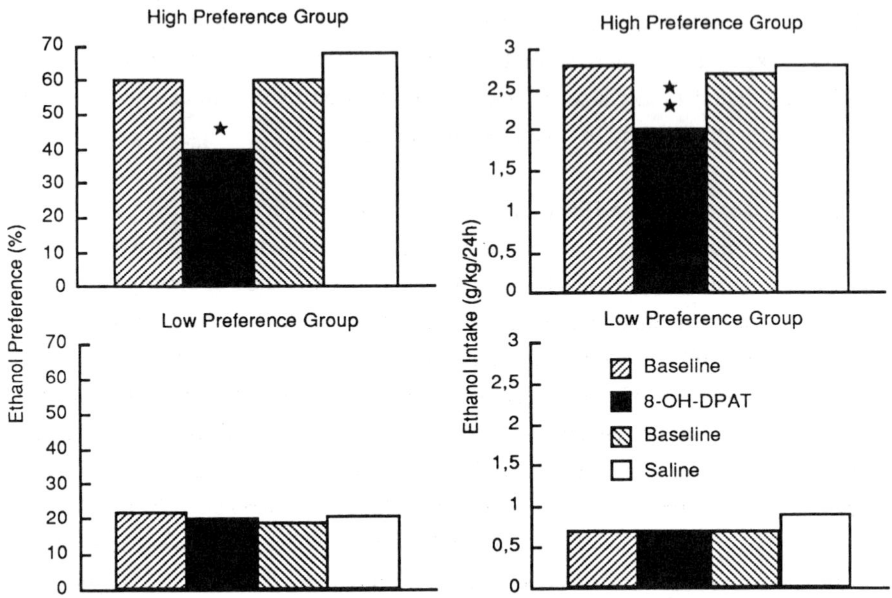

FIGURE 5. The effects of 8-OH-DPAT (0.125 mg/kg s.c.) on the preference and intake of ethanol in high (n=8) and low (n=9) preferring rats. Ethanol consumption in a free choice situation was recorded during a 3 day period in rats treated 2 times daily with 8-OH-DPAT. Comparisons with a 3 week baseline period. * $p<0.05$, ** $p<0.02$. (Data from Svensson et al. 1989)

the central 5-HT systems directly or indirectly alters the positive reinforcing effects of ethanol and thereby ethanol intake.

Over the years, we as well as others, have obtained data indicating that psychomotor activation and positive reinforcement of ethanol and other dependence producing drugs are homologous phenomena due to activation of common brain mechanisms (cf. Wise and Bozarth 1987). We therefore investigated if the locomotor stimulating effect of ethanol in mice could be influenced by the 5-HT_{1A} agonists. As shown in figure 6, locomotor stimulation was reduced by the 5-HT_{1A} agonist, 8-OH-DPAT, in doses that had little effect on locomotor activity per se, suggesting that 5-HT_{1A} mechanisms may be involved also in the mediation of ethanol induced locomotor stimulation.

Further support for an involvement of 5-HT_{1A} receptors in ethanol preference and intake is provided by the results from studies with another 5-HT_{1A} agonist, the azapirone ipsapirone. In order to more adequately study the effect of short-acting drugs on ethanol intake another procedure was used in these experiments. The rats were deprived daily of water and ethanol for the first four hours of the dark period between 10 a.m. and 2 p.m. After this period the animals were given free access to water and a

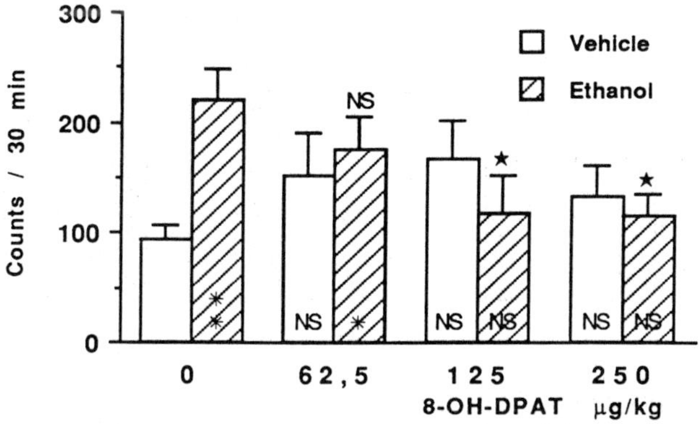

FIGURE 6. The effects of 8-OH-DPAT on ethanol (2.5 g/kg i.p) induced stimulation of locomotor activity in mice. Comparison with vehicle: ✱<0.05, ✱✱<0.01. Comparison with ethanol alone: ★<0.05.

deprived daily of water and ethanol for the first four hours of the dark period between 10 a.m. and 2 p.m. After this period the animals were given free access to water and a 6% ethanol solution. Water and ethanol consumption was measured for the following 60 minutes. This procedure was repeated several times until a stable level of ethanol intake/preference was established. One example of such a stability is shown in figure 7.

As shown in figure 8 the 5-HT_{1A} agonist ipsapirone dose-dependently reduced ethanol intake and preference for ethanol with a maximal reduction by more than 50%.

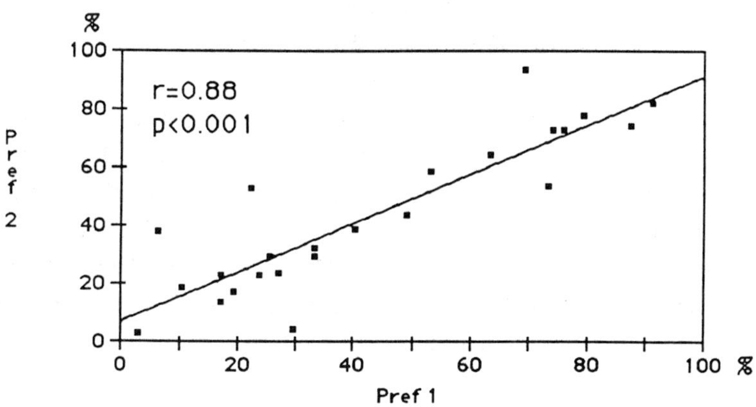

FIGURE 7. Correlation between the preference for ethanol estimated in 2 consecutive (Pref 1 and Pref 2) tests.

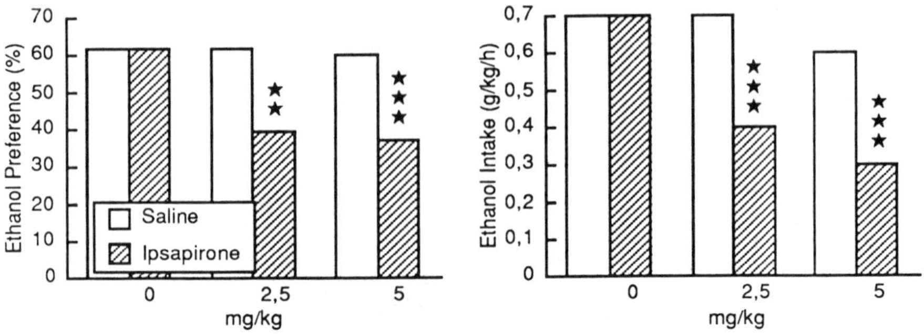

FIGURE 8. The effects of ipsapirone on the preference and intake of ethanol in rats. The consumption of ethanol was measured in a free choice situtation during a 1 hour recording period after 4 hours of fluid deprivation. Ipsapirone was administered i.p. 30 minutes before test. Comparisons with a 3 week baseline period. ** $p<0.01$, *** $p<0.001$.

In view of the validity of the free choice paradigm for the preclinical testing of drugs and that 5-HT uptake inhibitors consistently moderate ethanol intake in humans it would be of interest to test the potential of these 5-HT_{1A} agonists as treatments for moderating ethanol intake in problem drinkers.

In contrast to the effects of the 5-HT_{1A} agonists no effects of the 5-HT_3 antagonists ondansetron (GR 38032 F) or granisetron (BRL 43694) on ethanol intake or preference was observed in doses that are supposed to have adequate 5-HT_3 antagonistic properties (fig. 9). It should be noted, however, that the rewarding properties of other dependence producing drugs such as morphine and nicotine, measured in the place-preference conditioning paradigm, have been shown to be reduced by the 5-HT_3 antagonists ICS 205-930 and MDL 72222 (Carboni et al. 1988).

Taken together, these data provide further support for the notion that the serotonin system is involved in the regulation of ethanol intake. In addition we obtained results implicating specifically the 5-HT_{1A} system. Our findings are in substantial agreement with those of Wong et al. (1988) who found that there are quantitative differences in the 5-HT_1 but not 5-HT_2 receptors between the P and NP lines as measured by radioligand binding. Furthermore, using ^{3}H-8-OH-DPAT, McBride et al. (1990) recently reported, that specifically the 5-HT_{1A} receptor subtype may be involved in these lines of rats.

The 5-HT_{1A} receptors have been shown to be localized both presynaptically, somato/dendritic localization, and postsynaptically. From our data we cannot conclude if the effect of the 5-HT_{1A} agonists is mediated by pre- or postsynaptic receptors. which site/sites that is mediating the effect. However, considering published data showing that stimulation of 5-HT decreases alcohol intake whereas decreased influence

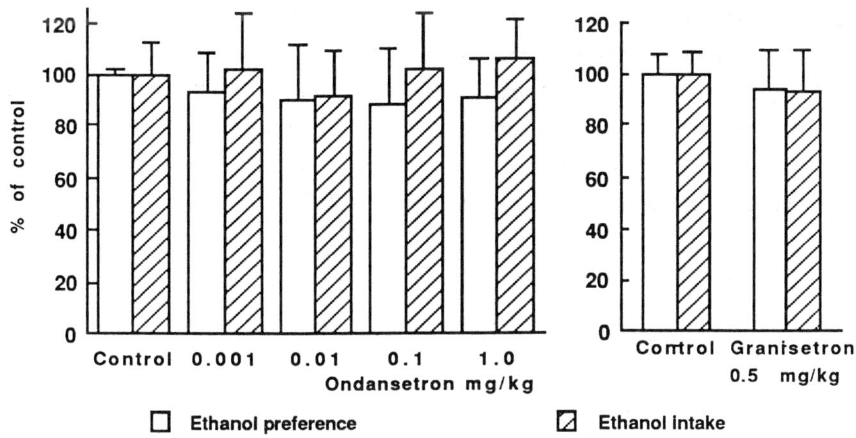

FIGURE 9. The effect of the $5HT_3$ antagonists ondansetron and granisetron on ethanol intake and preference in a two bottle choice paradigm.

of the 5-HT systems increases alcohol intake, it may be suggested that postsynaptic $5\text{-}HT_{1A}$ receptor subtypes are involved.

These findings do not a priori mean that the 5-HT system is directly involved in the reinforcing effects of ethanol consumption. It is well known that neurotransmitters do not operate independently. Thus changes in the 5-HT systems do not exclude possible interactions with other populations of neurotransmitters. The 5-HT systems are known to innervate a large number of structures in the central nervous system, most of the 5-HT neurons originating from the dorsal and median raphe nuclei. Thus for example, it has been shown that 5-HT exerts an inhibitory influence on some DA neurons (cf. Kelland et al. 1990) and consequently a decreased serotonergic activity could lead to a dopaminergic overactivity and vice versa. Tentatively, the 5-HT system could be regarded as a modulator of the DA reward system, and hence not directly involved in controlling the reward process. Accordingly, the basal 5-HT activity should be able to indirectly influence the effects of ethanol and other dependence producing drugs on the DA reward system. A high 5-HT tonus, drug-induced or physiological, would reduce the ability of ethanol and other dependence producing drugs to produce positive reinforcing effects. Alternatively, the 5-HT and DA systems could by a parallel organization be involved in the regulation of the reward systems.

Finally it should be emphasized that, as pointed out in the Introduction, ethanol also interacts with other neurotransmitter systems than the CA and 5-HT and which in all probability also are involved in the reward profile of ethanol. Therefore future research will undoubtedly have to identify subgroups of alcoholics possibly based i.a upon the neurochemical basis for their ethanol abuse. Consequently a pharmacological treatment strategy have to be tailored according to such a subdivision.

Acknowledgements

The present study was financially supported by grants from the Swedish Medical Research Council (no 4247, 7202), the Bank of Sweden Tercentenary Foundation, the Swedish Council for Research in the Humanities and Social Sciences, the Swdeish Alcohol Monopoly Foundation for Alcohol Research and Wilhelm and Martina Lundgren Foundation.

References

Carboni E, Acquas E, Leone P,Perezzani L, Di Chiara G. 5-HT_3 receptor antagonists block morphine- and nicotine-induced place-preference conditioning. Europ J Pharmacol, 1988, *151*, pp 159-160.

Collins DM, Myers RD. Buspirone attenuates volitional alcohol intake in the chronically drinking monkey Alcohol, 1987, *4*, pp 49-56.

Engel JA. Neurochemical aspects of the euphoria induced by dependence-producing drugs. In: Idesträm C-M (ed) Recent Advances in the Study of Alcoholism. Excerpta Medica, Amsterdam, International congress series no 407, 1977, pp 16-22.

Engel JA. Influence of age and hormones on the stimulatory and sedative effects of ethanol. In: Rydberg U, Alling C, Engel JA (eds) Alcohol and the Developing Brain. Raven Press, New York. 1985, pp 55-67.

Engel JA., Liljequist S. The involvement of different central neurotransmitters in mediating stimulatory and sedative effects of ethanol. In: Pohorecky L, Brick J (eds) Stress and Alcohol Use. Elsevier, New York, 1983, pp 153-169.

Engel JA, Oreland L, Ingvar DH, Pernow, Rössner S, Pellborn LÅ. Brain Reward Systems and Abuse. Raven Press, New York, 1985

Engel JA, Fahlke C, Hulthe P, Hård E, Johannessen K, Snape B, Svensson L. Biochemical and behavioral evidence for an interaction between ethanol and calcium channel antagonists. J Neural Transm, 1988, *74*, pp 181-193.

Fadda F, Mosca E, Colombo G, Gessa GL. Alcohol-preferring rats: Genetic sensitivity to alcohol-induced stimulation of dopamine metabolism. Physiol Behav, 1990, *47*, pp 727-729.

Gonon FG, Fombariet CM, Buda MJ, Pujol FJ. Electrochemical treatment of pyrolytic carbon fiber elctrodes. Anal Chem, 1981, *53*, pp 1386-1389.

Hjorth S, Carlsson A. Buspirone: effects on central monoaminergic transmission - possible relevance to animal experimental and clinical findings. Europ J Pharmacol, 1982, *83*, pp 299-303.

Imperato A, Di Chiara G. Preferential stimulation of dopmaine release in the nucleus accumbens offreely moving rats by ethanol. J Pharmacol Exp Ther, 1986, *239*, pp 219-228.

Kelland MD, Freeman AS, Chiodo LA. Serotonergic aferent regulation of the basic phsiology and pharmacological respponsiveness of nigrostriatal dopamine neurons. J Pharmacol exp Therap, 1990, *253*, pp 803-811.

McBride WJ, Murphy JM, Lumeng L, Li T-K. Serotonin and ethanol preference. Recent Dev Alcohol, 1989, *7*, pp 187-209.

McBride WJ, Murphy JM, Lumeng L, Li T-K. Serotonin dopamine and GABA involvement in alcohol drinking of selectiveley bred rats. Alcohol, 1990, *7*, pp 199-205.

Murphy JM, Waller MB, Gatto GJ, McBride WJ, Lumeng L, Li T-K. Monoamine uptake inhibitors attenuate ethanol intake in alcohol preferring (P) rats. Alcohol, 1985, *2*, pp 349-352.

Myers RD, Veale WL. Alcohol preference in the rat: Reduction following depletion of brain serotonin. Science, 1968, *160*, pp 1469-1471.

Naranjo CA, Sullivan J, Lawrin MO, Sellers EM. Strategies for the identification and testing of new pharmacological modulators of ethanol consumption. In: Engel J, Oreland L (eds) Brain reward systems and abuse. Raven Press, New York, 1987, pp 129-145.

Naranjo CA, Sellers EM. Serotonin uptake inhibitors attenuates ethanol intake in problem drinkers. Rec Develop Alc, 1989,*7*, pp 255-266.

Pileblad E, Carlsson A. In vivo effects of the Ca^{2+}-antagonist nimodipine on dopamine metabolism in mouse brain. J Neural Transm, 1986, *66*, pp 171-187.

Pileblad E, Carlsson A. The Ca^{2+}-antagonist nimodipine decreases and the Ca^{2+}-agonist Bay K 8644 incerase catecholamine synthesis in mouse brain. Neuropharmacol, 1987, *26*, pp 101-105.

Swanson TH, Green CL. Nifedipine: more than a calcium channel blocker. Gen Pharmacol, 1986, *17*, pp 255-260.

Svensson L, Engel JA, Hård E. Efects of the 5-HT receptor agonist 8-OH-DPAT, on the ethanol preference in the rat. Alcohol, 1989, *6*, pp 17-21.

Wise RE, Bozarth MA. Brain Reweard circuitry: Four circuit elements "wired" in apparent series. Brain Res Bull, 1984, *297*, pp 265-273.

Wise RE, Bozarth MA. A psychomotor stimulant theory of addiction. Psychol Rev, 1987, *94*, pp 469-492.

Wong DT, Lumeng L, Threlkeld PG, Reid LR,Li T-K.Serotonergic and adrenergic receptors in alcohol-preferring and -nonpreferring rats. J Neural Transm,1988, *71*, pp 207-218.

Zabik JE. Use of serotonin-active drugs in alcohol preference studuies. Rec Develop Alk 1989, *7*, pp 211-223.

7
Serotonin and Alcohol Consumption

G.A. Higgins, M.O. Lawrin, and E.M. Sellers

Overwhelming experimental evidence suggests that treatments which increase 5-HT availability in the CNS reduce ethanol consumption. For instance 5-HT precursors i.e tryptophan, 5-hydroxytryptophan (Zabik et al, 1985), 5-HT agonists e.g quipazine (Zabik et al, 1985), MK212 (Lawrin et al, 1986), intracerebrally-administered 5-HT (Hill, 1974), and selective 5-HT reuptake inhibitors e.g fluoxetine (Murphy et al, 1988; Haraguchi et al, 1990), zimelidine (Amit et al, 1984) all reduce alcohol intake in free choice paradigms. However these same treatments similarly effect food consumption (see Table 1 for summary). Interestingly, the effect of reducing central 5-HT tone fails to consistently elevate ethanol and food intake (see Table 1 for summary). This may imply that a low endogenous 5-HT tone is a prerequisite for ethanol consumption--a hypothesis supported by the fact that genetically derived rat strains which consume large quantities of ethanol show comparatively low forebrain serotonin function (see McBride et al, 1990; Rezvani et al, 1990).

The identification of drugs which selectively effect alcohol but not food consumption, would be of clinical value for the treatment of alcoholism and such approaches which could distinguish between a drugs effect on food and ethanol intake may be summarized as follows:

1. Dose response studies to identify the minimally effective doses of the test drug that affect food and ethanol intake. Furthermore, the magnitude of a drugs effect on each parameter can be determined and compared.
2. Microstructural analysis of the feeding/drinking parameters responsible for the observed consummatory response. Such studies have been instrumental in demonstrating that the hypophagic effect of both uptake blockers and fenfluramine are probably related to an enhancement of satiety (Blundell, 1984). Therefore these types of analyses can provide some insight into the mechanism behind the main response.
3. Pharmacological analysis of the 5-HT receptor subtypes involved. These experiments are especially relevant considering that 5-HT uptake blockers and releasers will, by enhancement of synaptic 5-HT, activate a multitude of 5-HT receptor subtypes (currently designated $5\text{-HT}_{1A\text{-}D}$, 5-HT_2, 5-HT_3; see Bradley et al, 1986; Peroutka, 1988). Identification of the subtypes effecting food and ethanol intake are of obvious interest.
4. Micro-injection studies to determine the central sites of action for 5-HT regulation of food and ethanol intake. With regard to food, the midbrain raphe-paraventricular hypothalamus axis appears to play a critical role (although a raphe-nucleus accumbens/striatal pathway may also be involved; see Fletcher, 1990; Muscat et al, 1989). Thus, injection of selective 5-HT_{1A} agonists either at low doses or directly into the midbrain raphe nuclei, increase food intake (Hutson et al, 1986; Fletcher and Davies, 1990). This effect is presumably mediated by activation of

inhibitory somatodendritic 5-HT_{1A} autoreceptors, producing a concommitant fall in terminal 5-HT release. Injection of 5-$HT_{1B/C}$ agonists into the paraventricular hypothalamus also reduces food intake, probably by activation of postsynaptic 5-HT receptors (Weiss et al, 1986; Kennett et al, 1987). As yet such studies have not been conducted with respect to ethanol, although it is noteworthy that low systemic doses of 5-HT_{1A} agonists e.g. 8-OH DPAT, gepirone, actually REDUCE alcohol drinking (Svensson et al, 1988; Knapp and Pohorecky, 1990). These observations may suggest different neuronal mechanisms are controlling each ingestional behaviour.

Table 1. Treatments Which Modify Serotonergic Function. Effects on Food and Ethanol Intake

a) Treatments Which Increase Central 5-HT

		Food Intake	Ethanol Intake
1.	Precursor Loading e.g. tryptophan, 5-HTP	**decreased** blocked by peripheral 5-HT_2 antagonist, (Fletcher & Burton, 1986)	**decreased** blocked by xylamidine (Zabik et al, 1985)
2.	5-HT Releasers e.g. fenfluramine	**decreased** (Blundell, 1977) via 5-HT_{1C} receptor activation? (Neill & Cooper, 1989; Thurlby et al, 1985)	**decreased** (Sellers et al, 1990) mechanism unknown
3.	5-HT Agonists e.g. quipazine, mCPP, MK212	**decreased** (Clineschmidt et al, 1977; Kennett et al, 1988; Hewson et al, 1988) antagonist studies suggest 5-$HT_{1C/2}$ or 5-HT_{1B}	**decreased** (Zabik et al, 1985; Lawrin et al, 1986) may suggest 5-$HT_{1C/2}$ receptor?
4.	5-HT Uptake Blockers e.g sertraline	**decreased** (Blundell, 1984; Lucki et al, 1988) antagonist studies suggest 5-HT_1 receptor	**decreased** (Gill et al, 1988; Sellers et al, 1990) mechanism unknown

b) Treatments Which Reduce Central 5-HT

		Food Intake	Ethanol Intake
1.	Synthesis Inhibition e.g. pCPA	**inconsistent** (see Blundell, 1984)	**inconsistent** possibly due to CTA (Holman et al, 1975; Walters, 1977)
2.	5-HT Neuronal Lesions e.g. 5,6 DHT, 5,7 DHT	**increased** (Saller & Stricker, 1976)	**increased** (Ho et al, 1974; Richardson & Novakoski, 1978)
3.	5-HT_{1A} Agonists (low dose) e.g. 8-OH DPAT, gepirone	**increased** (Dourish et al, Gilbert & Dourish, 1987)	**decreased** (Svensson et al, 1989; Knapp et al, 1990)
4.	5-$HT_{1/2}$ Antagonists e.g. metergoline, methysergide	**increased** (Dourish et al, 1989; Fletcher, 1988)	?
5.	5-HT_3 Antagonists	**inconsistent** (see Dourish et al, 1989; Van Der Hoek & Cooper, 1990)	**inconsistent** (Sellers et al, 1988; unpublished observations)

At the Addiction Research Foundation we have developed a computerised drinkometer system which continuously monitors drinking behaviour in rats. Variables such as the size of individual drinking episodes and the number of such episodes can be monitored, both with respect to ethanol and water consumption. This allows a microstructural analysis of drinking behaviour and the effect of various drugs on these parameters may be examined.

Previous results from our laboratory have shown that various 5-HT uptake blockers (e.g. fluoxetine, fluvoxamine, citalopram, zimelidine) and the 5-HT agonist (MK212) all dose-dependently reduce alcohol intake in Wistar rats (Lawrin et al, 1986; Lawrin, 1988) (see Figures 1a and 2). Fluoxetine produced a marked delay to the onset of ethanol drinking but not water drinking (Lawrin, 1988) (Figure 1b). This effect would suggest that this drug is in some way disrupting the initiation phase of ethanol drinking possibly by a blockade of its reinforcing properties (see Lawrin, 1988). Preliminary findings suggest that another 5-HT re-uptake blocker, sertraline, may similarly effect this initiation phase. Microstructural analysis also showed that fluoxetine reduced ethanol intake by reducing the number of drinking bouts, bout volume and duration (Lawrin, 1988). A comparison between the effects of some of these agents on ethanol and water intake, revealed that at certain doses water consumption was affected to a lesser degree, thus ethanol preference was reduced (Lawrin, 1988). Studies using the alcohol-preferring P-line of rat as well as rats trained to lever press for ethanol may support the contention that fluoxetine at least may show some selectivity for reducing ethanol intake (Murphy et al, 1988; Haraguchi et al, 1990). Thus fluoxetine markedly reduced the intragastric administration of a 20% ethanol solution (water intake was actually increased) at a dose that did not significantly effect food intake (Murphy et al, 1988). Similarly, fluoxetine showed a similar profile to haloperidol in that both drugs produced an early extinction of operant ethanol responding (Haraguchi et al, 1990). These workers have hypothesized that this commonality of response suggests that both drugs are inducing similar effects which may be associated with reduced ethanol reinforcement. The findings of Durcan et al (1988) showing that fluoxetine (but not fluvoxamine, desipramine or citalopram) attenuated that anxiolytic but not locomotor effects of ethanol in mice may give some clues as to the aspect of ethanol reinforcement effected. Also, the observations that fluoxetine reduces self-stimulation (Katz and Carroll, 1977) and zimeldine blocks amphetamine (but not morphine) place conditioning (Kruszewska et al, 1986) implies that under certain conditions 5-HT uptake blockers may modify drug reinforcement systems.

As reviewed earlier (see Table 1), enhancement of synaptic 5-HT reduces food intake by enhancing satiety and various groups have shown that a range of 5-HT uptake blockers including fluoxetine reduce food and palatable liquid consumption at ethanol effective doses (Gill et al, 1985, 1989; Leander, 1987; Lucki et al, 1988) leading to the conclusion that the effect on ethanol is non-specific. However, Gill and Amit (1989) reported that zimeldine had a more pronounced effect upon consumption of a 0.1% saccharin solution as compared to a 0.025% concentration and perhaps relevant to some of these studies are the findings of Montgomery and Burton (1986) who demonstrated that a peripheral serotonergic component may inhibit the "incentive" value of certain foods. Furthermore, Zabik et al (1985) have shown that peripheral 5-HT blockade will reverse 5-HTP-induced reductions in ethanol intake. Consequently, the involvement of peripheral as well as central 5-HT systems regulating a variety of independent processes may ultimately be involved in the ethanol reducing effects of 5-HT uptake blockers.

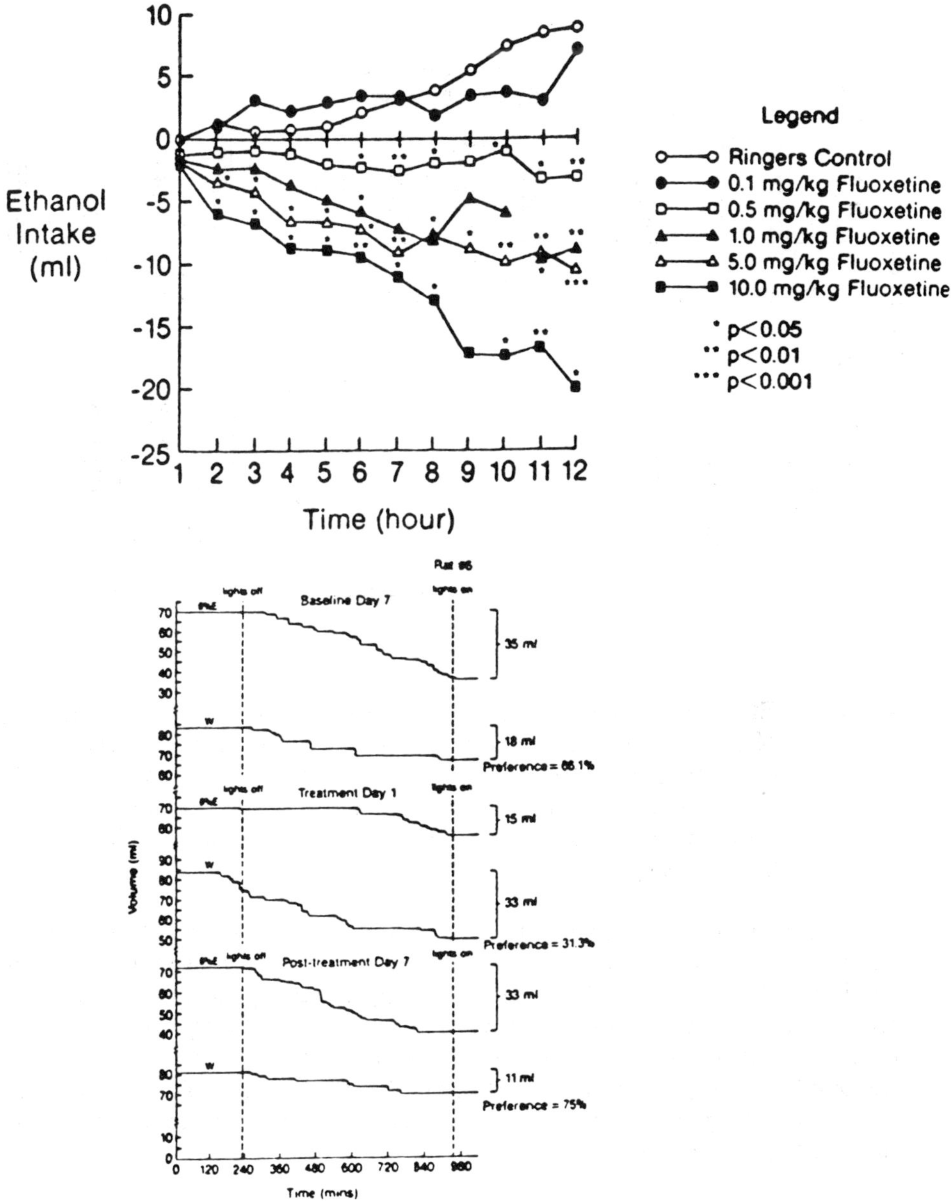

Figure 1 a) Effect of various doses of fluoxetine on ethanol intake. Data expressed as change in volume consumed with time by comparison to baseline intake. b) Temporal pattern of fluid intake by rat #6. Note during baseline and post-treatment that the rat preferentially consumes ethanol, however, following fluoxetine treatment (10 mg/kg) there is a marked delay to the onset of ethanol consumption and the total consumed is reduced. Since water intake shows a compensatory increase, ethanol preference is reduced. Data from Lawrin, 1988.

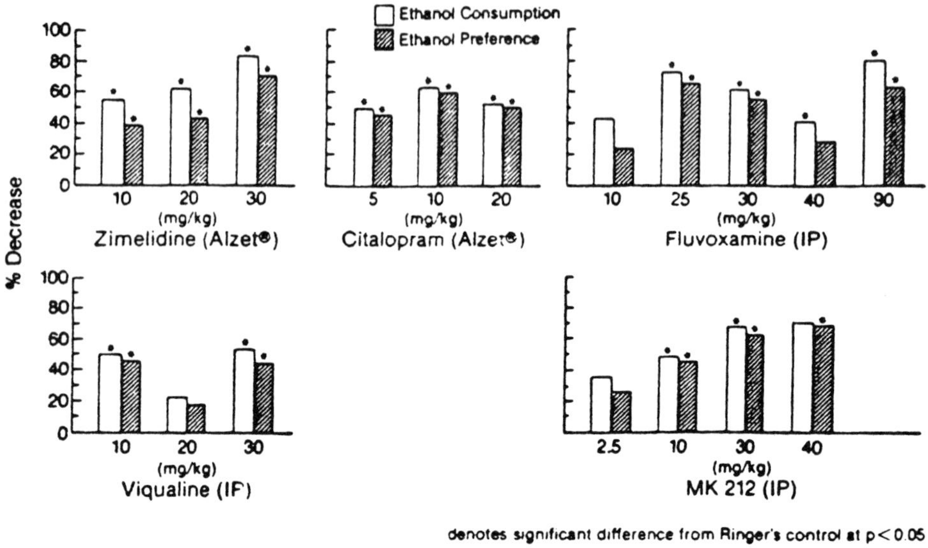

Figure 2. Effect of various 5-HT uptake blockers and the 5-HT agonist, MK212 on ethanol intake and preference. Data expressed as percentage decrease from baseline intake. All drugs given acutely via intraperitoneal injection, except zimelidine and citalopram which were administered chronically by Alzet(R) minipump. Data from Lawrin, 1988.

Recently, we have extended our studies to examine the 5-HT releaser d-fenfluramine. Male, Wistar rats selected for study showed stable self-administration of a 5% ethanol solution (approximately 2.4 g/kg/day) when allowed a free choice between ethanol and water. A Latin square design was used such that each rat received all treatments over two day periods surrounded by two day vehicle injections for washout. The results are shown by Table 2a; the percentage changes are expressed as differences from the surrounding washout days.

Table 2. a) Effect of d-Fenfluramine at Various Doses on 12 h Ethanol, Water and Food Intake (data are presented as percentage changes from surrounding washout days); b) Microstructural Changes in Drinking Behaviour Induced by d-Fenfluramine at 1 mg/kg (*p < 0.01 vs. controls)

	0.5 mg/kg	1 mg/kg	2.5 mg/kg
Ethanol	-9 ± 12	-42 ± 11*	-72 ± 5*
Water	- 3 ± 12	+21 ± 12	+13 ± 11
Food	-6 ± 2	-6 ± 3	-21 ± 3*

	Vehicle	1 mg/kg
Total Ethanol (ml)	25.8 ± 3.2	16.5 ± 2.8*
Total Ethanol (g/kg)	2.4 ± 0.3	1.4 ± 0.3*
Number of Drinks (N)	32.3 ± 4.5	20.9 ± 2.7*
Mean Drink Size (ml)	0.9 ± 0.1	0.8 ± 0.1
Total Water (ml)	25.4 ± 3.0	29.7 ± 3.1
Number of Drinks (N)	34.1 ± 3.7	35.4 ± 3.7
Mean Drink Size (ml)	0.8 ± 0.1	0.9 ± 0.1
Food Consumption (g)	32.5 ± 0.9	30.6 ± 0.8
Weight Gain (g)	4.5 ± 0.5	4.3 ± 0.5

These studies clearly show that at the 1mg/kg dose level, d-fenfluramine is producing a marked reduction in ethanol intake whilst food consumption is essentially unchanged. Water intake if anything is increased presumably to counter the reduced ethanol intake. At 2.5 mg/kg, d-fenfluramine significantly reduced both food and ethanol intake suggesting a non-specific action on consummatory behaviour. Microstructural analysis of the drinking patterns following the 1mg/kg dose yielded some interesting findings (see Table 2b). As stated earlier, fenfluramine does not effect the number of feeding bouts, instead the bout (or meal) size is reduced. This has lead to the popular concept that fenfluramine reduces food intake by an enhancement of satiety signals (Blundell, 1984), although inconsistent with this hypothesis is the observation that this treatment disrupts post-prandial behaviour (Montgomery and Willner, 1988). However the pattern of d-fenfluramine on ethanol consumption was entirely different; mean drink size was unaffected, instead there was a significant reduction in the number of discrete drinking bouts. These data suggest that ethanol intake may be effected by alternative factors to satiety. Hoebel and coworkers have recently provided evidence that d-fenfluramine (but not dl-fenfluramine) at doses around 1.5 mg/kg selectively depress lateral hypothalamic self-stimulation, a response consistent with an impairment of reward systems (Hoebel et al, 1988; McClelland et al, 1987). Further studies are clearly necessary to determine the mechanism behind the apparently selective effect of d-fenfluramine on ethanol intake. In future experiments we will attempt to address the issue of which 5-HT subtype underlies this response. Recent reports suggest that the 5-HT_{1C} receptor may be involved in the anorectic properties of d-fenfluramine (Neill and Cooper, 1989). The identification of an alternative 5-HT subtype to influence ethanol consumption would obviously support a dissociation of these effects, and also provide potential for the development of selective agonists as therapies for alcoholism.

In concluding, a role of 5-HT in regulating ethanol intake is obvious with a range of 5-HT agonists, uptake blockers and releasers markedly reducing ethanol consumption. However, the precise way in which these agents achieve this effect is complex and likely to involve factors relating to ethanol reinforcement, satiety, incentive value and anxiety as well as the motoric capacity of the animal.

ACKNOWLEDGEMENTS

We would like to thank Cathy Van Der Giessen for typing the manuscript and Jeff Tighe and Xiaoping Zhang for their excellent technical assistance.

REFERENCES

Amit Z (1984) Neurosci Biobehav Rev 8: 35-54.
Blundell JE (1984) Neuropharmacol 23: 1537-1551.
Bradley PB (1986) Neuropharmacol 25: 563-576.
Clineschmidt BV, et al (1977) Psychopharmacol 89: 216-220.
Dourish CT, et al (1985) Psychopharmacol 86: 197-204.
Dourish CT, et al (1989) Psychopharmacol 97: 54-58.
Durcan MJ, et al (1988) Psychopharmacol 96: 528-533.
Fletcher PJ (1988) Psychopharmacol 96: 237-242.
Fletcher PJ (1990) Soc Neurosci Abs. 311.1.
Fletcher PJ, Burton MJ (1986) Psychopharmacol 89: 216-220.
Fletcher PJ, Davies M (1990) Br J Pharmacol 99: 519-525.
Gilbert F, Dourish CT (1987) Psychopharmacol 93: 349-352.
Gill K, Amit Z (1989) In: Recent Developments in Alcoholism, Volume 7. Galanter M (ed.), Plenum Press, New York. pp. 225-248.

Gill K, et al (1985) Alcohol 2: 355-358.
Gill K, et al (1988) Alcohol 5: 349-354.
Haraguchi M, et al (1990) Pharmacol Biochem Behav 35: 259-262.
Hewson G, et al (1988) Br J Pharmacol 95: 598-604.
Hill SY (1974) Biol Psychiatry 8: 151-158.
Ho AKS, et al (1974) Psychopharmacol 40: 101-107.
Hoebel BG, et al (1988) Clin Neuropharmacol 11: S72-S85.
Holman RB, et al (1975) Br J Pharmacol 53: 299-304.
Hutson PH, et al (1986) Eur J Pharmacol 129: 347-352.
Katz RJ, Carroll BJ (1977) Psychopharmacol 51: 189-193.
Kennett GA, Curzon G (1988) Br J Pharmacol 94: 137-147.
Kennett GA, et al (1987) Eur J Pharmacol 141: 429-435.
Knapp DJ, Pohorecky LA (1990) P73 ISBRA Congress, Toronto, Canada.
Kruszewska A, et al (1986) Eur J Pharmacol 125: 283-286.
Lawrin MO (1988) Ph.D. Thesis, University of Toronto, Toronto, Canada.
Lawrin MO, et al (1986) Psychopharmacol Bull 22: 1020-1025.
Leander JD (1987) Psychopharmacol 91: 285-287.
Lucki I, et al (1988) Psychopharmacol 96: 289-295.
McBride WJ, et al (1990) Alcohol 7: 199-205.
McClelland RC, et al (1989) Pharmacol Biochem Behav 32: 411-414.
Montgomery AMJ, Burton MJ (1986) Psychopharamcology 88: 262-266.
Montgomery AMJ, Willner P (1988) Psychopharmacol 94: 397-401.
Murphy JM, et al (1988) Alcohol 5: 283-286.
Muscat R, et al (1989) Psychopharmacol 99: 402-408.
Neill JC, Cooper SJ (1989) Psychopharmacol 97: 213-218.
Peroutka SJ (1988) TINS 11: 496-500.
Rezvani AH, et al (1990) P83 5th ISBRA Congress, Toronto, Canada.
Richardson JS, Novakoski DM (1978) Drug Alcohol Depend 3: 253-264.
Saller CF, Stricker EM (1976) Science 192: 385-387.
Sellers EM, et al (1988) Soc Neurosci Abs. 21.4.
Svensson L, et al (1989) Alcohol 6: 17-21.
Thurlby PL, et al (1985) Pharmacol Res Commun 17: 1129-1139.
Van Der Hoek GA, Cooper SJ (1990) Br J Pharmacol 99: P82.
Walters JK (1977) Pharmacol Biochem Behav 6: 377-383.
Weiss GF, et al (1986) Pharmacol Biochem Behav 25: 1223-1230.
Zabik JE, et al (1985) In: Research Advances in New Psychopharmacological Treatments for Alcoholism. Naranjo CA, Sellers EM (eds.), Elsevier Science Publishers, Amsterdam. pp. 87-103.

8

Basic and Clinical Studies on Serotonin, Alcohol, and Alcoholism

D.T. George, K. Wozniak, and M. Linnoila

INTRODUCTION

Investigators in Laboratory of Clinical Studies, Division of Intramural Clinical and Biological Research of National Institute on Alcohol Abuse and Alcoholism have for the past several years explored the role of central nervous system serotonin in alcohol abuse and dependence. The following represents a progress report on these ongoing efforts as of the summer of 1990. This communication is not a comprehensive literature review rather it includes only citations directly pertinent to the work in progress.

ALCOHOLISM AND CENTRAL SEROTONIN METABOLISM

Several investigators [1-4] have reported that alcoholics or subgroups of alcoholics have on the average reduced cerebrospinal fluid (CSF) concentrations of 5-hydroxyindoleacetic acid (5-HIAA), the major metabolite of serotonin. The largest differences in CSF 5-HIAA concentrations between alcoholics and controls have been reported in young men. Early onset, male alcoholics have also peripheral indices of serotonin metabolism which are compatible with reduced turnover of central serotonin. [5] We have speculated that reduced central serotonin turnover is a biomedical characteristic of Type II alcoholics as originally described by Cloninger et al. [6] Thus, low CSF 5-HIAA concentration in alcoholics is over and beyond male gender and early age of onset probably associated with antisocial and criminal behavioral traits and a family history of paternal alcoholism.[7]

Alcoholics with a late age of onset (over 20 years of age) had higher CSF diazepam binding inhibitor (DBI) and corticotropin releasing hormone (CRH) concentrations than early onset alcoholics. [8] They are also thought to be more anxious than alcoholics with an early age of onset. [6] Alcoholics with a late age of onset have CSF 5-HIAA concentrations similar to age and sex matched healthy volunteers, [8] but they may lack the seasonal variation of CSF 5-HIAA we have described in healthy volunteers. [9] Furthermore, unlike healthy volunteers who have a relatively strong correlation between CSF 5-HIAA and thyrotropin releasing hormone (TRH) concentrations alcoholics as a group show no correlation between these two variables. [10] Because TRH is a cotransmitter with serotonin in certain central nervous system serotonergic neurones, the lack of a 5-HIAA and TRH correlation in CSF may be an additional sign of subtle serotonergic dysregulation even in late onset alcoholics.

In summary, our CSF studies have revealed a probable serotonergic deficit in early onset male alcoholics with antisocial and criminal behavioral traits and indications of subtle central serotonergic dysfunction even in late onset alcoholics.

SEROTONERGIC PHARMACOLOGICAL CHALLENGES IN ALCOHOLICS

Since direct measures of human brain function are limited by practical and ethical constraints, drug challenge paradigms are frequently employed as an indirect method to elucidate the role of various neurotransmitters in the pathogenesis of mental disorders. By comparing drug-induced neuroendocrine and behavioral responses in control and alcoholic populations, we may be able to make inferences concerning the functional state of neurotransmitter systems. Therefore, in order to explore the serotonin function in patients with alcohol dependence, we employed two relatively specific serotonergic agents: 1) clomipramine (a re-uptake inhibitor) and 2) m-chlorophenylpiperazine (mCPP) (a partial agonist). We report our preliminary findings on the behavioral effects of these drugs on subgroups of alcohol dependent patients.

Previous challenge studies, performed in animals, support the notion that serotonin may have a role in alcohol consumption. For example, the administration of the serotonin precursors, tryptophan and 5 HTP, to rats resulted in decreased alcohol consumption.[11,12,13] Conversely, administration of 5,6-dihydroxytryptamine, a serotonergic neurotoxin, increased alcohol consumption in rats[14,15]. However, when serotonin synthesis inhibitors were tested, the effects on alcohol consumption were mixed, owing perhaps to differences in study design.[13,16,17] Lastly, the administration of the serotonin reuptake inhibitors zimelidine and citalopram to humans significantly decreased alcohol consumption in a group of heavy social drinkers.[18,19]

In our studies, subjects with a DSM III-R diagnosis of alcohol dependence were admitted to the NIAAA research ward and were abstinent for at least three weeks prior to participating in research. Pertinent to our interests, we also investigated a subpopulation of alcoholics who additionally met DSM III-R diagnostic criteria for panic disorder. Subjects with physical illnesses or Axis I psychiatric diagnoses other than alcohol dependence were excluded. Our interest in panic disorder is based on literature suggesting that certain patients with this disorder may use or abuse alcohol to self-medicate anxiety symptoms[20,21] and, conversely, alcohol abuse may lead to an increased frequency and severity of panic attacks.[22] We reasoned that clomipramine could serve as a probe to explore the relationship between alcohol dependence and anxiety, given reports suggesting that a dysregulation of serotonin metabolism may be involved in both disorders.[23,24,25,26]

In our study all subjects were given 12.5 mg of clomipramine intravenously over 15 minutes. During the study, physiological, behavioral, and neuroendocrine measures were obtained at regular intervals. The subjective behavioral responses are summarized in Table 1.

Table 1. Clomipramine-Induced Behavioral Responses

Group	Anxiety	Panic	Depression
Alcoholic (n=18)	3	0	1
Alcoholic w/ panic (n=14)	6	5	7
Control (n=11)	4	0	0

Alcoholics with panic disorder were much more likely to experience severe anxiety or a panic attack following the clomipramine infusion than alcoholics without panic disorder or controls. Interestingly, 7 of 14 alcoholics with panic disorder became acutely depressed immediately following the infusion. The symptoms lasted from 15 to 60 minutes, and included tearfulness, hopelessness, suicidal ideation, and behavioral withdrawal. In several patients these symptoms were accompanied by feelings of panic and severe anxiety. In contrast, alcoholics without panic disorder (3 subjects experienced mild transient anxiety), had no prolonged clomipramine-induced mood changes. Although, serotonin dysfunction might have a role in the etiology of panic disorder, we conclude that these data do not support the hypothesis that overall central serotonin function is altered in alcoholics without panic disorder.

Since we observed essentially no behavioral effects of clomipramine in otherwise healthy alcohol dependent patients, we wondered whether a serotonin receptor agonist might yield different results. Therefore, we elected to challenge a different population of alcoholics with the serotonin agonist, m-chlorophenylpiperazine (mCPP). Our use of mCPP is based on a recent report showing that TFMPP, (a structural analogue of mCPP), generalized to ethanol when administered in a drug discrimination paradigm to rats. [27] Since laboratory studies have showed mCPP to have a relatively high affinity for the 5HT3 and $5HT1_c$ receptors, [28,29] we reasoned that action at one or both of these receptors could give rise to cues similar to alcohol.

In this paradigm mCPP was administered I.V. as a bolus (0.08 mg/kg) over 90 seconds and, as was done with clomipramine, behavioral responses were recorded. Because of recent interest in dividing alcoholics into subtypes, we elected to use von Knorring's criteria to classify the patients into Type I and Type II categories. [30] In von Knorring's typology, Type II alcoholics develop the onset of problem drinking before the age of 25 and have their first treatment before the age of 30. All patients not fulfilling criteria for Type II are considered to be Type I alcoholics.

mCPP gave rise to a number of behavioral responses (See Table 2). Members of all groups reported a "high" frequently likened to the effects of alcohol. As can be seen in Table 2, Type II alcoholics had the highest percentage (65%) of subjects reporting "high". A second finding, which was specific to the Type II alcoholic patients (with the exception of one Type I subject), was an expressed "urge to drink alcohol" following mCPP. When present, this phenomenon was quite striking and it represented a large change on the visual analog scale from "no urge to consume alcohol" reported following the placebo infusion. Those reporting an "urge to drink" also stated that "if I were not in a controlled setting I would definitely drink alcohol". This desire lasted between 5 to 60 minutes after the mCPP infusion and subsided gradually. By the end of the study all subjects returned to their baseline state and denied any further desire to drink alcohol. Roughly half of the subjects (independent of group) experienced anxiety. This feeling of anxiety did not appear to be related to the desire to drink produced by mCPP in the majority of Type II alcoholics.

Table 2. mCPP-Induced Behavioral Responses

Group	"Urge to drink"	High	Alcohol	Anxiety
Type I (n=15)	1	4	2	8
Type II (n=20)	12	13	11	9
Control (n=22)	0	8	5	11

Taken together both studies provide potential insights into the possible role of serotonin in alcoholism. Clomipramine had minimal behavioral effects on alcoholics (with the exception of alcoholics with panic disorder) whereas mCPP gave rise to a "high", frequently described as comparable to alcohol intoxication, and also stimulated an "urge to drink" in Type II alcoholics. This suggests that a role of serotonin in the etiology of alcoholism may best be further elucidated by focusing on serotonin receptor subtypes. The differential "urge to drink" response observed in Type I and Type II alcoholics supports the hypothesis that there are biologically different subtypes of alcoholics.

ANIMAL STUDIES ON ALCOHOL, DOPAMINE AND SEROTONIN

It is generally believed that ethanol, in common with other drugs of abuse, has positive reinforcing properties which account for the initiation and maintenance of its self-administration. The neurotransmitters 5-hydroxytryptamine (5-HT) and dopamine (DA) have, in particular, been implicated as playing a role in the mediation of these reinforcing properties of ethanol.

There is a large body of evidence to suggest a major role for dopaminergic systems in the stimulant and reinforcing properties of drugs of abuse, including ethanol [31-33]. Until recently, most of this evidence has been derived from in vitro studies of dopamine metabolites. These have generally reported that ethanol increases concentrations of the dopamine metabolites, 3,4- dihydroxy-phenylacetic acid (DOPAC) and homovanillic acid (HVA) in brain tissue [34-38]. In the absence of more direct measures these have been interpreted as reflecting an increase in synthesis, turnover or release of dopamine. Other in vitro studies more directly quantifying synthesis or release of dopamine concur with these findings [39-41] and generally suggest that ethanol increases dopaminergic function.

More recently, the development of sophisticated sampling techniques such as microdialysis, has allowed for direct measurements of extracellular dopamine concentrations in specific brain areas before, during, and after various pharmacological manipulations. In one such study, systemic ethanol was found to increase extracellular dopamine concentrations in both the corpus striatum and nucleus accumbens [42].

In an extension of this study, we have found that focal perfusion of specific brain areas with various concentrations of ethanol significantly elevated dopamine concentrations in both the corpus striatum and nucleus accumbens (Wozniak et al. in press). Specifically, dopamine concentrations in the striatum were elevated by an average of 150 to 500 percent of baseline, for a dose range of ethanol between 0.1 and 10 % v/v in the artificial cerebrospinal fluid, used for perfusing the microdialysis probe. Application of these concentrations of ethanol via the dialysis probe achieved a mean brain tissue concentration of between 1 and 10mM in the area of perfusion. The magnitude of the dopamine increase appeared to be dose-related.

Since it is well established that calcium is essential for physiological neurotransmitter release [43], it was important to ascertain the calcium dependency of this ethanol-induced dopamine release. This was derived from the finding that the removal of calcium from the perfusion medium and its replacement with magnesium (12.5 mM), a procedure that effectively blocks calcium channels, prevented or attenuated the ability of ethanol to increase extracellular dopamine. This finding indeed suggested that the increase in dopamine overflow following application of ethanol to brain tissue using this technique, is a result of exocytotic processes. Furthermore, it suggests that the mechanism conducive of the increased dopamine concentrations may be related to an enhancement of calcium dependent mechanisms, as has previously been suggested by other investigators [44-45].

Since different alcohols are known to possess varying degrees of pharmacological activity [46-47], the demonstration of any differential ability of various alcohols to increase dopamine would impart a possible pharmacological relevance for this observation. The results from a further study in our laboratory show that different alcohols do indeed differ in their potencies to increase extracellular dopamine concentrations (Wozniak et al., in press). The potency order for this effect related to the number of carbon atoms in the molecules i.e. butanol > ethanol > methanol. The exact reason for this rank order is unknown. The lipid solubility of alcohols is known to increase with additional carbon atoms [48] and parallel increases in potency with regard to membrane disordering [49], intoxication [47] and inhibition of NMDA activated ion currents [50], have been noted. Although differences in lipophilicity could result in differences in effective volume of distribution following systemic administration of the alcohols, this is unlikely to be a major factor following their direct focal application. Rather, the differences in lipophilicity might relate to the abilities of these alcohols to incorporate into membrane bilayers [51]. Increased fluidity of excitable membranes would reduce their excitability which could ultimately result in alterations in neurotransmitter function [52].

The mechanism of action of ethanol on dopamine function may, of course, be indirectly mediated via other systems (e.g. opiates), which in turn might alter DA neuronal activity [53-54]. Serotonin itself is thought to have a major role in alcoholism [55], as mentioned earlier. For example, it has been shown that administration of the 5-HT precursor, 5-hydroxytryptophan or of 5-HT itself produces a significant reduction in ethanol consumption in self-administering animals [13,56,57]. Other studies have found similar effects with specific 5-HT uptake inhibitors, such as fluoxetine and zimelidine [58]. Results from these studies support the general concept that 5-HT indeed appears to be involved in the mediation of ethanol consumption, either directly or indirectly.

In addition, there have been numerous biochemical, pharmacological and behavioral studies suggesting that 5-HT modulates DA transmission [59-61]. Serotonin itself causes an increased release of dopamine from superfused striatal slices [62]. Furthermore, selective agonists at 5-HT3 receptors, but not those acting at 5-HT2 or 5-HT1 receptor sites, have similar actions, suggesting a specific role for the serotonin3 receptor type. Recently an in vivo chronocoulometric study by Jiang et al. [63] has shown that intracerebroventricular administration of the 5-HT3 agonist, 2-methyl-serotonin induces dopamine release in the nucleus accumbens. In a recent study on the possible interactions between serotonergic and dopaminergic systems in the effects of ethanol, we investigated the effect of pretreatment with 5-HT3 antagonists on the ethanol-induced increases in extracellular dopamine, as previously described. The 5-HT3 antagonists, ICS 205-930 and MDL 72222, in a dose of 500 ug/kg effectively attenuated the increase in dopamine following subsequent application of ethanol, in both the corpus striatum and the nucleus accumbens [64]. This finding, together with previously reported data from various groups utilizing antagonists of 5-HT3 receptors against drug-induced dopamine release or dopamine-related behaviors, support the notion that many dependence producing substances act to stimulate dopamine release and that 5-HT might have important modifying actions on this effect, specifically via 5-HT3 receptors. Interestingly, 5-HT3 antagonists have also been recently shown to attenuate ethanol's discriminative stimulus properties in pigeons [65].

These findings support the notion that both dopamine and 5-HT are important in the mediation of ethanol's effects on neurotransmitter function. It is conceivable that both 5-HT and dopamine are released following ethanol application, and interact with each other to produce the net effect on neurotransmission. Of possible relevance to this is a recent study by Nakahara et al. [66], in which they demonstrated increases in both dopamine and serotonin in the nucleus accumbens following intracranial self-stimulation.

Finally, the data suggest a possible function for the 5-HT3 receptors which have been localized in both rat [67] and human brain [68]. Furthermore, the reported data have implications for the possible use of 5-HT3 antagonists in the treatment of alcoholism and other substance abuse.

In summary, patients with alcohol dependence have biochemical signs of reduced or altered central serotonergic functioning. Such alterations may be quite subtle as indicated by the possible lack of seasonal variation in CSF 5HIAA concentrations and lack of correlation between CSF 5HIAA and TRH concentrations. Furthermore, pharmacological challenge studies show that serotonergic dysfunction in alcoholics may be limited to specific serotonin receptor subtypes. Animal studies show that serotonin3 receptors have an important role in regulating ethanol-induced dopamine release in the nucleus accumbens. These receptors could, therefore, affect rewarding effects of ethanol which may be important for the development of alcohol dependence.

REFERENCES

1. Takahashi S, Yamane H, Kondo H, Tani M (1974). CSF monoamine metabolites in alcoholism, a comparative study with depression. *Folia. Psychiat. Neurol. Japan,* 28, 347-354.

2. Ballenger J, Goodwin F, Major L, Brown G (1979). Alcohol and central serotonin metabolism in man. *Arch. Gen. Psychiatry,* 36, 224-227.

3. Banki C (1981). Factors influencing monoamine metabolites and tryptophan in patients with alcohol dependence. *J. Neural Transm.,* 50, 98-101.

4. Linnoila M, Virkkunen M, Scheinin M, Rimon R, Goodwin FK (1983). Low cerebrospinal fluid 5-hydroxyindoleacetic acid concentration differentiates impulsive from nonimpulsive violent behavior. *Life Sci.,* 33, 2609-2614.

5. Buydens-Branchey L, Branchey M, Noumair D, Lieber C (1989). Age of alcoholism onset. II. Relationship to susceptibility to serotonin precursor availability. *Arch Gen Psychiatry,* 46, 231-236.

6. Cloninger C, Bohman M, Sigvardsson S (1981). Inheritance of alcohol abuse: cross fostering analysis of alcoholic men. *Arch. Gen. Psychiatry,* 38, 861-868.

7. Linnoila M, DeJong J, Virkkunen M (1989). Family history of alcoholism in violent offenders and impulsive fire setters. *Arch Gen Psychiatry,* 46, 613-616.

8. Roy A, DeJong J, Lamparski D, Adinoff B, George DT, Moore V, Garnett D, Kerich M, Linnoila M (in press). Mental disorders among alcoholics: Relationship to age of onset and cerebrospinal fluid neuropeptides. *Arch Gen Psychiatry.*

9. Brewerton RD, Berrettini WH, Nurnberger JI, Linnoila M (1988). Analysis of seasonal fluctuations of CSF monoamine metabolites and neuropeptides in normal controls: findings with 5-HIAA and HVA. *Psychiatry Res.,* 232, 257-265.

10. Roy A, Bissette G, Nemeroff CB, DeJong J, Ravitz B, Adinoff B, Linnoila M (1990). Cerebrospinal fluid thyrotropin-releasing hormone concentrations in alcoholics and normal controls. *Biol. Psychiatry,* 28, 767-772.

11. Sprince H, Parker CM, Smith GG, Gonzales LJ (1972). Alcoholism: Biochemical and nutritional aspects of brain amines, aldehydes and amino acids. *Nutr. Report. Int.,* 5, 185-200.

12. Zabik JE, Binkerd K, and Roache JD (1985). Serotonin and ethanol aversion in the rat. In: Research Advances in New Psychopharmacological Treatments for Alcoholism, (C.A. Naranjo, E.M. Sellers, Eds.), Elsevier Science Publishers B.V., Amsterdam, pp. 23-41.

13. Geller I (1973). Effects of para-chlorophenylalanine and 5-hydroxytrypotophan on alcohol intake in the rat. *Pharmacol. Biochem. Behav.*, 1, 361-365.

14. Ho AKS, Tsai CS, Chen RCA, Begleiter H, Kissin B (1974). Experimental studies on alcoholism I. Increased alcohol preference by 5, 6-dihydroxytryptamine and brain acetylcholine. *Psychopharmacologia*, 40, 101-107.

15. Melchior CL, Myers RD (1976). Genetic differences in ethanol drinking of the rat following injection of 5-OHDA, 5, 6-DHT or 5, 7-DHT into the cerebral ventricles. *Pharamacol. Biochem. Behav.*, 5, 63-72.

16. Stein JM, Wayner MJ, Tilson HA (1977). The effect of parachlorophenylalanine on the intake of ethanol and saccharin solutions. *Pharmacol. Biochem. Behav.*, 6, 117-122.

17. Parker LF, Radow BL (1976). Effects of para-chlorphenylalanine on ethanol self-selection in the rat. *Pharmacol. Biochem. Behav.*, 4, 535-540.

18. Naranjo CA, Sellers EM, Roach CA, Woodley DV, Sanchez-Craig M, Sykora K (1984). Zimelidine-induced variations in alcohol intake by nondepressed heavy drinkers. *Clin. Pharmacol. Ther.*, 35, 374-381.

19. Naranjo CA, Sellers EM, Sullivan JT, Woodley DV, Kadle K, Sykora K (1987). The serotonin uptake inhibitor citolopram atten-uates ethanol intake. *Clin. Pharmacol. Ther.*, 41, 266-274.

20. Bibb JL, Chambless DL. (1986). Alcohol use and abuse among diagnosed agoraphobics. *Behav. Res. Ther.*, 24, 49-58.

21. Smail P, Stockwell T, Canter S, Hodgson R (1984). Alcohol dependence and phobic anxiety states, I. A prevalence study. *Br. J. Psychiatry.*, 144, 53-47.

22. Stockwell T, Snail P, Hodgson R, Carter S (1984). Alcohol dependence and phobic states. II. A retrospective study. *Br. J. Psychiatry.*, 144, 58-63.

23. Kahn RS and Van Praag HM (1988). A serotonin hypothesis of panic disorder. *Hum. Psychopharm.*, 3, 285-288.

24. Charney DS, Woods SW, Goodman WK, Heninger GR (1987). Serotonin function in anxiety. II. Effects of the serotonin agonist mCPP in panic disorder patients and healthy subjects. *Psychopharmacology,* 92, 14-24.

25. Ballenger JC, Goodwin FK, Major LF, Brown GL (1979). Alcohol and central serotonin metabolism in man. Arch. Gen. Psychiat

26. Wong DT, Lumerg L, Threlkeld PG, Reid LR, Li T-K (1988). Serotonergic and adrenergic receptors in alcohol preferring and non-preferring rats. *J. Neurol. Transm.,* 71, 207-218.

27. Schechter MD (1988). Use of TFMPP stimulus properties as a model of 5-HT1B receptor activation. *Pharm. Biochem. Beh.,* 31, 53-57.

28. Hoyer D (1988). Functional correlates of serotonin 5HT1 recognition sites. *J. Receptor Res.,* 8, 59-81.

29. Kilpatrick GJ, Jones BJ, Tyers MB (1987). Identification and distribution of 5HT3 receptors in rat brain using radioligand binding. *Nature,* 330, 746-748.

30. von Knorring AL, Bohman M, von Knorring L, Oreland L (1985). Platelet MAO activity as a biological marker in subgroups of alcoholism. *Acta Psychiatr. Scand.,* 72, 51-58.

31. Fibiger HC, and Phillips AG (1979). Dopamine and the neural mechanisms of reinforcement. In: The Neurobiology of Dopamine, (AS Horn, J Korf, BHC Westerink, Eds.), Academic Press, New York, Academic Press, 1979.

32. Wise RA, Bozarth MA (1982). Action of drugs of abuse on brain reward systems: an update with specific attention to opiates. *Pharmacol. Biochem. Behav.,* 17, 239-243.

33. Rogers J, Siggins GR, Schulman JA, Bloom FE (1980). Physiological correlates of ethanol intoxication, tolerance and dependence in rat cerebellar Purkinje cells. *Brain Research,* 196, 183-198.

34. Bustos G, Roth RH (1976). Effect of acute ethanol treatment on transmitter synthesis and metabolism in central dopaminergic neurones. *J. Pharm. Pharmacol.,* 28, 580-582.

35. Dar SM, Wooles WR (1984). The effect of acute ethanol on dopamine metabolism and other transmitters in the hypothalamus and corpus straitum of mice. *J. Neural Transm.,* 60, 283-294.

36. Fadda F, Argiolas A, Melis MR, Serra G, Gessa GL (1980). Differential effect of acute and chronic ethanol on dopamine metabolism in frontal cortex, caudate nucleus and substantia nigra. *Life Sci.,* 27, 979-986.

37. Karoum F, Wyatt RJ, Majchrowicz E (1976). Brain concentrations of biogenic amines in acutely treated and ethanol dependent rats. *Br. J. Pharmacol.*, 56, 403–411l.

38. Reggiani A, Barbaccia ML, Spano PF, Trabucchi M (1980). Dopamine metabolism and receptor function after acute and chronic ethanol. *J. Neurochem.*, 35, 34–37.

39. Carlsson A, Lindqvist M (1973). Effect of ethanol on the hydroxylation of tyrosine and tryptophan in rat brain in vivo. *J. Pharm. Pharmacol.*, 25, 437–440.

40. Tabakoff B, Hoffman PL 1979). Alterations in receptors controlling dopamine synthesis after chronic ethanol ingestion. *J. Neurochem.*, 208, 216–222.

41. Carlsson A, Magnusson T, Svensson TH, Waldeck B (1973). Effects of ethanol on the metabolism of brain catecholamines. *Psychopharmacology*, 30, 27–36.

42. Imperato A, Di Chiara G (1986). Preferential stimulation of dopamine release in the nucleus accumbens of freely moving rats by ethanol. *J. Pharmacol. Exp. Ther.*, 239, 219–228.

43. Blaustein MP, Nachshen DA, Drapeau P (1981). Excitation–secretion coupling: the role of calcium. In: Chemical Neurotransmission, L Stjarne, P Hedqvist, H Lanercrantz, A Wennmalm Eds), Academic Press, London.

44. Carlen PI, Gurevich N, Durand D (1982). Ethanol in low doses augments calcium–mediated mechanisms measured intracellularly in hippocampal neurones. *Science*, 215, 306–309.

45. Engel JA, Fahlke C, Hulthe P, Hard E, Johannessen K, Snape B, Svensson L (1988). Biochemical and behavioral evidence for an interaction between ethanol and calcium channel agonists. *J. Neural. Transm.*, 74, 181–193.

46. Lyon AC, McComb JA, Schreurs J, Goldstein DB (1981). Relationship between alcohol intoxication and the disordering of brain membranes by a series of short–chain alcohols. *J. Pharmacol. Exp. Ther.*, 218, 669–675.

47. McCreery MJ, Hunt WA (1978). Physico–chemical correlates of alcohol intoxication. *Neuropharmacology*, 17, 451–461.

48. Lindenberg BA (1951). P Sur la solubilite des substances organiques amohitatiques dans les glycerides neutres et hydroxyles. *J. Chim. Phys.*, 48, 350–355.

49. Goldstein DB: The effects of drugs on membrane fluidity. *Ann. Rev. Pharmacol. Toxicol.* 24:43–64, 1984.

50. Lovinger DM, White G, Wright FF (1989). Ethanol inhibits NMDA-activated ion current in hippocampal neurones. *Science,* 243, 1721-1724.

51. Lyon AC, Mc Comb JA, Schreurs J, Goldstein DB (1981). Relationship between alcohol intoxication and the disordering of brain membranes by a series of short-chain alcohols. *J. Pharmacol. Exp. Ther.,* 218, 669-675.

52. Hunt WA (1981). Neurotransmitter function in the basal ganglia after acute and chronic ethanol treatment. *Fed. Proc.,* 40, 2077-2081.

53. Ducobu J (1984). Naloxone and alcohol intoxication. *Ann. Intern. Med.,* 100, 617-618.

54. Holman RB, Snape BM, Widdowson S (1987). Naloxone elicits dose-dependent changes in alcohol-induced increases in endogenous dopamine release from rat striatum. *Alcohol and Alcoholism,* (Suppl. 1), 737-741.

55. Myers RD, Melchior CL: Alcohol and alcoholism (1977). Role of serotonin. In: Serotonin in Health and Disease, Vol. II, (WB Essman, Eds), Spectrum, New York.

56. Myers RD, Veale WL (1968). Alcohol preference in the rat: reduction following depletion of brain serotonin. *Science,,* 160, 1469-1471.

57. Myers RD, Martin GE (1973). The role of cerebral serotonin in the ethanol preference of animals. *Ann. N.Y. Acad. Sci.,* 215, 135-144.

58. Rockman GE, Amit Z, Carr G, Brown ZW, Ogren SO (1979). Attenuation of ethanol intake by 5-hydroxytryptamine uptake blockade in laboratory rats. 1. Involvement of brain 5-hydroxytryptamine in the mediation of the positive reinforcing properties of ethanol. *Arch. Int. Pharmacodyn. Ther.,* 241, 245-259.

59. Carter CJ, Pycock CJ (1979). The effects of 5,7-dihydroxy-tryptamine lesions of extrapyramidal and mesolimbic sites on spontaneous motor activity and amphetamine-induced stereotypy, *Naunyn Schmiedebergs Arch. Pharmacol.,* 208, 51-54.

60. Jackson EA, Kelly PH, Schultz A (1985). Effects of serotonergic activity in nucleus accumbens septa on drug-induced circling. *Neuropharmacology,* 24, 721-727.

61. Chesselet MF (1984). Presynaptic regulation of neurotransmitter release in the brain: facts and hypotheses. *Neuroscience,* 12, 1347-1375.

62. Blandina P, Goldfarb J, Craddock-Royal B, Green JP (1989). Release of endogenous dopamine by stimulation of 5-hydroxytryptamine3 receptors in rat striatum. *J. Pharmacol. Exp. Ther.,* 251 803-809.

63. Jiang LH, Ashby CR, Kasser RJ, Wang R (1990). The effect of intraventricular administration of the 5-HT3 receptor agonist 2-methylserotonin on the release of dopamine in the nucleus accumbens : an in vivo chronocoulometric study. *Brain Research,* 513, 156-160.

64. Wozniak KM, Pert A, Linnoila M (1990). Antagonism of 5-HT3 receptors attenuates the effects of ethanol on extracellular dopamine. *Eur. J. Pharmacol.,* 187, 287-289.

65. Grant, KA, Lovinger DM, White G, Barret JE (1990). Blockade of the discriminative stimulus properties of ethanol by 5-HT3 antagonists. *FASEB,* 14A, 989.

66. Nakahara D, Ozaki N, Miura Y, Miura H, Nagatsu T (1989). Increased dopamine and serotonin in rat nucleus accumbens produced by intracranial self-stimulation of medial forebrain bundle as measured by in vivo microdialysis. *Brain Research,* 495, 178-181.

67. Kilpatrick GJ, Jones BJ, Tyers MB (1987). Identification and distribution of 5-HT3 receptors in rat brain using radioligand binding. *Nature,* 330, 746-748.

68. Barnes JM, Barnes NM, Costall B, Ironside JW, Naylor RJ (1989). Identification and characterization of 5-hydroxytryptamine3 recognition sites in human brain tissue. *J. Neurochem.,* 1787-1793.

9

Evaluation of the Effects of Serotonin Uptake Inhibitors in Alcoholics: A Review

C.A. Naranjo and K.E. Bremner

1. ABSTRACT

Preclinical studies, using various models, have consistently shown that serotonin uptake inhibitors (SUI) decrease alcohol consumption in rats in a dose-related manner. Similarly, in four (zimeldine, citalopram, viqualine, fluoxetine) short-term (2 to 4 weeks of treatment) randomized, double-blind studies, patients with moderate dependence on alcohol showed a dose-dependent decrease in alcohol consumption. Number of drinks decreased from baseline by averages of 15% to 20%, with some subjects showing a 60% decrease. The effect on alcohol consumption is not due to toxicity, antianxiety or antidepressant effects of SUI or to aversive interactions with alcohol. Side effects have generally been mild and few. Subjects who correctly believed that they received a SUI did not respond differently than those who believed they received placebo, so expectation was not responsible for SUI effects. SUI (e.g. citalopram) decrease the desire and liking for alcohol as well as consumption. Changes in these variables correlated, suggesting a possible mechanism of action. SUI seem to have a differential effect on addictive behaviors since cigarette smoking did not decrease and consumption of nonalcoholic beverages was unaltered. Slight weight losses were observed, probably due to decreased appetite and food intake, since variations in alcohol intake were not correlated with changes in body weight. SUI are one of the most promising psychopharmacological agents available for treating alcoholics. They may act by decreasing desire to drink and the reinforcing properties of alcohol making them uniquely suitable for relapse prevention strategies. Evaluation of their long-term effects in conjunction with behavioral interventions continues.

2. INTRODUCTION

A series of consistent results in rodents indicate that serotonin uptake inhibitors decrease the ethanol intake of rats (Lawrin et al, 1986; Naranjo

---

Parts of this manuscript have been published in abstracts and other articles by the authors.

et al, 1987b; Amit and Smith, 1991). Once the effectiveness of a medication has been shown in animals, it must be confirmed in humans. Initial human studies must also determine the dose-response relationship and possible mechanism of action (Naranjo and Kadlec, 1991). Subsequent pivotal human studies must be undertaken (Naranjo et al, 1987b). Since selective and safe drugs which inhibit serotonin uptake are available for human use, clinical trials were first conducted with the serotonin uptake inhibitor, zimeldine (Amit et al, 1985; Naranjo et al, 1984a). Although zimeldine was withdrawn from the market because of serious hepatic and neurologic toxicity in Swedish patients (Fagius et al, 1985; Naranjo et al, 1990b) these studies indicated the therapeutic potential of serotonin uptake inhibitors. We, therefore, developed a research program to systematically evaluate the clinical effects of other serotonin uptake inhibitors, citalopram, viqualine, and fluoxetine, on ethanol intake and other addictive behaviors in humans.

3. CLINICAL TRIALS WITH SEROTONIN UPTAKE INHIBITORS

The effects of four serotonin uptake inhibitors, zimeldine, citalopram, viqualine and fluoxetine on alcohol intake and other addictive behaviors were assessed in randomized, placebo-controlled, double-blind trials.

3.1 Subjects and Methods

Subjects were volunteers, recruited by advertisement and compensated for their participation. They were screened for depression, anxiety, social stability and physical and emotional health (Naranjo et al, 1984a, 1987a, 1989, 1990a). Subjects met the criteria for the DSM-III-R diagnosis of mild to moderate alcohol dependence (American Psychiatric Association, 1987); (i.e., they usually drank alcohol in larger amounts or over longer periods than intended, desired or had attempted to decrease or stop drinking, spent a great deal of time drinking or recovering from its effects, had developed some degree of tolerance for alcohol, and/or had reduced some activities because of alcohol use). Mild intoxication, withdrawal symptoms or social, psychological or medical problems were occasionally encountered in the subjects. Subjects for all studies were assessed to be non-depressed and socially stable, and they did not abuse or only occasionally abused other drugs (other than cigarette smoking). They reported drinking 28 or more standard drinks (each containing 13.6 g absolute ethanol) per week before the study.

Testing procedures were similar in all studies. During the two-week baseline periods, subjects recorded their daily alcohol consumption, intake of non-alcoholic beverages and cigarettes smoked (daily smokers only) on a self-monitoring form and took evening urine samples which were returned and analyzed for ethanol and riboflavin concentrations. Those who complied with these procedures and met the entrance criteria were randomized to receive a serotonin uptake inhibitor (zimeldine, citalopram, viqualine or fluoxetine) or placebo (identical-looking capsules with a riboflavin 20 mg marker) for two or four weeks according to the study protocols. No other treatment or advice was offered. Subjects continued to record their alcohol intake and to provide urine samples. Biweekly assessments included depression and anxiety scales, laboratory tests and a physical examination. In the studies with viqualine and fluoxetine subjects were asked to indicate their interest, desire, and liking for alcohol on a 5-point scale, from "not at all" to "an awful lot", (Naranjo et al, 1989, 1990). Compliance with medication was confirmed by measurements of riboflavin in daily urine samples, drug and metabolite concentrations in plasma, serotonin concentration in blood and serotonin uptake inhibition by platelets. The self-reports of ethanol intake (daily standard drinks) were correlated with ethanol concentrations in the daily urine samples.

Three studies had a cross-over design. Thirteen subjects were assigned to receive zimeldine (Z) 200 mg/day and placebo (P) in four two-week periods (ZPZP or PZPZ), but only 10 completed all four periods. Thirty-nine subjects received citalopram (C) 20 mg/day (n=20) or 40 mg/day (n=19) and respective placebos for four consecutive weeks each, separated by a two-week washout (CP or PC), and 29 subjects received viqualine (V) 100 mg/day (n=15) or 200 mg/day (n=14) and respective placebos for two weeks each, separated by a one-week washout (VP or PV). The long half-life of fluoxetine necessitated a parallel design study. Twenty-nine subjects received either fluoxetine 40 mg/day (n=8), fluoxetine 60 mg/day (n=11) or placebo (n=10) for four consecutive weeks.

The effects of the serotonin uptake inhibitors on alcohol intake (number of daily drinks, drinks per drinking day, total drinks per period, and number or percent of abstinent days per period), non-alcoholic drinks and cigarettes were tested by analysis of covariance with baseline measures as the covariates and treatment (serotonin uptake inhibitor or placebo) and order of treatment allocation (crossover studies only) as independent variables. A repeated measures design was used for the crossover studies. Also, the main dependent variables were analyzed in repeated measures analysis of variance tests comparing each treatment, drug and placebo, with baseline. Intent-to-treat analyses were performed when there was sufficient data.

3.2 Results

All measures of compliance indicated that subjects took the experimental drugs as required and that they reported their alcohol consumption accurately. They attended all of the study visits and returned over 95% of the expected urine samples.

None of the lower doses of serotonin uptake inhibitor significantly changed any of the measures of alcohol intake compared with placebo or baseline. However, zimeldine 200 mg/day, citalopram 40 mg/day, viqualine 200 mg/day and fluoxetine 60 mg/day all decreased alcohol intake. Order of treatment (drug or placebo first) had no effects. Mean daily drinks during serotonin uptake inhibitor treatment and placebo depended on baseline values (all $p<0.01$).

The effects of zimeldine 200 mg/day were tested in the 13 subjects who completed only the first two two-week experimental periods. In these subjects, zimeldine decreased mean daily drinks compared with placebo, from 6.0 ± 0.8 ($\bar{x} \pm SEM$) to 5.5 ± 0.9 ($p<0.05$) (Table 1). Days of abstinence increased from 1.5 ± 0.4 days during the 14-day placebo period to 3.7 ± 0.8 days during zimeldine ($p<0.005$). In the 10 subjects who completed all 4 treatment periods, zimeldine had no effect on mean daily drinks, but it increased abstinent days.

Citalopram 40 mg/day decreased mean daily drinks to 6.0 ± 0.8 ($\bar{x} \pm SEM$) compared with placebo (6.7 ± 0.7) ($p<0.05$) (Table 1). Subjects also reported a greater number of abstinent days during the 28-day citalopram treatment period than during placebo (3.2 ± 0.8 vs 1.3 ± 0.5, $p<0.005$).

Alcohol intake also decreased during viqualine 200 mg/day compared with placebo. Mean daily drinks ($\bar{x} \pm SEM$) were 7.7 ± 0.8 during placebo and only 6.4 ± 0.8 during viqualine ($p<0.05$) (Table 1). However, viqualine had no significant effect on the number of abstinent days per 14-day period, (1.4 ± 0.5 during placebo and 1.8 ± 0.6 during viqualine, n.s.).

In the parallel design study, mean daily drinks during fluoxetine 60 mg/day ($\bar{x} \pm SEM = 6.9 \pm 0.7$) were not significantly different than during placebo (7.5 ± 0.7). However, fluoxetine 60 mg/day decreased mean daily drinks compared with its own baseline (8.3 ± 0.7) ($p<0.05$) (Table 1). In contrast, the baseline to treatment differences were not significant for fluoxetine 40 mg/day (7.2±0.5 [baseline] vs 7.4±0.9, n.s.) or placebo (7.9±0.8 vs 7.5±0.7). Because only 7 of the 11 subjects who received fluoxetine 60 mg/day had any abstinent days during the two-week baseline or four-week treatment period, average values for abstinent days, calculated as percent of days abstinent, were very low (2.6 and 3.9 for baseline and treatment, respectively), and not significantly different.

Table 1: Effects of Serotonin Uptake Inhibitors (SUI) on Alcohol Intake

Serotonin Uptake Inhibitor	Mean Daily Drinks ($\bar{x}$±SEM) Baseline	Placebo	SUI)	p[1]
Zimeldine 200 mg/day (n=13)	6.2±0.9	6.0±0.8	5.5±0.9	<0.05
Citalopram 40 mg/day (n=19)	7.1±0.6	6.7±0.7	6.0±0.8	<0.05
Viqualine 200 mg/day (n=14)	7.9±0.6	7.7±0.8	6.4±0.8	<0.05
Fluoxetine 60 mg/day (n=11)	8.3±0.7	-	6.9±0.7	<0.05

1 In repeated measures analysis of covariance tests comparing drug and placebo with baseline as covariate, except for fluoxetine, for which drug and baseline were compared in repeated measures ANOVA.

Figure 1 shows the average decrease in alcoholic drinks during each serotonin uptake inhibitor compared with their own baselines. The average response for the four drugs was a 17% decrease in alcoholic drinks. The placebos did not change alcohol intake significantly (less than 2% average). There was some variation in response to the drugs but 92% of zimeldine subjects decreased their alcoholic drinks and/or increased their abstinent days by at least 25% compared with placebo, as did 63% of the citalopram 40 mg/day subjects and 64% of the viqualine 200 mg/day subjects. Of the subjects who received fluoxetine 60 mg/day, 36% decreased daily drinks and/or increased abstinent days by at least 25% compared with their own baseline. The size of the effect in the responders is encouraging - a 33% to 39% decrease in alcoholic drinks and two- to three-fold increase in days of abstinence.

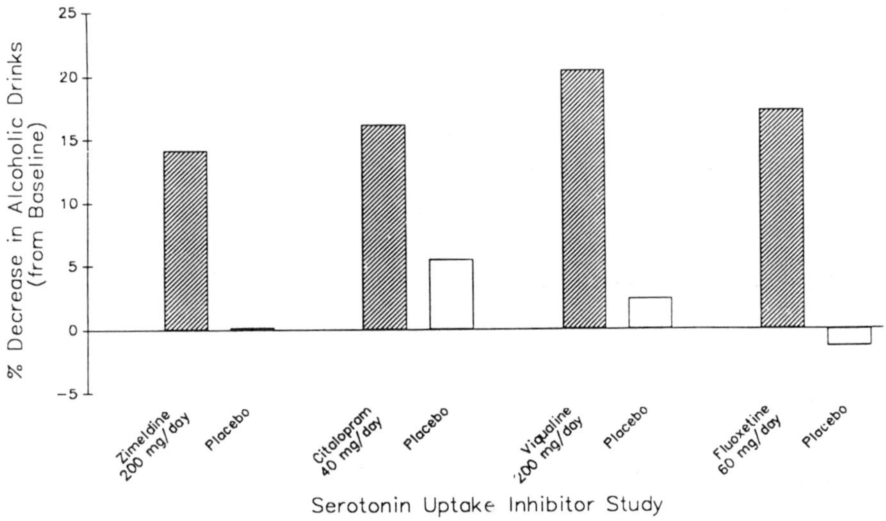

Figure 1. Response to serotonin uptake inhibitors

A few subjects dropped out of the study before completing both pharmacological treatments (in the crossover studies) or completing the 4-week fluoxetine or placebo treatments. When these subjects were included in intent-to-treat analyses, the conclusions with respect to the effects of serotonin uptake inhibitors on alcohol intake and other consummatory behaviors did not change.

3.3 Possible Mechanisms of Action

Frequent side effects, changes in depression or anxiety or alcohol-sensitizing reactions were not observed and therefore could not account for the effect of serotonin uptake inhibitors on alcohol intake. No consistent temporal relationship between the few side effects and decreases in drinking could be discerned. Studies which were specifically designed to determine the behavioral, pharmacokinetic and dynamic interactions of the drugs with alcohol concluded that the effects of alcohol (at blood concentrations approximating the legal limit for driving a motor vehicle in Canada) on performance, and self-ratings of intoxication, sedation, and performance were not accentuated or diminished by viqualine (Sullivan et al, 1989) or fluoxetine (Shaw et al, 1989). No interactions between ethanol and citalopram were found (Lader et al, 1986), but zimeldine was found to enhance the psychomotor impairment produced by ethanol (Naranjo et al, 1984b) and attenuate ethanol deleterious effect on memory (Weingartner et al, 1983). Therefore, serotonin uptake inhibitors do not have any important, harmful or detrimental interactions with alcohol. In addition, no pharmacokinetic interactions were detected between ethanol and serotonin uptake inhibitors.

The modulating effects of citalopram, viqualine and fluoxetine were specific to alcohol intake (Naranjo et al, 1987a, 1989, 1990). No significant changes in consumption of non-alcoholic drinks or cigarette smoking (Sellers et al, 1987; Kadlec and Naranjo, 1991) were detected. Therefore, there is no evidence that these drugs decrease all fluid intake or other addictive behaviors.

However, small weight losses were observed in most of the male heavy drinkers who received citalopram 40 mg/day, viqualine 200 mg/day and fluoxetine 60 mg/day. Average weight losses per 2 weeks during serotonin uptake inhibitor treatment were 0.4 to 1.2 kg, compared with weight gains of 0.1 to 0.3 kg during placebo treatment ($p<0.05$). Decreases in calories from alcohol were not related to the weight losses. Furthermore, citalopram 20 mg/day, viqulaine 100 mg/day and fluoxetine 40 mg/day decreased body weight by averages of 0.3 to 1.0 kg per 2 weeks, but did not significantly decrease alcohol intake (Sellers et al, 1988). Subjects were of normal weight and not trying to diet. Since loss of appetite was frequently reported during citalopram 40 mg/day and fluoxetine 60 mg/day ($p<0.05$ compared with placebo), food intake probably decreased. Fluoxetine has been shown to be efficacious for weight loss in obese patients who were given advice to decrease their caloric intake (Levine et al, 1987) and it also reduced weight and binge eating in patients with bulimia nervosa (Enas et al, 1989). Therefore, serotonin uptake inhibitors may decrease appetite or desire to eat.

A similar mechanism may mediate the effect of these drugs on alcohol intake. Interest, desire and liking for alcohol were assessed in the viqualine and fluoxetine studies, in order to determine if variations in urge to drink and/or the reinforcing properties of alcohol could be observed. Decreases in interest, desire and liking for alcohol were detected in the subjects who received viqualine 200 mg/day, compared with placebo. No significant variations were detected with fluoxetine 60 mg/day. However, in a more recent study, 16 subjects reduced their alcohol intake and increased their abstinent days during one week of treatment with citalopram 40 mg/day compared with placebo and concomitant decreases in interest, craving, desire and liking for alcohol were observed. Changes in these variables correlated with number of drinks (Naranjo et al, 1991). Further research is needed to determine the effects of serotonin uptake inhibitors on desire to drink.

Placebo treatment was administered in all of our randomized, double-blind studies in order to control for non-pharmacological effects, such as expectancies, motivation or beliefs. Subjects in the citalopram, viqualine and fluoxetine studies were asked to indicate, at the end of each treatment period, their perception of which treatment, drug or placebo, they had been receiving. Perception of treatment has been reported to be a significant factor determining response in one study; among the subjects who received the drug, those who believed they received drug reduced their alcohol consumption to a significantly greater degree than those who believed they had received placebo (Toneatto et al, 1991). However, we did not find any evidence for the effect of a psychological factor such as expectancy in our studies with citalopram, viqualine or fluoxetine. During the drug treatments the subjects who correctly perceived that they had received drug did not respond differently from those who perceived they had received placebo. Table 2 shows that perception of treatment received had no consistent or significant effects on decrease in alcohol intake from baseline, even when all the subjects (n=44) are analyzed together. Also, subjects who correctly perceived that they had received placebo during placebo treatment did not respond differently from those who believed they had received drug.

4. FUTURE CLINICAL APPLICATIONS

An increase in abstinent days was the main effect of two serotonin uptake inhibitors, zimeldine and citalopram, indicating that subjects decreased their alcohol intake by drinking on fewer days, rather than by drinking fewer drinks per drinking occasion. Therefore, these drugs may exert

Table 2: Response (% decrease in alcohol intake from baseline [$\bar{x}\pm$SEM]) and perception of whether drug or placebo had been administered during treatment with serotonin uptake inhibitors.

Serotonin Uptake Inhibitor	Perceived drug n	Perceived drug % decrease	Perceived Placebo n	Perceived Placebo % decrease	p
Citalopram 40 mg/day (n=19)	6	28.7±5.0	13	10.4±7.0	n.s.
Viqualine 200 mg/day (n=14)	7	12.7±9.5	7	28.2±10.2	n.s.
Fluoxetine 60 mg/day (n=11)	11	17.3±5.0	0*	-	-
Total (n=44)	24	18.8±3.8	20	16.6±6.0	n.s.

*all subjects correctly perceived fluoxetine treatment.

their main effect on the initiation of drinking. In addition, decreases in interest, desire and liking for alcohol were observed in some of our studies and may have mediated this effect. Modification of the urge to drink, desire for alcohol and liking (reinforcing effects) of alcohol may mediate the effects of serotonin uptake inhibitors and this mechanisms of action should be applied to direct the focus of treatments to initiate the reduction of alcohol intake and prevent relapse.

Further studies are underway using various strategies to maximize the drug effect: a) by combining pharmacotherapy with a brief psychosocial intervention, such as advice and guidelines to modify alcohol consumption (Naranjo et al, 1988); b) by adjusting the dose for individual patients; c) by stressing relapse prevention: because relapse is a common problem for recovered alcoholics, the long-term effects of the combination of treatments are also important (Naranjo and Kadlec, 1991). Serotonin uptake inhibitors are, therefore, one of the most promising psychopharmacological agents available for treating alcoholics and their clinical effects continue to be evaluated.

5. ACKNOWLEDGEMENTS

We wish to thank Drs. E.M. Sellers, J.T. Sullivan, V. Khouw, P. Sanhueza, H. Valencia, and S.L. Lee, Mrs. Theresa Fan, Mr. Walter Juzytsch, Mrs. D. Woodley-Remus, Mrs. G. Kennedy, Miss M. McPhee and Mr. M. Paunil for their help in conducting the human studies. We also thank Mrs. Linda Neuman for preparing the manuscript. These studies have been supported by the Intramural Grant Program of the Addiction Research Foundation of Ontario.

The views expressed in this publication are those of the authors and do not necessarily reflect those of the Addiction Research Foundation.

6. REFERENCES

American Psychiatric Association (1987). DSM-III-R Diagnostic and Statistical Manual of Mental Disorders (Third Edition-Revised), Washington, D.C.

Amit, Z., Z. Brown, A. Sutherland, G. Rockman, K. Gill and N. Selvaggi (1985). Reduction in alcohol intake in humans as a function of treatment with zimelidine: implications for treatment. In: *Research Advances in New Psychopharmacological Treatments for Alcoholism*, (C.A. Naranjo, E.M. Sellers, Eds.), Elsevier Science Publishers B.V., Amsterdam, pp. 189-198.

Amit, Z., and B.R. Smith (1991). Neurotransmitter systems regulating alcohol intake. In: *Novel Pharmacological Interventions for Alcoholism*, (C.A. Naranjo, E.M. Sellers, Eds.), Springer-Verlag, New York (in press).

Enas, G., H.G. Pope, L.R. Levine et al (1989). Fluoxetine in bulimia nervosa: a double-blind study. Presented at the 142nd annual meeting of the American Psychiatric Association, San Francisco.

Fagius, J., P.O. Osterman, A. Siden, and B.-E. Wiholm (1985). Guillain-Barre syndrome following zimeldine treatment. *Neurol. Neurosurg. Psychiatry*, 48, 65-69.

Kadlec, K.E. and C.A. Naranjo (1991). Differential effects of serotonin uptake inhibitors (SUI) on addictive behaviors in alcoholics [abstract]. (Committee on Problems in Drug Dependence, Palm Beach, Florida, June 16-20, 1991) (in press).

Lader, M., A. Melhuish, G. Freka, K.F. Overo, and V. Christensen (1986). The effect of citalopram in single and repeated doses and with alcohol on physiological and psychological measures in healthy subjects. *Eur. J. Clin. Pharmacol.*, 31, 183-190.

Lawrin, M.O., C.A. Naranjo, and E.M. Sellers (1986). Identification and testing of new drugs for modulating alcohol consumption. *Psychopharmacol. Bull.*, 22, 1020-1025.

Levine, L.R., S. Rosenblatt and J. Bosomworth (1987). Use of a serotonin re-uptake inhibitor, fluoxetine, in the treatment of obesity. *Int. J. Obesity*, 11 (Suppl. 3), 185-190.

Naranjo, C.A., E.M. Sellers, C.A. Roach, D.V. Woodley, M. Sanchez-Craig, and K. Sykora (1984a). Zimelidine-induced variations in alcohol intake by non-depressed heavy drinkers. *Clin. Pharm. Ther.*, 35, 374-381.

Naranjo, C.A., E.M. Sellers, H.L. Kaplan, C. Hamilton, and V. Khouw (1984b). Acute kinetic and dynamic interactions of zimelidine and ethanol. *Clin. Pharmacol. Ther.*, 36, 654-660.

Naranjo, C.A., E.M. Sellers, P.H. Wu and M.O Lawrin (1985). Moderation of ethanol drinking: role of enhanced serotonergic neurotransmission. In: *Research Advances in New Psychopharmacological Treatments for Alcoholism*, (C.A. Naranjo, E.M. Sellers, Eds.), Elsevier Science Publishers B.V., Amsterdam, pp. 171-186.

Naranjo, C.A., E.M. Sellers, J.T. Sullivan, D.V. Woodley, K. Kadlec, and K. Sykora (1987a). The serotonin uptake inhibitor citalopram attenuates ethanol intake. *Clin. Pharm. Ther.*, 41 266-274.

Naranjo, C.A., J.T. Sullivan, M.O. Lawrin and E.M. Sellers (1987b). Strategies for the identification and testing of new pharmacological modulators of ethanol consumption. In: *Brain Reward Systems and Abuse*, (J. Engel, L. Oreland, D.H. Ingvar, B. Pernow, S. Rossner, L.A. Pellborn, Eds.), Raven Press, New York, pp. 129-145.

Naranjo C.A., P. Sanhueza and E.M. Sellers (1988). An evaluation of the efficacy of citalopram, a very selective and specific serotonin uptake inhibitor, in problem drinkers. Research protocol, Addiction Research Foundation.

Naranjo, C.A., J.T. Sullivan, K.E. Kadlec, D.V. Woodley-Remus, G. Kennedy, and E.M. Sellers (1989). Differential effects of viqualine on alcohol intake and other consummatory behaviors. *Clin. Pharmacol. Ther.*, 46, 301-309.

Naranjo, C.A., K.E. Kadlec, P. Sanhueza, D. Woodley-Remus, and E.M. Sellers (1990a). Fluoxetine differentially alters alcohol intake and other consummatory behaviors in problem drinkers. *Clin. Pharmacol. Ther.*, 47, 490-498.

Naranjo, C.A., D. Lane, M. Ho-Asjoe, and K.L. Lanctot (1990b). A Bayesian assessment of idiosyncratic adverse reactions to new drugs: Guillain-Barre syndrome and zimeldine. *J. Clin. Pharmacol.*, 30, 174-180.

Naranjo, C.A., C.X. Poulos, K.E. Kadlec, K.L. Lanctot and E.M. Sellers (1991). Citalopram decreases desirability, liking and consumption of alcohol. *Clin. Pharmacol. Ther.*, 49, 138.

Naranjo, C.A., and K.E. Kadlec (1991). Possible pharmacological probes for predicting and preventing relapse in treated alcoholics. *Alcohol & Alcoholism*, Suppl. 1, 523-526.

Sellers, E.M., C.A. Naranjo and K. Kadlec (1987). Do serotonin uptake inhibitors decrease smoking? Observations in a group of heavy drinkers. *J. Clin. Psychopharmacol.*, 7, 417-420.

Sellers, E.M., C.A. Naranjo, K.E. Kadlec and D.V. Woodley-Remus (1988). Weight loss induced by serotonin uptake inhibitors (SUI) in male heavy drinkers [abstract]. *Psychopharmacology*, 96 (suppl.), 311.

Shaw, C.A., J.T. Sullivan, K.E. Kadlec, H.L. Kaplan, C.A. Naranjo and E.M. Sellers (1989). Ethanol interactions with serotonin uptake selective and non-selective antidepressents: fluoxetine and amitriptyline. *Human Psychopharmacology*, 4, 113-120.

Sullivan, J.T., C.A. Naranjo, C.A. Shaw, H.L. Kaplan, K.E. Kadlec and E.M. Sellers (1989). Kinetic and dynamic interactions of oral viqualine and ethanol in man. *Eur. J. Clin. Pharmacol.*, 36, 93-96.

Toneatto, T., E.M. Sellers, L.C. Sobell and M.B. Sobell (1991). Perception of whether drug or placebo had been administered as a determinant of drinking reduction. In: *Novel Pharmacological Interventions for Alcoholism*, (C.A. Naranjo, E.M. Sellers eds.), Springer-Verlag New York Publishers, New York (in press).

Weingartner, H., M.V. Rudorfer, M.S. Buchsbaum, and M. Linnoila (1983). Effects of serotonin on memory impairment produced by ethanol. *Science*, 221, 472-474.

Part III
Opioids and Alcohol Consumption

10
Opioids Modulate Rats' Propensities to Take Alcoholic Beverages

L.D. Reid and C.L. Hubbell

The prime question of alcohol abuse and alcoholism is why do some people drink too much, too often. Given that alcoholism has been a problem throughout history, there has been ample opportunity for many kinds of answers to be posed to the prime question. Given that problems of addiction to opium have also been extant for a long time; given that there are, at least, some gross similarities between the addictions to alcohol and opium; and given that there has been rapid progress in understanding how opium achieves its effects; it is not surprising that there are both old [1] and new [2] speculations concerning how opioids might be involved in alcoholism. Recently, a review of these considerations has appeared [3].

Despite considerable speculation about how addictions to the active ingredient of alcoholic beverages, ethanol, and to the active ingredient of opium, morphine, are related, there is only a small experimental literature relating how morphine might effect intake of alcoholic beverages. There is also only a small literature describing the effects of naloxone, the classic antagonist of morphine's effects, on intake of alcoholic beverages. In this particular paper, and in papers of this section, there are presentations relating the gist of the relevant literature as well as some flavor of the extant controversies.

Across the last 15 years, there has been rapid and extensive progress made in describing the substrates by which morphine, and related drugs (opioids), achieve their effects. In brief, there are a number of kinds of specialized receptors on neurons that selectively bind opioids. Furthermore, these receptors are part of information processing systems that interact with the products of, at least, 3 genes. Those products are known as the endogenous opioids (or endogenous opioid peptides or previously endorphins) and include two pentapeptides; Leu- and Met-enkephalin. These systems are widely distributed in brain as well as peripheral organs such as the gut and adrenal (for a review, see [4]).

The endogenous opioids have a variety of functions including those associated with modulation of pain, and reactivity to stress. Also, there is a growing consensus that opioids are involved with control of ingestive processes. An emerging concept that is particularly relevant to our topic is that opioids are somehow involved with the maintenance of ingestive behaviors once begun [5].

From what we now know, morphine is a drug which mimics the effects of endogenous opioids. Naloxone is an antagonist not only to the effects of morphine, but also to the effects of the endogenous opioids. Consequently, the study of the effects of naloxone, and related antagonists, is apt to reveal something about the functioning of the endogenous opioids [6].

Given the extensive discussions of the relationships between the addictions to morphine and ethanol, many of which involved direct speculation about how opioidergic events affected propensity to drink alcoholic beverages, it is, indeed, interesting that there is such a small and controversial literature germane to the topic. The acquisition of knowledge of how morphine, for example, might affect intake of alcoholic beverages could, on the surface, be acquired by simple experimental procedures, say by getting rats to take alcoholic beverages and then by giving them injections of morphine. This apparently straightforward approach, however, is complicated by an inordinate array of conceptual concerns.

The study of rats' drinking of alcoholic beverages has been, for example, extraordinarily controversial. There just is no consensus that it is reasonable to use rats to model people's alcoholism. Given that rats are the experimental subjects of choice (because they are inexpensive, easy to use and we have considerable knowledge of them) [7], not having such a consensus is, indeed, a problem. The controversy is whether or not rats evidence alcoholism. The approach was to first decide that A, B, C, D, and E were essential aspects of people's alcoholism and then demonstrate that rats' manifest A, B, C, D and E. It was apparently only after the experimental model was established that it was possible to use rats to study variables related to alcoholism.

It turned out that it was difficult to arrange for rats to show all of the supposedly essential features of people's alcoholism and, therefore, the approach of using rats was stymied. Of course, if one was going to study which features of people's alcoholism were essential, the initial approach taken with rats was not helpful, since the decision of what was essential was made before the issues were studied. One of the supposedly essential features of people's alcoholism, for example, was the development of physical dependence, i.e., the appearance of withdrawal symptoms such as proneness to seizures when intake of alcohol was abruptly halted. Rats do not, however, across just a few months, voluntarily drink alcoholic beverages in sufficiently high doses to remain intoxicated for a sufficiently long period of time to develop physical dependence. The conclusion was reached, therefore, that rats' drinking was not a reasonable model of people's alcoholism and, furthermore, they were not appropriate for studying other variables that might affect their drinking (if the goal was to make generalizations that were applicable to the human condition).

One can make rats dependent upon ethanol by keeping them constantly intoxicated across a 4-day period [8]. Making rats dependent, however, does not lead rats to drink large amounts of alcoholic beverages. People usually drink extensively for years before they develop severe withdrawal symptoms. The question that might be asked is what sustains drinking prior to the time of onset of withdrawal symptoms.

Modern theories of addiction, in fact, do not emphasize the processes involved with the development of physical dependence as a critical part of the addiction syndrome [9]. So, the arbitrary establishment of a criterion of physical dependence, due to voluntary drinking of an alcoholic beverage by rats as a first step in studying what variables might affect rats' drinking, does not seem reasonable from a modern perspective. Yet, presence of physical dependence was one of the criterion usually mentioned as a necessary condition for the establishment of an animal model of alcoholism. By rigidly holding to these arbitrary criteria, the careful study of rats' drinking which, in turn, might have lead to applicable theory of people's drinking may have been hindered.

An experimental model of a condition such as alcohol abuse and alcoholism does not have to be isomorphic with the human condition. Obviously, exact equivalence is worthless. For a model to be useful, it must be simpler and easier to study. The criterion of utility is whether or not it generates useful information, and not its exact similarity to the human condition. The utility of the information is determined, in turn, by whether or not the model is useful in predicting how certain variables will affect the human condition [10] and whether or not features of germane theories can be assessed [11].

Although one can attribute the lack of careful study of opioids on propensity to drink alcoholic beverages to a lack of consensus about the value of studying rats' drinking (it was surely not based on a lack of commentary about the relevance of such study), the controversy may have been more argumentive than substantial. Rats will drink alcoholic beverages in sufficient amounts to produce behavioral effects. Furthermore, they are apt to drink quite large amounts across a short period of time under certain circumstances. The fact that rats will drink alcoholic beverages, in amounts producing behavioral effects, is sufficient to begin the process of determining what variables might affect that drinking. The codification of those variables could lead to an applicable theory.

With the goal of having a moderate (but meaningful) level of intake of ethanol across a period of time during which a number of interesting drugs might be tested, the following procedures were instigated. Daily, rats were deprived of water for 22 hr and then for 2 hr presented with (a) a sweetened solution containing 12% pure ethanol and (b) water. The individually housed rats always had food available; but, since they were deprived of water, they were probably somewhat deprived of food. The 2-hr sessions usually occurred during the lighted portion of a light-dark cycle, at the same time each day. The daily regimen was continued day after day.

Under the influence of the daily regimen of 2 hr a day to take alcoholic beverage and water, rats appear healthy and grow at nearly the same rate as rats without a schedule of deprivation. At first, they take hardly any ethanol; but across days, they escalate their intakes until they are taking, on average, about 2.0 g of pure ethanol per kilogram of body weight (g/kg) a day. This daily regimen involves a number of setting conditions potentiating the intake of alcoholic beverage.

The daily regimen of deprivation and presentation of water and alcoholic beverage, but not water deprivation by itself, potentiates intakes (i.e., if water is provided just before the session, the same amount of ethanol is taken) [12]. Provisioning a palatable solution is an important setting condition potentiating higher levels of drinking. The fact that the session is during the rats' ordinary period for sleep also seems to provide some slight potentiation of intake [13]. Also, importantly, days on the regimen is an important setting condition across the first 3 weeks of the daily regimen. There are considerable individual differences in rats' intake of ethanol; some rats take, day after day, large amounts of ethanol whereas others take very little.

As mentioned, at first, a rat takes hardly any alcohol. After about 3 weeks, a rat's intake becomes somewhat stable. A good predictor of what a rat will take on any given day (without any further manipulation) is the mean of what it has taken across the previous few days.

Rats on the daily regimen are alert and active just prior to their daily presentation of fluids. They usually drink some water first. They then groom and may eat. Then, they usually take alcoholic beverage. They then take more water, groom more, eat some, and take more beverage. The intake of beverage for most rats is sufficient to produce behavioral signs of intoxication, for example, an increased amount of time to turn over when placed on their backs.

Even though most of the intake of ethanol solution and water, on the daily regimen, occurs during the 1st half hour, this is too short a period to use to test the effects of certain drugs. Some drugs of interest may increase intakes by prolonging the period during which ethanol is taken. If the session is only 30 min in duration, then the actions of these drugs will not be manifest. This is particularly salient when studying the intake of alcoholic beverages, since alcohol abuse and alcoholism may be characterized by continuing to drink beyond what is ordinary.

This kind of a daily regimen has some features making it potentially useful for assessing the effects of drugs on the intake of ethanol. First, it involves the voluntary ingestion of ethanol in sufficient amounts to clearly produce behavioral effects. The propensity to take alcoholic beverage is, in turn, motivated by a number of setting conditions, thereby making it a robust phenomena. (People's excessive drinking is also probably multidetermined by a variety of kinds of setting conditions.) Second, the concurrent intake of water provides a metric that helps in the interpretation of how a drug affects propensity to take ethanol. If intakes of alcoholic beverage and water are both decreased by a manipulation, then it is possible that the manipulation is debilitating or is merely affecting the propensity to take fluids. If intakes of alcoholic beverage and water are both increased by a manipulation, then it is possible that the manipulation is not specific to alcoholic solutions. Third, as mentioned, the duration of the period of measurement (2 hr) is about the correct length to test most drugs of interest and to not confound the effects of drugs with the after effects of drugs.

In summary, the procedures of the daily regimen involving 22 hr of water deprivation followed by a 2-hr opportunity to take a palatable alcoholic beverage and water has a number of setting conditions that motivate rats to consume considerable amounts of ethanol daily. This voluntary consumption of an alcoholic beverage has some features that make it useful for studying how a drug like morphine might modify intake of ethanol.

Although we are convinced on rational grounds that motivated drinking of an alcoholic beverage (by programming a number of setting conditions) is potentially a reasonable model for studying the psychopharmacology of an essential feature of alcohol abuse and alcoholism (i.e., propensity to drink alcoholic beverages), it has its limitations. A drug, for example, might modify rats' reactivity to the flavoring of the alcoholic beverage rather than rats' reactivity to the ethanol.

Palatability is a factor in the oral intake of any kind of alcoholic beverage. Merely providing ethanol in water as the alcoholic beverage, as some have suggested to control for palatability, does not eliminate palatability as a factor. Initially, ethanol in water is evidently aversive to rats [14,15]. Consequently, such a solution is apt to make palatability highly salient, rather than inconsequential. Adding flavoring is apt to reduce the salience of palatability. It is impossible to eliminate palatability as a factor when studying voluntary oral intake of alcoholic beverages, but it is not impossible to reduce its salience when studying how other variables might affect propensity to take alcoholic beverages.

To see if any particular flavoring used in an alcoholic beverage is critical, it is necessary to use other flavorings and see if the manipulation in question produces similar results. In other words, it takes more than one test to come to the firm conclusion about how a drug affects rats' propensity to take ethanol regardless of the particular kind of alcoholic beverage used initially.

Although we are convinced that our procedures have the potential to be a reasonable model to use for initially assessing the effects of agents on propensity to take ethanol, we do not believe it is the only model that will be useful. Indeed, when results are concordant from a number of procedures, there is more confidence that the manipulation in question is one that is meaningful. Indeed, the ultimate test of a conclusion from any model (or group of models) is whether or not that conclusion is predictive. There have been only limited tests with rats and people of the same psychopharmacological agents, and, therefore, we have only limited information to assess any model. What information is available supports the conclusion that the way a drug affects rats' intakes using the procedures outlined also affects people's intakes similarly.

Prior to recent tests, there had been limited testing of morphine and naloxone's effects on intake of an alcoholic beverages. The results of those initial tests were, indeed, confusing. Large doses of morphine were shown to decrease intake of an alcoholic beverage (ethanol and water provided across a 24-hr period) among rats [16,17]. Doses of naloxone often, but not always, decreased intakes of alcohol. A dose of naltrexone, a longer acting antagonist similar to naloxone, decreased intravenous administration of alcohol by monkeys [18]. Generally, it was shown that both morphine and naloxone decreased intake of alcohol. These agents, since they produce opposite results on opioidergic systems, should produce opposite effects on propensity to take alcoholic beverages, if opioidergic events were specifically related to intake of ethanol, but they did not.

Figure 1 presents a summary of data from a number of experiments and depicts the effect of doses of morphine and naloxone on propensity to take alcoholic beverage when rats were on the daily regimen described above of 2 hr a day to take sweetened alcoholic beverage and water. Small doses of morphine increase intake and large doses tend to decrease intakes. If one looks at the effects of small doses, the conclusion is reached that morphine increases intake of alcohol; but,if one looks at the effects of large doses, the opposite conclusion is reached. Naloxone reduces intakes.

The effects of large doses of morphine on propensity to take alcoholic beverage are due in part to the fact that these doses produce a malaise that is incompatible with drinking. Large doses of morphine also reduce intake of water. When, however, the narcotic effects of large doses are blocked by a partial antagonist (diprenorphine), even large doses tend to increase intakes [19]. Also, relevant to deriving theory concerning how endogenous opioids might affect propensity to take alcoholic beverages, it should be noted that the large doses of morphine that might decrease intakes are so large that it is difficult to imagine how they could be duplicated by the body's own opioidergic systems.

With the initial assessments of a full dose-response relationship, it became clear that morphine could increase intake of alcoholic beverages and that naloxone decreased intakes providing the necessary bipolar effects expected of these compounds. The bipolar effect supports a general conclusion that opioidergic systems can be involved in the control of propensity to take alcoholic beverages.

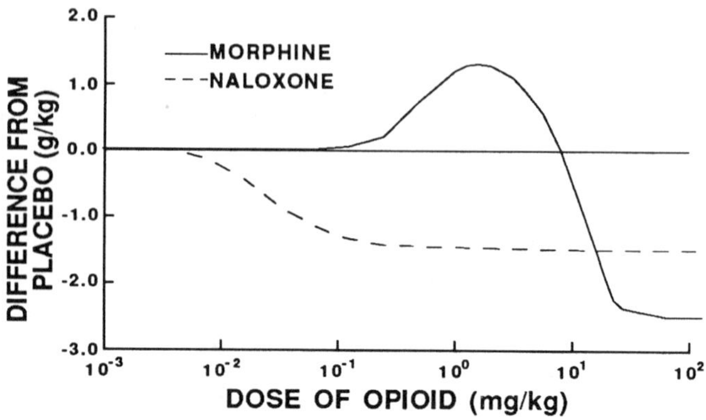

FIGURE 1. A summary of outcomes of giving rats various doses of morphine and naloxone in terms of differences from intake when given placebo. Intake under placebo differed across various groups but generally was about 2.25 g of pure ethanol taken per kg of body weight (g/kg) during a 2-hr test-period.

A number of questions remained concerning the specificity of the small-dose morphine-effect. Were the effects of small doses of morphine limited to the particular procedural arrangements of the initial experiments: For example, do small doses of morphine increase intake only when rats are deprived of nutrients? Only when presented palatable alcoholic beverages? Only when male rats are the subjects? etc.? Experiments were then done to assess the generality of the effect.

In summary, no one or two of the setting conditions (deprivation, kind of beverage, daytime sessions, or days of opportunity to take fluids provided rats are taking some alcoholic beverage) used to elicit moderate to high levels of intake of ethanol is critical. Small doses of morphine increased intakes in every circumstance. Furthermore, other variables such as sex of subjects, their age (excluding very young and very old which have not been tested), or previous history of morphine or naloxone administration did not affect, in any apparent consequential way, the small-dose-morphine-effect. There is one variable that is of consequence. The session cannot be short (say, 30 min) and the effect still be observed. Morphine tends to lengthen the period of taking alcoholic beverage. With a short session, the effect is just not observable. As will be shown subsequently, the session can also be too long.

An interesting feature of these results is that the various setting conditions have additive effects. Rats take more alcoholic beverages with instigation of each setting condition. Small doses of morphine increase intakes with each combination of setting conditions. A small dose of morphine produces an increment in intakes, it does not drive intakes to some maximum.

For the small-dose-morphine-effect to be meaningful to developing theories of alcohol abuse and alcoholism, a number of other conditions must be met. The effect, for example, should not wane, i.e., there should not be tolerance of the effect with respect to increasing intake of alcohol. In brief, there is no diminution of the effect with repeated administrations of morphine [20,21,22]. Furthermore, when rats are fixed with osmotic pumps delivering constant infusion of morphine, their intakes are increased and, even further, an injection of a small dose of morphine in addition to the infused morphine produces an even further increment in intake [20,22].

Rats show tolerance to the analgesic effects of morphine with constant infusion of morphine. It follows, therefore, with the observation that infusions do not diminish the effects of small doses of morphine, that the analgesic actions of morphine are not critical to morphine's ability to increase intakes. In fact, many of morphine's classic effects are not related to its ability to increase intakes, for examples, its ability to produce analgesia, narcosis, or catatonia. This is shown, also, in the data presented in Table 1. Some opioids that do not produce analgesia and, in fact, are antagonists to other opioids' analgesia (and a number of other effects of morphine), increase intakes. Opioids that produce signs of eliciting positive affect are among those that increase intakes.

The opioidergic effect that accounts for increasing intakes of alcoholic beverages is a central neural effect. Very small doses of morphine delivered to the ventricles of the brain also increase intake [24,25]. Opioids that do not cross the blood-brain barrier do not modulate intake of alcoholic beverages [26,27].

TABLE 1

OPIOID (dose range, SC)	Analgesia	Intake
Etonitazene (0.2 to 2.0 microg/kg)	+	+
Fentanyl (20 to 40 microg/kg)	+	+
Morphine (0.5 to 2.5 mg/kg)	0+	+
Morphine (> 10 mg/kg)	+	0-
Morphine-3-B-glucuronide (0.3 to 3.0 mg/kg)	0	0
Morphine-6-B-glucuronide (0.3 to 1.0 mg/kg)	+	+
Methadone (1.0 to 2.0 mg/kg)	+	+
Methadone (> 4.0 mg/kg)	+	-
Ethylketocyclazocine (0.02 to 0.08 mg/kg)	+	0
U 50,488-H (1.0 to 3.0 mg/kg)	+	+
LY 117413 (> 0.1 mg/kg)	0(At)	-
LY 255582 (> 0.01 mg/kg)	0(At)	-
MR 2266 (> 0.15 mg/kg)	0(At)	-
Naloxone (> 1.0 mg/kg)	0(At)	-
(+)-Naloxone (0.1 to 10.0 mg/kg)	0	0
Naltrexone (> 5.0 mg/kg)	0(At)	-
Diprenorphine (25 to 100 microg/kg)	0(At)	+
WIN 44,441-3 (0.03 to 10.0 mg/kg)	0(At)	+

Note: The table is a summary of the effects of various opioids on intake of ethanol and on analgesia. There is no relationship between analgesia and intake. Doses are given SC, about 15 min before a test. Analgesia refers to suppression of a response, say a tail-flick, that usually follows an aversive stimulus, say radiant heat. Intake refers to voluntary ingestion of a sweetened alcoholic beverage across a brief period. In both columns, 0 = no effect. When in the column of Analgesia, + = the opioid produces analgesia. At stands for antagonist, i.e., the opioid antagonizes other opioids' analgesia. When in the column of Intake: + = increase in intake; and - = decrease in intake. Portions of this table are reprinted, with permission, from [23].

As the observations were being made concerning the specificity and generality of the small-dose-morphine-effect, the idea emerged that surfeits of opioidergic activity might be particularly related to the often observed characteristic of alcoholics' inability to maintain control over their drinking, i.e., loss of control [20,28]. The idea is that the equivalent of a small-dose-morphine-effect would potentiate drinking once begun. Such an effect would augment other setting conditions promoting drinking. The net effect of a surfeit of opioidergic activity would be enhanced motivation to take alcoholic beverage once drinking had begun and the apparent inability to stop drinking.

The concept that loss of control involved opioidergic systems of brain can be independent of the idea that ethanol achieves some of its reinforcing effects by way of its action on central opioidergic systems. Although we have evidence that opioidergic effects are related to ethanol's reinforcement [29], ethanol could achieve its reinforcement by way of other neural systems and the resulting activity be augmented in terms of its reinforcing value or be sustained by way of opioidergic systems.

The frequency of drinking and the extent of drinking once begun could both be related to a surfeit in opioidergic activity. Such a surfeit could be a result of ordinary variations seen with nearly all biological systems (a genetic variation) or could be a result of events that could potentiate the activity of these systems. This broad generalization that surfeits could be the product of genetic variation or experience is, however, so broad as to be vacuous and adds little to the basic idea that surfeits of opioidergic activity lead to loss of control. What is needed is more specificity about what potentially relevant variables might lead to surfeits of opioidergic activity which, in turn, might be related to excessive intake of alcoholic beverages.

The concept of loss of control is applicable to the level of drinking seen in an early history of problematic drinking, but is often used to describe the drinking of persons who are clearly alcoholic. Erickson, for example, relates his view of the progression of the problems this way: The potential alcoholic is "... abstinent early in life, then becomes a social drinker, and then an alcohol abuser. An alcohol abuser may drink large amounts of alcohol for a large portion of his/her life, but not be an alcoholic. Then at some point in life, there is a transition to the disease of alcohol addiction or alcoholism, which is characterized by loss of control over alcohol drinking" [30, p. 558]. Erickson goes on to ask what neurochemical systems might be critical to that transition from alcohol abuser to alcoholic, i.e., what system is related to loss of control.

The data from rats showing that small doses of morphine increase intake of alcoholic beverages can be combined with data showing how damage to the liver leads to surfeits of circulating endogenous opioids to produce a hypothesis concerning the dramatic loss of control alluded to by Erickson. The liver, evidently, plays a major role in the enzymatic degradation of blood born opioid peptides. Consequently, individuals with disease of the liver have increased levels of circulating opioids. Since ethanol is clearly a hepatotoxin, the following series of events could occur. Heavy social drinking may impair the liver which, in turn, leads to high levels of circulating peptides. High levels of circulating opioidergic peptides would lead to higher levels of the peptides in the brain. Higher central levels of opioids would promote greater drinking (loss of control) which, in turn, would cause more toxicity of the liver, more circulating opioids, more drinking, more toxicity, and so on. It is evidently well-established that disease of the liver leads to a marked increase in circulating opioids particularly the enkephalins [31,32,33,34] and that these higher levels are manifest in morphine-like effects [31]. Our data strongly supports the idea that increased levels of opioidergic activity would combine with other setting conditions to promote more drinking.

There are surely other events that could lead to increased levels of opioidergic activity in brain. Certain kinds of stress, apparently, can lead to changes in opioidergic activity. The intake of ethanol itself could lead to a variety of events (increased release, modification of receptors, etc.) that would have the net effect of providing an increment in opioidergic activity. Consequently, there are a number of ways in which a surfeit of opioidergic activity could be a setting condition for increased intakes. Relatedly, some of the setting conditions that we use to promote drinking prior to injections of drugs, such as the daily regimen of opportunity to drink, might have opioidergic components [35].

Regardless of whether or not a surfeit of opioidergic activity is a product of inherently high levels of opioids, or a product of peripheral events such as damage to the liver, it seems that a treatment for alcoholism that would suppress the motivation to drink excessively would be a treatment reducing or blocking the effects of opioids. Naltrexone, the longer acting opioid antagonist, would achieve these effects [2]. Figure 2 presents the outcomes of giving doses of naltrexone to rats that are taking alcoholic beverages on the daily regimen described above (2 hr to chose to drink palatable alcoholic beverage daily following water-deprivation). Naltrexone effectively reduces rats' propensity to take alcoholic beverage in a dose-related manner.

The idea that an excess, or surfeit, of opioidergic activity is the critical event that enhances the frequency and extent of intake of alcoholic beverage (or loss of control) is the opposite of most theories [1,2,36,37,38,39,40,41,42,43,44,45] about the relationship between opioids and propensity to drink alcohol. Most theories postulate that alcoholics suffer from a deficit in opioidergic activity and that somehow the intake of ethanol compensates for the deficiency. One example of such a theory is presented in Figure 3.

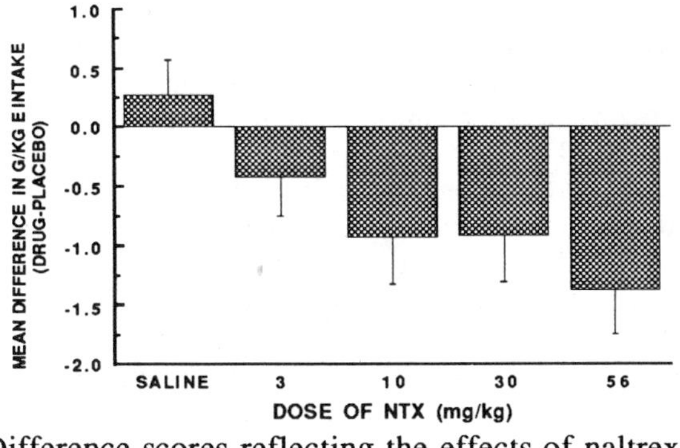

FIGURE 2. Difference scores reflecting the effects of naltrexone on intake of ethanol (E) are depicted. Under placebo, rats drank about 2.5 g/kg. A negative score indicates reduced intake. When intake of alcoholic beverage was decreased, intake of water was increased. Error Bars represent standard errors of the means.

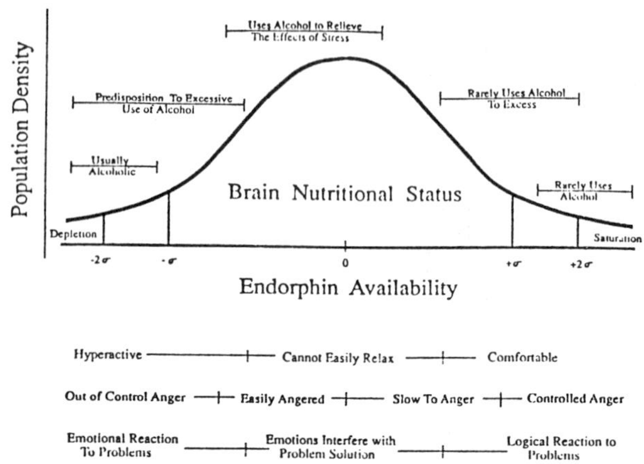

FIGURE 3. The figure summarizes one theory of the putative relationship between level of opioidergic activity and propensity to drink alcoholic beverages. This figure is also an advertisement for the nutritional supplement SAAVE which has an enkephalinase inhibitor that leads to greater enkephalin levels and, hence, from this view a remediation of the cause of excessive drinking. Figure reprinted with the permission of MATRIX Technologies, Inc.

The general idea of a deficit in opioidergic activity as a primary setting condition for alcoholism has even lead some (e.g., [1]) to suggest that methadone is the appropriate treatment for alcoholism. Such an idea follows directly from the premise that alcoholics suffer a deficiency. If they do, then provide a treatment clearly overcoming that deficiency. The same premise leads to the suggestion that blockade of the metabolism of enkephalins, for example with a "nutrient" [38], will overcome the supposed deficit and, therefore, be helpful (if not a cure).

Until we have better ways of measuring basal levels of opioidergic activity and, therefore, deviations from that basal level, how can we test the two opposing ideas about the relationship of levels of opioids to propensity to drink alcoholic beverages? With some simple assumptions, a test is possible. We can assume that (a) a period shortly after an injection of morphine is a period of extraordinarily high levels of opioidergic activity and (b) a period that is subsequent to morphine's metabolism is a period of suppressed endogenous opioidergic activity. The assumption of high opioidergic activity during morphine's presence in the brain is hardly controversial. The assumption of low opioidergic activity, even a deficit in activity, following morphine's actions fits with a considerable body of knowledge concerning the way a system responds to high levels of activity. Negative feedback and opponent processes are common biological processes. Given these assumptions, a test of the two rival hypotheses is possible by giving rats, that are accustomed to voluntarily taking alcohol 2 hr a day, an opportunity to take alcoholic beverage during the period of putative higher and lower levels of opioidergic activity. The relationships are presented in Figure 4.

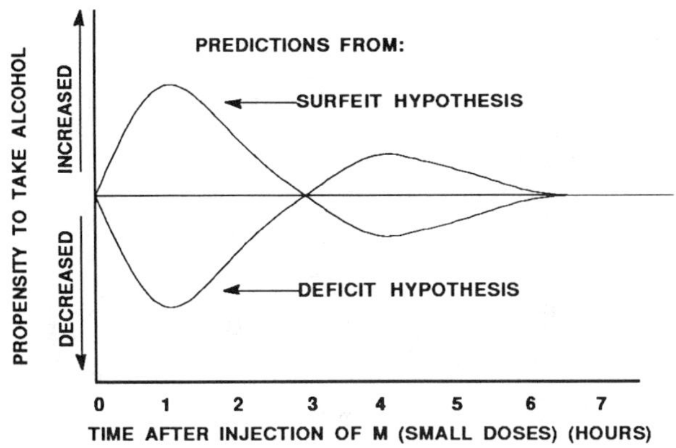

FIGURE 4. Predictions made by the two hypotheses concerning the level of opioidergic activity and propensity to take alcoholic beverage. The predictions are in terms of a change from a baseline level of drinking. The time immediately after a dose of morphine (M) is a time of high levels of opioidergic activity whereas the time after morphine is metabolized is a period of low levels of activity (about 3 to 6 hr after injections).

Figures 5 and 6 presents the outcomes of tests described in Figure 4 and the accompanying text. The test was made, as outlined, with morphine as well as with naloxone. When morphine was given 4.0 hr before the session during which an alcoholic beverage was presented, a period of reduced levels of opioidergic activity, intakes were actually decreased compared to baseline. The observed effects are concordant with the idea that surfeits in opioidergic activity lead to extraordinarily high levels of intake and that periods of supposed deficits in opioidergic activity (when naloxone is in the brain and after morphine has been metabolized) actually lead to lower levels of intakes.

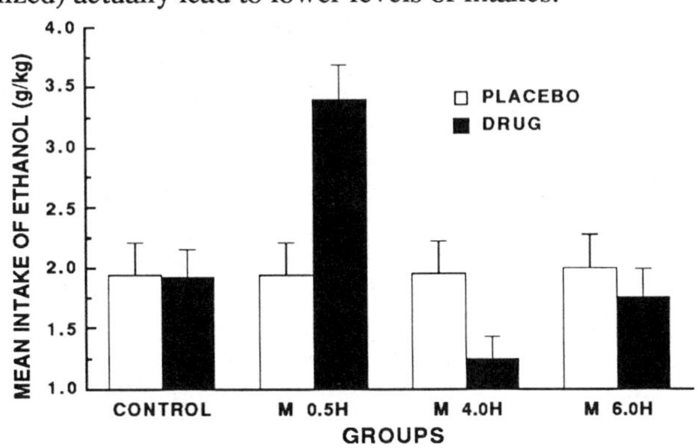

FIGURE 5. The effects of giving placebo or morphine, 2 mg/kg subcutaneously, at various times prior to a 2-hr opportunity to drink a sweetened alcoholic beverage are depicted. The group designated M 0.5H, for example, got morphine 0.5 hr before the session. The group designated "control" got carrier of morphine on both days. Error bars represent standard errors of the means.

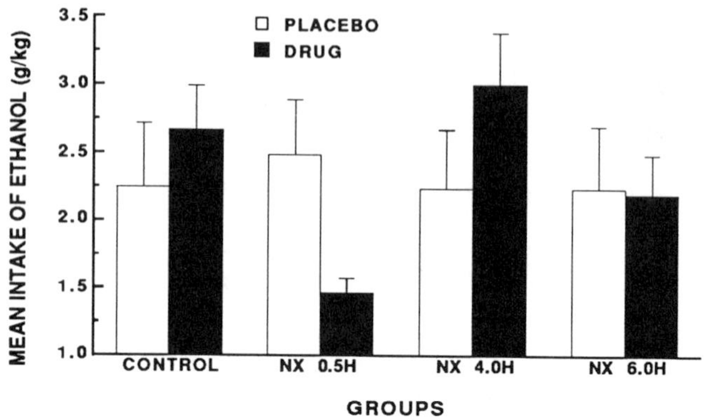

FIGURE 6. The effects of giving placebo or naloxone, 4 mg/kg subcutaneously, at various times prior to a 2-hr opportunity to drink a sweetened alcoholic beverage are depicted. The group designated NX 0.5H, for example, got naloxone 0.5 hr before the session. Error bars represent standard errors of the means.

Aside from an inherently high level of opioidergic activity, there are a number of possible ways that an extraordinarily high level of opioidergic activity might occur among people. Stress is known to increase levels of opioids [46]. Damage to the liver will increase levels [30]. Also, some property of ethanol itself, by a number of means [20], could increase levels.

Erickson [30, p. 558] in his commentary about the neurochemistry of compulsive loss of control, and relating the extant literature, indicated that " a deficiency of endorphins" is one of the "defects" or "dysfunctions" that is possibly related to loss of control. It seems that this traditional view of the putative relationship between endogenous opioidergic processes and propensity to take alcoholic beverage needs to be modified. It is not a deficiency of opioidergic activity that potentiates drinking, but a surfeit (excess). There are a number of implications to this new theory.

One of the clearest implications is that any treatment that might lead to an increase in levels of opioidergic activity, particularly those that might be the equivalent of a small dose of morphine in rats, is a treatment that will tend to exacerbate alcohol abuse and alcoholism. There are two current situations, involving people, that might fit the circumstance of being similar to small doses of morphine in rats: (a) the situation in which methadone is used to treat heroin addicts and when it is systematically reduced across a period of days (eventually a small dose is administered) [47], and (b) the situation recommended by Matrix Technologies in which the advice is for persons being treated for alcoholism to take a nutritional "supplement" that blocks the breakdown of opioids (an enkephalinase inhibitor) [38].

If as Erickson theorizes that there is an abrupt transition from alcohol abuse to alcoholism characterized by extremes of "loss of control" [30], if these people have damage to their liver that results in increased enkephalin levels [31], and if the neurochemical basis of "loss of control" is a surfeit in opioidergic activity [20], then we have available a treatment that should remediate part of the problem. Individuals suffering from loss of control can be treated with naltrexone. This will block the effects of surfeits in opioidergic activity resulting from the liver's inability to metabolize opioid peptides which, in turn, should lead to less extensive drinking. With less drinking, hopefully, the condition of the liver will return to a more normal state thereby obviating the necessity to continue to take naltrexone. Indeed, in the first controlled trials of naltrexone as a treatment for alcoholism [2], the signs of damage to the liver common to alcoholics did improve. Naltrexone is not the only longer acting opioid antagonist. Other antagonists might accomplish the same effects with respect to intake of alcoholic beverages, but be safer [23]. In general, the new way to think about opioids and alcoholism leads to the optimistic prediction that the prescription of opioid antagonists will be very helpful to many alcoholics.

REFERENCES

1. Siegel, S. In: Cappell, H.D., Glaser, F.B., Israel, Y., Kalant, H., Schmidt, W., Sellers, E.M., & Smart, R.G. (Eds.), Research Advances in Alcohol and Drug Problems 9:279-314; 1986.
2. Volpicelli, J.R., et al. In: Reid, L.D. (Ed.), Opioids, Bulimia, and Alcohol Abuse & Alcoholism. New York: Springer-Verlag, pp. 195-214, 1990.
3. Reid, L.D. (Ed.). Opioids, Bulimia, and Alcohol Abuse & Alcoholism. New York: Springer-Verlag. 1990.
4. Unterwald, E.M., & Zukin, R.S. In: Reid, L.D. (Ed.), Opioids, Bulimia, and Alcohol Abuse & Alcoholism. New York: Springer-Verlag, pp. 49-72, 1990.
5. Cooper, S.J., & Kirkham, T.C. In: Reid, L.D. (Ed.), Opioids, Bulimia, and Alcohol Abuse & Alcoholism. New York: Springer-Verlag, pp. 91-110, 1990.
6. Goldstein, A. In: Lipton, M.A., Dimascio, A., & Killam, K.F. (Eds.), Psychopharmacology: A Generation of Progress. New York: Raven Press, pp. 1557-1563, 1978.
7. Reid, L.D. American Psychologist 24:956-958; 1969.
8. Majchrowicz, E. Psychopharmacoligia 45:245-254; 1975.
9. Reid, L.D. In Bozarth, M.A. (Ed.), Methods of Assessing the Reinforcing Properties of Abused Drugs. New York: Springer-Verlag, pp. 391-440, 1987.
10. Carlton, P.L. A Primer of Behavioral Pharmacology. New York: W.H. Freeman and Company, 1983.
11. Mook, D.G. American Psychologist 38:379-387; 1983.
12. Czirr, S.A., et al. Alcohol 4:117-120; 1987.
13. Choi, H.W., et al. Alcohol 7:7-10; 1990.
14. Kiefer, S.W., & Dopp, J.M. Behavioral Neuroscience 103:1318-1326; 1989.
15. Kiefer, S.W., et al. Alcohol 7:115-120; 1990.
16. Sinclair, J.D. Pharmacology Biochemistry & Behavior 2:409-412; 1974.
17. Sinclair, J.D., et al. Nature 246:425-427; 1973.
18. Altshuler, H.L., et al. Life Sciences 26:679-688; 1980.
19. Reid, L.D., et al. Alcohol 4:161-168; 1987.
20. Hubbell, C.L., & Reid, L.D. In: Reid, L.D. (Ed.), Opioids, Bulimia, and Alcohol Abuse & Alcoholism. New York: Springer-Verlag, pp. 145-174, 1990.

21. Hubbell, C.L., et al. Alcohol 4:149-156; 1987.
22. Hubbell, C.L., et al. Alcohol 5:141-146; 1988.
23. Reid, L.D. In: Reid, L.D. (Ed.), Opioids, Bulimia, and Alcohol Abuse & Alcoholism. New York: Springer-Verlag, pp. 275-280, 1990.
24. Lineseman, M.A., & Harding, S. Pharmacology Biochemistry & Behavior 36:405-408; 1990.
25. Wild, K.D. & Reid, L.D. Life Sciences 47:PL49-PL54; 1990.
26. Hubbell, C.L., et al. Alcohol 3:39-54; 1986.
27. Linesman, M.A. Pharmacology Biochemistry & Behavior 33:407-413; 1989.
28. Beaman, C.M., et al. Alcohol 1:39-42; 1984.
29. Marglin, S.H., & Reid, L.D. In: Reid, L.D. (Ed.), Opioids, Bulimia, and Alcohol Abuse & Alcoholism. New York: Springer-Verlag, pp. 145-191, 1990.
30. Erickson, C.K. Alcohol 7:557-558; 1990.
31. Jones, E.A., & Bergasa, N.V. Hepatology 11:884-887; 1990.
32. Thornton, J.R., et al. Gut 29:1167-1172; 1988.
33. Thornton, J.R., & Losowsky, M.S. British Medical Journal 297:1501-1504; 1988.
34. Thornton, J.R., & Losowsky, M.S. British Medical Journal 297:1241-1242; 1988.
35. Przewlocki, R., et al. Science 219:71-73; 1983.
36. Blum, K., et al. In: Rigter, H., & Crabbe, J.C. (Eds.), Alcohol Tolerance and Dependence. New York: Elsevier Biomedical Press, pp. 371-391, 1980.
37. Blum, K., et al. Alcohol 4:449-456; 1987.
38. Blum, K., et al. Alcohol 5:481-493; 1989.
39. Blum, K., et al. Journal of the American Medical Association 362:2055-2060; 1990.
40. Davis, V.E., & Walsh, M.J. Science 167:1005-1007; 1970.
41. Gianoulakis, C. In: Reid, L.D. (Ed.), Opioids, Bulimia, and Alcohol Abuse & Alcoholism. New York: Springer-Verlag, pp. 229-246, 1990.
42. Myers, R.D., & Melchior, C.L. Science 196:554-556; 1977.
43. Trachtenberg, M.C., & Blum, K. American Journal of Drug and Alcohol Abuse 13:365-372; 1987.
44. Volpicelli, J.R. British Journal of Addiction 82:381-392; 1987.
45. Volpicelli, J.R., et al. In: Reid, L.D. (Ed.), Opioids, Bulimia, and Alcohol Abuse & Alcoholism. New York: Springer-Verlag, pp. 195-214, 1990.
46. Akil, H., et al. In: Kosterlitz, K. (Ed.), Opiates and Endogenous Opiate Peptides. Amsterdam: Elsevier/North Holland Biomedical Press, 1976.
47. Mudar, P.J., et al. Alcohol 3:303-308; 1986.

ACKNOWLEDGEMENTS

This work was supported, in part, by a grant from NIDA (DA04440). We thank Edward J. Bilsky for his help in preparing this manuscript, and for collecting the data associated with Figure 2.

11
The Enkephalinergic System and Maintenance of Ethanol Drinking

J.C. Froelich and T.-K. Li

Many behavioral and physiological effects of opiates and ethanol are very similar including induction of euphoria, sedation, acquisition of tolerance and development of physical dependence (1). These similarities have led to the hypothesis that the reinforcing properties of ethanol may be due, in part, to an interaction between ethanol and the endogenous opioid system. Specifically, consumption of ethanol may stimulate increased activity in the opioid system which, in turn, leads to further ethanol drinking. If this hypothesis is correct, antagonists which block the action of endogenous opioids might be expected to decrease ethanol intake. Rats of the alcohol-preferring (P) and high alcohol drinking (HAD) lines, which have been genetically selected for oral ethanol preference, were used to determine whether activation of the endogenous opioid system is important for the maintenance of ethanol drinking. Initial experiments explored the effects of nonspecific opioid receptor antagonists, such as naloxone and naltrexone on ethanol drinking. Naloxone, in doses of 0.075-18.0 mg/kg, significantly suppressed ethanol drinking in a dose-dependent manner without altering water intake in rats of the HAD line when ethanol and water were presented concurrently (2,3). These results suggest that the stimulation of the endogenous opioid system and occupation of opioid receptors may be necessary for the maintenance of ethanol drinking.

In order to begin identifying the specific opioid receptor subtypes which may be important in mediating ethanol drinking, selective mu and delta opioid receptor antagonists were tested for their efficacy in reducing ethanol intake in rats of the P and HAD lines. The selective mu receptor antagonist, B-funaltrexamine (B-FNA), did not alter either ethanol or water intake in rats of the P line (4). In contrast, specific delta opioid receptor antagonists (ICI 174864 and naltrindole hydrochloride or NTI), were found to be very potent in suppressing voluntary ethanol drinking in a dose-dependent manner without significantly altering water intake in rats of the P and HAD lines (4,5). For instance, ICI 174864, in doses of 3.0, 5.0, and 8.0 mg/kg BW, suppressed ethanol consumption by 24.7%, 39.7% and 77.6%, respectively, without altering water intake. Given that the endogenous ligands with the highest affinity for delta opioid receptors are enkephalins (6,7,8), the results indicate that activation of the endogenous enkephalinergic system, and occupation of delta opioid receptors, may be important for maintaining ethanol drinking. This conclusion is supported by our recent findings that prolonging the duration of action of endogenous enkephalins, by blocking enkephalin degradation, produces a significant increase in ethanol consumption (5).

We have recently begun to explore whether a genetic predisposition toward ethanol drinking is accompanied by increased activity in the central enkephalinergic system. We have compared Met-enkephalin content in the hypothalamus and striatum of rats which have been genetically selected for high (alcohol-preferring or P) or low (alcohol-nonpreferring or NP) ethanol preference. The results indicate a trend toward higher Met-enkephalin levels in the hypothalamus, anterior striatum and posterior striatum of rats from the P line compared with the NP line, which may indicate that a genetic predisposition toward voluntary ethanol drinking is associated with increased activity in the central enkephalinergic system (2). However, tissue levels of a peptide reflect the sum of four processes: synthesis, processing, release and degradation. A more accurate assessment of central enkephalinergic activity will be achieved by simultaneous measurement of genetic message for enkephalin synthesis together with post-translational product formation. Hence, future experiments will include measurements of preproenkephalin mRNA and enkephalin content in discrete brain regions of rats that differ in their genetic predisposition toward ethanol drinking.

REFERENCES

1. Kalant, H. (1977) Comparative aspects of tolerance to, and dependence on, alcohol, barbiturates and opiates. Adv. Exp. Med. Biol. 85:169-186.
2. Froehlich, J.C., Harts, J., Lumeng, L. and Li, T.K. (1987) Naloxone attenuation of voluntary alcohol consumption. Alcohol and Alcoholism, Suppl. 1:333-337.
3. Froehlich, J.C., Harts, J., Lumeng, L. and Li, T.K. (1990) Naloxone attenuates ethanol intake in rats selectively bred for high ethanol preference. Pharmacology, Biochemistry and Behaviour 35:385-390.
4. Froehlich, J.C., Zweifel, M., Kurtz, D. and Li, T.K. (1990) Opioid antagonists selectively suppress ethanol intake. Alcoholism: Clinical and Experimental Research 14:289.
5. Froehlich, J.C., Harts, J., Zweifel, M., Lumeng, L. and Li, T.K. (1990) Importance of delta opioid receptors in maintaining high alcohol drinking. Psychopharmacology, in Press.
6. Chang, K.J., Cooper, B.R., Hazum, E. and Cuatrecasas, P. (1979) Multiple opiate receptors: Different regional distribution in the brain and differential binding of opiates and opioid peptides. Molecular Pharmacology 16:91-104.
7. Snyder, S.H. and Goodman, R.R. (1980) Multiple neurotransmitter receptors. Journal of Neurochemistry 35:5-15.
8. Chang, K.J. and Cuatrecasas, P. (1981) Heterogeneity and properties of opiate receptors. Federation Proceedings 40:2729-2734.

12

The Relationship of Alcohol Drinking and Endogenous Opioids: The Opioid Compensation Hypothesis

B.J. Berg, J.R. Volpicelli, A.I. Alterman, and C.P. O'Brien

INTRODUCTION

Alcohol has been used and abused by man as long as recorded history. As much as we know about how alcohol affects various organs and body systems to exert its acute and chronic effects, we are still a long way from understanding why it is that some people can drink alcohol without losing control while others cannot.

There are a variety of etiological mechanisms that culminate in alcohol dependence and any comprehensive model for understanding alcoholism needs to consider the multifactorial nature of the disorder. Without question, genetic, cultural, environmental, and psychological forces all play a major role in determining whether a particular individual will develop the syndrome of alcohol dependence. This chapter focuses on the relationship between alcohol drinking and endogenous opioid activity, one important biological factor in the biopsychosocial understanding of alcohol dependence.

This chapter presents evidence to support the hypothesis that some people are predisposed to alcoholism because of a genetic or environmentally induced deficiency in opiate receptor activity. The basic tenet of the Opioid Compensation Hypothesis is that alcohol drinking stimulates opiate receptor activity and it is the increase in opiate receptor activity that reinforces alcohol drinking and leads to alcohol dependence. This theory suggests that: (1) alcohol drinking is influenced by the level of opiate receptor activity; (2) alcohol can compensate for a relative deficiency of opiate receptor activity; and (3) alcohol drinking can be reduced by blocking alcohol's stimulation of opiate receptors.

ALCOHOL DRINKING AND OPIATE AGONISTS

The starting point for considering the Opioid Compensation Hypothesis is to show that alcohol consumption is related to alcohol's effects on opiate receptors. If the reinforcing properties of alcohol are related to its ability to stimulate opiate receptors, then one would predict that deficiencies of opiate receptor activity might be associated with a greater propensity to drink alcohol and that excessive levels of opioidergic activity might suppress alcohol drinking (Volpicelli, 1987).

In a recent study we found that morphine produced a dose dependent decrease in alcohol preference (Volpicelli & Ulm, 1991). Rats given free access to food, water, and five percent alcohol were randomized to receive subcutaneous injections of saline or two different dose levels of morphine sulfate. In comparison to the saline treated rats, rats treated with high doses of morphine (10 mg/kg) had a 60 percent reduction in alcohol self-administration during the last four days of morphine administration, while rats treated with low doses (2.5 mg/kg) had approximately a 20 percent reduction in alcohol consumption (See Figure 1). The doses of morphine used in this study did not affect general activity and had only modest effects in reducing total fluid consumption and body weight relative to the saline injected rats. Ho and Chen, using morphine injections of 10, 30, and 60 mg/kg, also derived a dose response curve that demonstrated an inverse relationship between alcohol preference and opiate receptor activity (Ho & Chen, 1975).

During the post-morphine or opiate withdrawal phase, when opiate receptor activity is presumed to be deficient, investigators have uniformly found that rats increase alcohol preference relative to placebo treated rats (Ho & Chen, 1975; Volpicelli & Ulm, 1991). In our study, a dramatic increase in alcohol preference occurred in the morphine treated rats when the injections were discontinued, whereas alcohol preference remained constant in the saline treated rats (Figure 1). The low dose morphine group drank nearly twice as much alcohol as the saline-injected subjects over the last three trials. Although the high dose morphine group had very low levels of alcohol preference initially, once injections stopped, their alcohol preference progressively increased until it approximated the alcohol preference of the low dose group. In summary, these results support an interaction between alcohol drinking and opiate receptor activity.

Studies in humans also show an inverse relationship between opiate use and alcohol drinking. Confirmed opiate addicts, when administered a regular, stable dose of methadone, show a reliable decrease in their alcohol consumption (Siegel, 1986). Similarly, narcotic abusers regularly increase their alcohol consumption when they do not have a stable opiate supply. In fact, the pharmacological cross-tolerance between alcohol and opiates was recognized in the 19th century when it was common to prescribe opiates for the treatment of alcohol dependence and vice versa (Siegel, 1986). In such cases, the alcoholic typically found that opiates not only relieved the symptoms of alcohol withdrawal but also reduced their proclivity to drink excessively. At that point, many alcoholics were converted into opiate addicts. Although the hazards of opiate dependence were not unrecognized in the 19th century, it was the near unanimous opinion of physicians of that era (and perhaps now as well) that if a choice of evils were to be made, opiate dependence seems "by far the lesser" (Black, 1889).

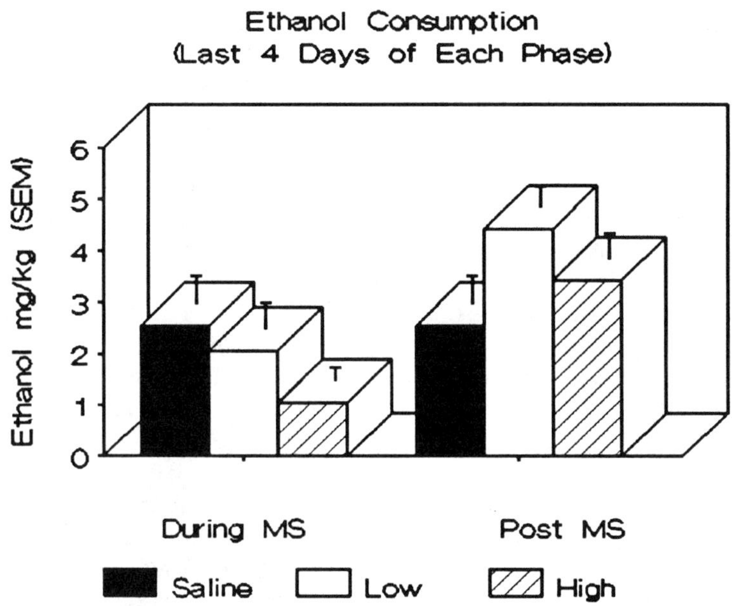

Figure 1. Mean ethanol consumption in rats during the last four days (out of eight) during and following daily injections of saline and two dose levels of morphine sulfate (low dose = 2.5 mg/kg; high dose = 10 mg/kg).

While these data clearly support a relationship between alcohol drinking and opiate receptor activity, it is not clear how alcohol might interact with opiate receptors. In contrast to opiates, alcohol does not seem to have specific agonist effects in stimulating opiate receptors directly. Rather, it is believed that alcohol has nonspecific effects on the lipid components of cellular membranes such that alcohol influences the activity of membrane-bound proteins (enzymes, receptors) which may cause the release of certain hormones and neurotransmitters contained within the cell (Eskelson, Hameroff & Kanel, 1980). In fact, it has been determined that acute alcohol administration can stimulate the release of glucocorticoids such as ACTH in both rats and humans (Bellet, Roman, Delastro & Herra, 1970; Ellis, 1966). This finding, combined with the fact that both ACTH and beta-endorphin are derived from a common precursor (proopiomelanocortin) (Epper & Mains, 1978), lends support to the theory that alcohol stimulates the release of beta-endorphin which may then account for some of the reinforcing effects of alcohol drinking. This is not to imply that alcohol's effects on the endogenous opioid system are its only effects or that the reinforcing properties of alcohol are only mediated through opiate receptors. However, the interaction between alcohol and the endogenous opioid system seems important enough that changes in opioid system activity can significantly influence alcohol drinking.

OPIATE ANTAGONISTS DECREASE ALCOHOL DRINKING

If drinking alcohol increases opiate receptor activity, then opiate antagonists should block the reinforcing effects of alcohol and thus lead to reduced alcohol use over time. This prediction is supported by several animal studies that show that alcohol consumption decreases when opiate receptors are blocked by opiate antagonists (Ho & Chen, 1975; Reid & Hunter, 1984; Hubbell, Czirr, Hunter, et al., 1986). Monkeys barpressing for IV alcohol decreased their barpress responses by 50 percent when they were administered naltrexone at a dose of 20 mg/kg (Altshuler, Phillips & Feinhandler, 1980). Furthermore, it has been found that opiate antagonists block many of the effects of alcohol and that they increase the lethal dose (LD_{50}) of alcohol approximately twofold (Ho & Ho, 1979).

The use of opiate antagonists to decrease alcohol drinking in humans is being investigated at the Philadelphia Veterans Affairs Medical Center in male subjects who meet DSM-III-R criteria for alcohol dependence. Subjects enter detoxification and then are randomized to receive either naltrexone (50 mg/day) or placebo for 12 weeks as an adjunct to outpatient rehabilitation. Each subject is followed weekly to assess the amount and frequency of any alcohol use in the preceding week. Subject's self report of alcohol use is compared with the results of breathalyzer readings and urine drug screens. Liver enzyme levels are assessed monthly as an additional objective measure used to detect alcohol use. In addition, each subject is asked to complete a self-administered scale of craving for alcohol at each visit.

In this double-blind, placebo-controlled study, relapse to drinking is arbitrarily distinguished from a "slip" by a subject's report of drinking five or more days within one week, by having five or more drinks in a day, or by a blood alcohol concentration greater than 100 mg/percent. Theoretically, naltrexone might not prevent subjects from craving or sampling alcohol. Once subjects sample alcohol, however, they would discover that alcohol is no longer reinforcing. This should reduce subsequent alcohol drinking.

Preliminary results, compiled thus far on the first 30 subjects, indicate that naltrexone was, as expected, only marginally effective in preventing sampling of alcohol (Volpicelli, O'Brien, Alterman, and Hayashida, 1990). Alcohol sampling occured in 36% (5 of 14) of naltrexone subjects during the 12 week study period, in comparison to 75% (12 of 16) of placebo subjects. More importantly, naltrexone treatment significantly reduced the mean number of days per week in which alcohol was sampled, 0.07 days per week for the naltrexone group as compared to 0.81 days per week for the placebo group. This difference is statistically significant when controlling for baseline drinking days.

Relapse rates for the entire sample showed a dramatic effect in favor of naltrexone treatment. An impressive 93% (13 of 14) of all naltrexone treated subjects were able to remain sober or retain control over their drinking such that they did not meet the criteria for relapse by the end of the 12 week study. In contrast, only 37% (6 of 16) of placebo treated subjects were able to maintain control over their drinking. A relapse rate of 63% within the first 12 weeks of outpatient treatment is not unusual, according to other reports of relapse rates (Miller & Hester, 1986; Nathan, 1986). In contrast, a relapse rate of only 7% is considered excellent, particularly in a V.A. population. Subjects taking placebo who sampled alcohol nearly always went on to lose control over their drinking and relapse (83% or 10 of 12 subjects), whereas only 20% (1 of 5) of naltrexone subjects who sampled alcohol went on to meet the criteria for relapse. The finding that relapse did not generally occur among naltrexone subjects and that sampling of alcohol did not invariably lead to relapse in the naltrexone group as it did in the placebo group suggests that naltrexone may indeed be effective in blocking the reinforcing effects of drinking alcohol.

Further support for this interpretation was found when craving was examined. Using a subjective rating scale for craving and controlling for baseline scores, craving was found to be significantly lower in the naltrexone group (as a whole) than in the placebo group (as a whole). Among naltrexone-treated subjects who sampled alcohol, craving was comparable to those subjects who did not sample alcohol, whereas craving was significantly higher in the subgroup of placebo subjects who sampled alcohol. The effects of naltrexone on craving seem similar to the effects of naltrexone on drinking and these effects are perhaps most dramatic in subjects who have a slip from abstinence.

In summary, these results suggest that naltrexone may be an effective adjunct in the treatment of alcohol dependence. In our preliminary study, naltrexone appeared to decrease craving, mean days of drinking, and relapse rates. It seemed to be particularly effective in preventing loss of control over drinking after a slip from abstinence. The efficacy of naltrexone in preventing relapse, particularly among alcoholics who have a slip, is supported by the preliminary results of a similar study conducted by O'Malley and colleagues at Yale University (personal communication; preliminary results presented at the ISBRA '90 Satellite Symposium in Toronto, Ontario, Canada, June 1990). The results of both these studies lend further support to the hypothesis that the reinforcing effects of alcohol are mediated to a significant degree through the opioid system.

The findings presented above could be interpreted to be antithetical to the previously stated theory. If the efficacy of naltrexone was due to blockade of the opiate receptor and concomitantly the reinforcing effects of alcohol, how can one explain the finding that naltrexone may have been effective in reducing craving and, if anything, may have reduced the incidence of "slips"? If naltrexone were to have any effect, it might be expected to increase craving and increase the incidence of slips because of its effects in blocking endogenous opioid activity. One could postulate that alcoholics might try to override the effects of naltrexone by drinking larger quantities of alcohol. It was pointed out earlier that when opioid receptor activity is low, alcohol drinking generally increases.

Since our study only included people who met DSM-III-R criteria for alcohol dependence, one can postulate that these individuals had low endogenous opioid activity at baseline and so the additional antagonism provided by naltrexone had little effect in increasing craving. It has been shown that human alcoholics have decreased levels of central beta-endorphin during early alcohol withdrawal (Genazzani, Nappi, Eacchinetti, et al., 1982). This suppression of endorphin levels may reflect an effect of alcohol (in depleting or reducing production of endogenous opioids) or may reflect a genetic predisposition to have lower levels of endogenous opioid system activity.

DIFFERENTIAL OPIOID RESPONSES TO ALCOHOL DRINKING IN INDIVIDUALS GENETICALLY PREDISPOSED TO ALCOHOLISM

Are some individuals predisposed to alcoholism because of an enhanced opioid system response to alcohol drinking? Studies of alcoholics which have examined measures of opioid system activity have not been able to determine whether significant deviations from normal are due to an underlying predisposition or are the result of the alcohol abuse itself. One approach is to study beta-endorphin levels in non-alcoholic individuals from families with a strong history of alcoholism and compare them with non-alcoholic individuals who do not have a family history for alcoholism (Gianoulakis, Angelogianni, Meaney, et al., 1990). Gianoulakis and colleagues took a three generational family history and divided subjects into either a high risk (HR) or low risk (LR) group based upon whether the family history was strongly positive or strongly negative for alcoholism. Gianoulakis also considered a third group of known alcoholics who had been abstinent and matched these subjects in age and sex with the nonalcoholic HR and LR subjects. Gianoulakis' research produced several significant findings. First, it provided evidence that there are physiological differences which might explain the finding that family members of identified alcoholics are at increased risk of developing alcoholism themselves. Mean baseline plasma levels of immunoreactive beta-endorphin were significantly lower in both the HR and the abstinent alcoholic groups in comparison to the LR subjects. Thus, non-alcoholic individuals with genetic loading for alcoholism as well as abstinent alcoholic subjects were potentially endorphin deficient during basal non-stress, non-drug conditions in comparison to individuals who were not alcoholic and who did not have such genetic loading. Second, the HR and the LR groups differed significantly in their plasma levels of immunoreactive beta-endorphin when such levels were measured for 120 minutes after intake of alcohol (0.5 g/kg) (for ethical reasons, the abstinent alcoholic subjects received placebo but not alcohol). Forty minutes after the administration of alcohol, the HR subjects had a marked *increase* (nearly two-fold) in their plasma beta-endorphin level whereas the LR group exhibited a small *decrease* in their beta-endorphin level, which continued to decline over time. Interestingly, the absolute value of plasma beta-endorphin levels rose in the HR subjects following administration of alcohol to a level close to, but not exceeding, the plasma levels of the LR subjects.

One has to be careful in interpreting Gianoulakis' findings however because of the fact that she measured *plasma* levels of beta-endorphin and such levels may not accurately reflect *central* endorphin activity. Nevertheless, her data provide compelling evidence that alcohol does have effects on individuals who are genetically predisposed to the development of alcoholism that are different from its effects on individuals who are not predisposed. Furthermore, it provides direct evidence that alcohol does in fact increase beta-endorphin levels, at least peripherally, in non-alcoholic subjects with genetic loading for alcoholism. Prior to this study, only indirect evidence existed that alcohol could boost endorphin levels. Studies of alcoholic subjects which have measured beta-endorphin levels in specific areas of the central nervous system have found increased beta-endorphin levels following acute administration of alcohol (2.5 g/kg) and a reduction in beta-endorphin levels following chronic alcohol consumption (Schulz, Wister, Duka & Herz, 1980). However, such studies have not been able to determine whether such findings are a cause of, or a result of, the chronic abuse of alcohol.

Gianoulakis' findings show that there are physiological differences between the high and low risk subjects which are not the result of the abuse of alcohol and which can explain the positively reinforcing effects of alcohol on some people while not on others. It provides evidence that alcohol may act differentially on individuals with high familial risk for the development of alcoholism by pharmacologically stimulating their opiate receptors. In comparison to the low risk subjects, high risk subjects were found to have significant differences in both their baseline beta-endorphin levels and their response to alcohol such that endorphin levels were temporarily increased by drinking. This provides a mechanism for explaining how naltrexone might reduce craving for alcohol, reduce use of alcohol, and block the reinforcing effects of alcohol such that rates of relapse are reduced.

ALCOHOL DRINKING AND ENVIRONMENTAL STRESS

There is another possible mechanism by which naltrexone might reduce craving and sampling of alcohol. Just as opiate receptor stimulation by exogenous opiates leads to compensatory changes such that discontinuation of the opiates produces craving and a characteristic withdrawal syndrome, there is the potential for endogenous opioids to produce similar compensatory changes and craving upon withdrawal. In essence, one can perhaps become "dependent" on an increased level of one's own endogenous opioids. Animal research supports this phenomena in that signs of opiate withdrawal can be observed after opioid release is stimulated by uncontrollable aversive stimuli (Volpicelli & Ulm, 1990). In addition, recent studies of post-traumatic stress disorder have suggested that such symptoms as increased arousal and autonomic instability may be the result of an endogenous opioid withdrawal syndrome after endogenous opioids are released during the re-experiencing of the trauma (Kolk, Greenberg & Boyd, 1985). Therefore, if stress-induced opioid release is blocked by an opiate antagonist, then the post-stress (relative) opioid depletion and the craving associated with this depletion might also be blocked. In this way, naltrexone could prevent or attenuate the urge to drink following a stressful life event.

An assumption underlying the alcohol-endogenous opioid theory presented here is that the strongest desire to drink occurs after, rather than during, a stress. This idea runs counter to the tension reduction hypothesis for alcohol dependence which holds that alcohol is used during times of stress because of its efficacy in reducing tension. In actuality, alcohol's effects in relieving subjective, behavioral and physiological indices of tension have been shown to be inconsistent and quite variable (Volpicelli, 1987). Consideration of the times when humans are most likely to drink - at the end of the workday or workweek, on vacation and during times of leisure, and after a crisis or important life event - supports the notion that individuals increase alcohol drinking upon relief from a stress and not during the actual stress. One can test this hypothesis by returning to the animal laboratory. We have in fact done this and have data to show that it is not that alcohol reduces tension but rather tension reduction that elicits alcohol drinking. Rats exposed to 4 days of inescapable shock did not show an increase in alcohol consumption until after the shock was discontinued (Volpicelli, Ulm & Hopson, 1990). When naltrexone was administered following the shock stimulus, it proved to be effective in blocking the increase in alcohol consumption which was observed among placebo treated rats (Volpicelli, Davis & Olgin, 1986).

IMPLICATIONS FOR TREATMENT

If reinforcement of alcohol drinking is mediated in part by the endogenous opioid system, this opens the way for new potential treatment approaches. The data presented provide evidence that opiate antagonists might have clinical utility in reducing not only the high relapse rates that often occur early in treatment, but also in reducing the quantity of alcohol consumed. Thus, naltrexone may be effective in breaking the vicious cycle whereby the first drink leads to a heightened desire for further alcohol consumption. While we certainly do not want to suggest that naltrexone could allow an alcohol dependent individual to drink socially, the evidence presented here does suggest that treatment with naltrexone can give patients a "second chance" after a slip from abstinence. Since outcome studies have shown that approximately one-half of alcohol dependent individuals relapse to drinking and terminate treatment within three months of completing an intensive inpatient or residential treatment program (Miller & Hester, 1986; Nathan, 1986), the availability of a pharmacological agent which is efficacious in reducing craving, quantity of alcohol imbibed, and relapse rates would represent an important advance in the treatment of alcohol dependence.

SUMMARY

Our consideration of the Opioid Compensation Hypothesis began with a review of the data which demonstrate that alcohol does interact with the endogenous opioid system. Gianoulakis' study provides evidence suggesting that there are differences between persons genetically predisposed to develop alcoholism and persons not predisposed in their baseline beta-endorphin levels. Her study also provides evidence that alcohol affects individuals with a genetic predisposition for alcoholism differently from those without such a predisposition. We have also presented a set of experimentally derived hypotheses which tie together the differences found between alcoholics and non-alcoholics and the different patterns of drinking behavior which are observed clinically.

To summarize, our hypothesis is that there are at least two distinct conditions which can predispose one to develop alcoholism. Some people may have a genetic predisposition which renders them opioid deficient at baseline. Other individuals may develop a (post)stress-induced opioid deficiency and thus may exhibit alcoholic behavior only at certain times. These two conditions are not mutually exclusive. Individuals who have low levels of opioid activity at baseline and/or who are rendered functionally opioid deficient by stress may respond to small doses of alcohol by experiencing an opioid surge which serves to reinforce the drinking behavior. Continued drinking leads to an adaptation to high opioid activity or perhaps opioid depletion such that the "high" experienced is not sustained and if the person decreases alcohol drinking, a relative deficiency in opioid activity exists. It is this relative opioid deficient state which produces a craving for alcohol and sets the stage for the next opioid boost. Hence a vicious cycle is created whereby drinking alcohol sets the occasion for more alcohol drinking. Opiate antagonists are thus effective in breaking this vicious cycle by inhibiting both the craving for alcohol and the reinforcing effects of drinking alcohol. By blocking the increase in opiate receptor activity, the rebound opioid deficient state is also blocked or attenuated and therefore craving for alcohol is reduced.

REFERENCES

Altshuler, H.L., Phillips, P.E. and Feinhandler, D.A. (1980) Alterations of ethanol self-administration by naltrexone. *Life Sciences*, 26, 679-688.

Bellet, S., Roman, 1., Delastro, O. and Herra, M. (1970) Effect of acute ethanol intake on plasma 11-hydroxycorticosteroid levels. *Metabolism*, 19, 664-667.

Black, J.R. (1889) Advantages of substituting the morphia habit for the incurably alcoholic. *Cincinnati Lancet-Clinic*, 22, 537-541.

Ellis, F.W. (1966) Effect of ethanol on plasma corticosterone levels. *Journal of Pharmacology and Experimental Therapeutics*, 153, 121-127.

Epper, B.A. and Mains, R.E. (1978) Existence of a common precursor to ACTH and endorphin in the anterior and intermediate lobe of the rat pituitary. *Journal of Supramolecular Research*, 8, 247-262.

Eskelson, C.D., Hameroff, S.R. and Kanel, J.S. (1980) Ethanol increases serum beta-endorphin levels in rats. *Anesthesia and Analgesia*, 7, 537-538.

Genazzani, A.R., Nappi, G., Eacchinetti, F., Mezzella, G.L., Parrini, D., Sinforiani, E., Petraglia, F. and Savoldi, F. (1982) Central deficiency of beta-endorphin in alcohol addicts. *Journal of Clinical Endocrinology and Metabolism*, 55, 583-586.

Gianoulakis, C., Angelogianni, P., Meaney, M., Thavundayil, J. and Tawar, V. (1990) Endorphins in Individuals with high and Low Risk for Development of Alcoholism in *Opioids, Bulimia, and Alcohol Abuse & Alcoholism.* Reid, L.D., Ed., Springer-Verlag, New York

Ho, A.K.S. and Chen, C.A.(1975) Interactions of narcotics, narcotic antagonists, and ethanol during acute, chronic and withdrawal states. *Annals of New York Academy of Sciences*, 260, 247-310.

Ho, A.K. and Ho, C.C. (1979) Toxic interactions of ethanol with other central depressants: antagonism by naloxone to narcosis and lethality. *Pharmacology, Biochemistry and Behavior*, 11, 111-114.

Hubbell, C.L., Czirr, S.A., Hunter, G.A., Beaman, C.M., LeCann, N.C. and Reid, L.D. (1986) Consumption of ethanol solution is potentiated by morphine and attenuated by naloxone persistently across repeated daily administrations. *Alcohol*, 3, 39-54.

Kolk, B., Greenberg, M. and Boyd, H. (1985) Inescapable shock, neurotransmitters and addiction to trauma: Toward a psychobiology of post-traumatic stress. *Biological Psychiatry*, 20, 314.

Miller, W.R. and Hester, R.K. (1986) The effectiveness of alcoholism treatment methods: What research reveals in *Treating Addictive Behaviors: Process of Change*, Miller, W.R. and Heather, N. (Eds.) Plenum Press, New York.

Nathan, P.E. (1986) Outcomes of treatment for alcoholism: Current Data. *Annals of Behavioral Medicine*, 8, 40-46.

Reid, L.D. and Hunter, G.A.(1984) Morphine and naloxone modulate intake of ethanol. *Alcohol*, 1, 33-37.

Schulz, R., Wister, M., Duka, T. and Herz, A. (1980) Acute and chronic ethanol treatment changes endorphin levels in brain and pituitary. *Psychopharmacology*, 68, 221-227.

Siegel, S. (1986) Alcohol and Opiate Dependence: Re-evaluation of the Victorian Perspective in *Research Advances in Alcohol and Drug Problems*, Vol. 9, Cappell, H.D., Glaser, F.B., Israel,Y., Kalant, H., Schmidt, W., Sellers, E.M. and Smart, R.C., Eds., Plenum Publishing Corp., New York.

Volpicelli, J.R. (1987). Uncontrollable Events and Alcohol Drinking. *British Journal of Addiction*, 82(4), 381-392.

Volpicelli, J.R., O'Brien, C.P., Alterman, A.I. and Hayashida, M. (1990) Naltrexone and the Treatment of Alcohol Dependence: Initial Observations, in *Opioids, Bulimia, and Alcohol Abuse & Alcoholism*. Reid, L.D., Ed., Springer-Verlag, New York.

Volpicelli, J.R., Davis, M.A. and Olgin, J.E. (1986) Naltrexone blocks the post-shock increase of ethanol consumption. *Life Sciences*, 38, 841-847.

Volpicelli, J.R. and Ulm, R.R. (1991) Alcohol drinking in rats during and following morphine injections. *Alcohol*, in press, 1991.

Volpicelli, J.R., Ulm, R.R. and Hopson, N. (1990) The bidirectional effects of shock on alcohol preference in rats. *Alcoholism: Clinical and Experimental Research*, 14, 913-916.

13

Naltrexone in the Treatment of Alcohol Dependence: Preliminary Findings

S.S. O'Malley, A. Jaffe, G. Chang, G. Witte, R.S. Schottenfeld, and B.J. Rounsaville

INTRODUCTION

To date, there are no clearly efficacious pharmacotherapies for alcoholism (Meyer, 1989). In a large multi-center controlled study, disulfiram, the only medication marketed specifically for alcoholism, was found to be no better than an inactive dose of disulfiram (1 mg) or no medication in affecting rates of abstinence, time to first drink, employment, or social stability (Fuller et al., 1986). A recent double blind placebo controlled trial of lithium (Dorus et al., in press) also failed to demonstrate greater efficacy for active medication over placebo.

More recently, the potential value of narcotic antagonists in the treatment of alcohol dependence has been suggested by preclinical and clinical studies. Several converging lines of evidence provide support for similarities between the pharmacological properties of alcohol and opiate stimulation. In rodents, pharmacological cross tolerance between alcohol and opiates such as morphine has been identified (Blum, Wallace, Schweter, & Eubanks, 1976; Jones & Spratto, 1970). In addition, opiate antagonists have been shown to block some of the effects of alcohol, including behavioral symptoms of alcohol withdrawl (Blum, Futterman, Wallace, & Schwetner, 1979; Berman, Lee, Olson, & Goldman, 1984), alcohol-elicited increases in motor activity (Middaugh, Read, & Boggon, 1978), and alcohol induced sleep and lethality (Ho & Ho, 1979).

With regard to voluntary alcohol consumption in animals, small doses of morphine have been shown to stimulate alcohol consumption (Hubbell, Czirr & Reid, 1987; Reid & Hunter, 1984). Conversely, opiate antagonists such as naloxone and naltrexone have been shown to reliably reduce ethanol consumption under a variety of circumstance (DeWitte, 1984; Hubbell et al., 1986; Samson & Doyle, 1985; Volpicelli, Davis, & Olgin, 1986).

Acknowledgments: This research was supported in part by grant AA-P50-03-510 from the National Institute of Alcohol Abuse and Alcoholism.

In humans, the potential value of opiate antagonists in treating alcohol dependence was first evaluated by Volpicelli (1990), who used naltrexone as an adjunctive treatment to standard psychotherapy in a placebo-controlled double-blind study of 58 recently detoxified alcohol dependent subjects. The preliminary results of this study revealed that naltrexone treated patients reported lower levels of alcohol craving, fewer drinks consumed per drinking occasion, fewer drinking days, and lower rates of relapse than did placebo treated patients.

In light of the promise shown by naltrexone, we are currently undertaking a large scale study of 120 alcohol dependent patient that attempts to replicate and extend Volpicelli's findings (1990). In particular, we are interested in evaluating the efficacy of naltrexone alone and in combination with a 12-week program of coping skills training based on the principles of social learning theory (Marlatt & Gordon, 1985). Coping skills training is designed to increase the patient's ability to avoid or cope with high risk situations and to reduce the rate of relapse. The effectiveness of this structured treatment will be contrasted with a supportive nondirective therapy designed to support the patient's own efforts at abstinence without providing skills training. Using a standard factorial design, the following four conditions will be compared: (1) coping skills therapy and naltrexone; (2) coping skills therapy and placebo; (3) supportive psychotherapy and naltrexone; and (4) supportive psychotherapy and placebo. It is hypothesized that the combination of naltrexone and coping skills therapy will be particularly effective in reducing relapse to drinking. Using the first 33 subjects completing the trial, the present paper reports on preliminary analyses comparing the effectiveness of naltrexone and placebo on drinking related measures.

METHODS

Subjects

Thirty-three subjects meeting DSM-III-R criteria for alcohol dependence were recruited into the study. Two patients placed on naltrexone were withdrawn from the study because of side effects experienced after their first dose. Of the remaining 31 subjects, eighteen received naltrexone; 15 received placebo. The two groups were comparable in their demographic characteristics which are presented in Table 1.

Table 1. Demographic Characteristics

Variable	Naltrexone	Placebo
Age (M + SD)	43.0 + 11.0	37.7 + 11.2
Male (%)	88	60
Caucasian (%)	81	93
High School (%)	86	93
Married (%)	63	80

Subjects were recruited from among patients seeking treatment at the outpatient Alcohol Treatment Unit of the Connecticut Mental Health Center and from individuals resonding to study advertisements in the New Haven paper. Prior to entering the study, subjects were screened according to a number of inclusion and exclusion criteria:

Inclusion Criteria: (1) 18-65 years old; (2) abstinent from alcohol for a period of 7-30 days; and (3) able to read English and complete study evaluations.

Exclusion Criteria: (1) currently meets DSM-III-R criteria for abuse or dependence on substances other than alcohol; (2) regular use of psychoactive drugs including anxiolytics and antidepressants; (3) current use of disulfiram; (4) psychosis or other severe psychiatric symptoms such as suicidality or mania; (5) significant cerebral, renal, thyroid, or cardiac pathology; (6) laboratory evidence of significant hepatocellular injury as evidenced by SGOT, SGPT or GGT levels three times normal or elevated bilirubin; (7) past history of opiate abuse; and (8) female patients who are pregnant, nursing, or refuse to use a reliable method of birth control.

Procedures

Pre-induction week. Subjects who reported abstinence from alcohol for at least seven days were screened by a research assistant for inclusion and exclusion criteria. Subjects appropriate for the study were invited to participate, and informed consent was obtained. An intake battery of assessments was then completed in one to two sessions, and the patient received a physical exam. The intake battery included extensive measures of drinking behaviors, psychological symptoms, social and occupational functioning, and other patient attributes. Alcohol and substance abuse disorders were diagnosed with the Structured Clinical Interview for DSM-III-R (Spitzer & Williams, 1985).

The study psychiatrist reviewed the patient's medical records for eligibility criteria and met with the patient to discuss the study medication and the research protocol. The patient was then randomly assigned to one of the study cells. The patient began the medication on the day of their first session with their individual therapist. The psychiatrist, therapist, research assistant, and patient were all blind to the study medication. The research assistant and the psychiatrist were blind to the psychotherapy condition.

Pharmacotherapy Conditions. In order to relicate the findings of Volpicelli (1990), as well as comply with standard clinical doses of naltrexone, the dosage level for the study was 50 mg naltrexone or inert placebo. Riboflavin 50 mg was also incorporated into all capsules in order to evaluate patient compliance. Urine samples were inspected bi-weekly using an ultraviolet light to detect the presence of riboflavin. Compliance was also assessed by conducting a count of remaining capsules at each visit during the 12 week medication period.

Therapy Phase. Patients participated in weekly individual coping skills relapse prevention sessions or supportive psychotherapy sessions with a Ph.D. level therapist for 12 weeks. Prior to meeting with the therapist each week, the patient completed the Beck Depression Scale and the Speilberger State Anxiety Scale. They were also asked to report on the amount of alcohol and other drugs used each day during the previous week, to rate their overall level of craving for the week and their present level of craving, and to rate their satisfaction with the study medication and the degree of change in their condition.

During each session, the therapist completed a side effects questionnaire with the patient. Following the session, the therapist completed the Global Assessment Scale (Endicott et al., 1976) and measures assessing the type of psychotherapy provided. After sessions 4, 8, and 12, the independent clinical evaluator interviewed the patient with the Addiction Severity Index (McClellan et al., 1980).

At the final therapy session held at the end of week 12, the research assistant completed a termination interview which addressed the patient's level of functioning and the reasons for termination. The patient also provided measures of satisfaction with the treatment received.

Follow-up. Although not analyzed for the present paper, a 6 month follow-up evaluation was conducted with patients to evaluate enduring and/or delayed treatment effects.

RESULTS

Side Effects

Side effects reported at each week by naltrexone and placebo treated subjects were compared using chi-square analyses. The groups differed significantly on the occurence of nausea at one week ($p < .05$). Fifteen percent of naltrexone subjects reported nausea in contrast to none of the placebo treated patients. Naltrexone treated patients also tended to report decreased libido (12%; week 4) and panic anxiety (12%; week 1) more often than placebo treated patients (0%).

Although naltrexone was tolerated well by most patients, two patients experienced panic anxiety after the first dose of naltrexone and discontinued the medication. The first patient, a male in his forties, described an "acute" anxiety reaction within two hours of taking the medication which was accompanied by dry mouth, extreme subjective anxiety, and irritability. The second patient, a male in his mid-thirties, described feelings of panic, irritability, shakiness, nausea, flushing and derealization.

SGOT and SGPT Levels

Liver function tests at termination were compared for the two groups using analysis of covariance controlling for baseline values. Because alcohol abuse is associated with elevated SGOT and SGPT levels, these measures were examined as an indirect measure of alcohol use. In addition, this assessment was undertaken in light of reports of naltrexone induced hepatotoxicity at doses (300 mg/daily) substantially higher than used in the current study (Pfohl et al., 1986). The results of these analyses indicated that there were no significant differences between the groups on SGOT or SGPT.

Retention in Treatment

One measure of the effectiveness of treatment is the proportion of patients successfully completing therapy. Of the original 33 patients recruited into the study, eighty-three percent of the naltrexone treated patients completed the study in contrast to 67% of placebo treated patients. Of the placebo treated patients, 27% dropped out presumably due to relapse to alcohol, whereas only 6% of naltrexone treated patients dropped out. One placebo patient was withdrawn from the study due to elevated liver enzymes. As noted earlier, two naltrexone patients, but none of the placebo treated patients, discontinued the study because of side effects.

Alcohol Consumption

The most stingent measure of outcome is abstinence. Fifty percent of the naltrexone treated patients were abstinent in contrast to 33 percent of the placebo treated patients, although these differences were not statistically significant [*chi-square* (1, N = 31) = .88, p = .35]

The two groups were found to be comparable on the percentage of days on which alcohol was consumed [t (30) = -1.37, p = .19]. In this regard, naltrexone patients drank on 4.2 percent of the days (*SD* = 6.8) compared to placebo patients who drank on 9.4 percent of the days (*SD* = 12.9).

When the number of drinks consumed per drinking day were compared for those naltrexone patients (N = 8) and placebo patients (N = 10) who drank during the protocol, there was a trend for naltrexone treated patients to drink less than placebo treated patients [t (17) = -1.91, p = .08]. Naltrexone patients drank 3.2 standard drinks on average (*SD* = 1.9) compared to 6.4 drinks (*SD* = 4.8) for placebo treated patients.

Relapse Rates

The final analysis of alcohol consumption measures examined rates of relapse, defined by drinking more than 5 drinks per drinking day. When the entire sample was considered, 46.7 percent of the placebo treated patients relapsed compared to 12.5 percent of the naltrexone treated patients [*chi-square* (1, N = 31) = 4.39, $p < .05$]. When only those patients who drank were examined, only 25% of the naltrexone treated patients relapsed after the initiation of drinking in contrast to 70 percent of the placebo treated patients (*Fisher's Exact Test*, p = .15).

Craving Ratings

Patients rated their craving weekly on a likert scale ranging from 1 ("not at all") to 20 ("more than ever"). Using endpoint ratings, the mean craving scores for the two groups did not differ significantly [t (30) = -.79, p = .44). Mean craving ratings for the naltrexone treated patients and the placebo treated patients were 3.5 (*SD* = 3.1) and 4.7 (*SD* = 5.3) respectively.

DISCUSSION

The results of this preliminary study are consistent with previous research by Volpicelli (1990), suggesting that naltrexone may be a useful pharmacological adjunct in the treatment of alcohol dependence. The major findings are that naltrexone treatment was associated with better patient retention, lower levels of alcohol consumption and reduced rates of relapse. Although naltrexone did not appear to prevent the initiation of alcohol consumption in this sample, the difference in alcohol consumption levels noted for naltrexone and placebo treated patients is clinically significant. Naltrexone patients drank on average three drinks per occasion, whereas placebo treated patients drank over six drinks per occasion. At these doses, placebo patients were more likely to achieve significiant levels of alcohol intoxication, thereby placing them at greater risk of psychosocial and medical consequences of alcohol use. Similarly, placebo treated patients were less likely to remain in treatment where occasions of drinking could be addressed and strategies for resuming abstinence developed.

Another important finding is that naltrexone appears to be well tolerated by subjects. With the exception of marked anxiety reported by two subjects, other side effects such as nausea were minimal and acceptable to patients. Given this, it is likely that patient acceptance and compliance for naltrexone will be substantially higher than the most widely used medication, disulfiram, which produces a disulfiram-ethanol interaction consisting of severe nausea, vomiting, flushing, light-headedness, abdominal pain, and tachycardia. Unlike medications such as lithium, tricyclic antidepressants, and MAO-Inhibitors which have the potential for adverse reactions precipitated by interactions between alcohol consumption and medication, naltrexone appears to be a relatively safe drug provided that subjects with significant liver disease are screened out.

In considering the finding that naltrexone is associated with lower levels of alcohol consumption per drinking occasion, questions arise about how the experience of alcohol consumption is modified while on the medication. In our study, a number of patients have spontaneously remarked that their preferred alcoholic beverage tasted different and less pleasant while on naltrexone. Consistent with these reports, naltrexone has been shown to produce a significant decrease in pleasureable evaluations of sweetened solutions among healthy nonobese subjects (Fantino, Hosotte, & Apfelbaum, 1986).

Another hypothesis is that naltrexone blocks other rewarding effects of alcohol that may be mediated by the opiate receptor system. It is well established, for example, that the pleasureable effects of alcohol such as stimulation and euphoria occur on the ascending limb of the blood alcohol curve shortly after initial consumption of alcohol. Given that naltrexone treated patients discontinue drinking at relatively low levels of alcohol consumption rather than continuing to drink to intoxication suggests that naltrexone may reduce these pleasureable and reinforcing aspects of alcohol consumption that under normal circumstance prime further drinking. In order to refine hypotheses about the interaction of alcohol and naltrexone, we recently added a self-report measure to be completed after an episode of drinking that assesses how the experience of alcohol consumption is modified while on medication. Additional laboratory research is needed, however, that directly tests these hypotheses by challenging naltrexone and placebo maintained subjects with alcohol and measuring their subjective and objective responses to intoxication.

In conclusion, the results of these preliminary analyses provide evidence for the potential value of naltrexone as a pharmacotherapy for alcohol dependence. Future analyses will examine the differential efficacy of naltrexone in combination with coping skills relapse prevention therapy and a supportive psychotherapy. Given that comprehensive assessments are being obtained on patients, we will also attempt to delineate the characteristics of patients for whom naltrexone and the different forms of psychotherapy are particularly particularly effective.

REFERENCES

Bernam RF, Lee JA, Olsen KL, Goldman MS: Effect of naloxone on ethanol dependence in rats. *Drug and Alcohol Dependence* 1984; 13: 245-254.

Blum K, Futterman S, Wallace JE, Schwertner HA: Naloxone-induced inhibition of ethanol dependence in mice. *Nature* 1977; 265: 49-51.

Blum K, Wallace JE, Eubanks J, Schwertner HA: Effects of naloxone on ethanol withdrawal, preference and narcosis. *The Pharmacologist* 1975; 17: 197.

DeWitte P: Naloxone reduces alcohol intake in a free-choice procedure even when both drinking bottles contain saccharin sodium or guinine substances. *Neuropsychobiology* 1984; 12: 73-77.

Dorus W, Ostrow DG, Anton R, Kushman P, Collins JF: Lithium carbonate treatment of depressed and nondepressed alcohlics in a double-blind, placebo controlled study. *JAMA* 1989; 262: 1646-1652.

Fantino M, Hosotte J, Apfelbaum M: An opioid antagonist, naltrexone, reduces preference for sucrose in humans. *Am J of Physiology* 1986; 251: 91-96.

Fuller RK, Branchey L, Brightwell DR, et al: Disulfiram treatment of alcoholism: A Veterans Administration cooperative study. *JAMA* 1986; 256: 1449-1455.

Ho AK, Ho CC: Toxic interactions of ethanol with other central depressants: Antagonism by naloxone to narcosis and lethality. *Pharmacology Biochemistry & Behavior* 1979; 11: 111-114.

Hubbell CL, Czirr SA, Reid LD: Persistence and specificity of small doses of morphine on intake of alcoholic beverages. *Alcohol* 1987; 4: 149-156.

Hubbell CL, Czirr SA, Hunter GA, Beaman CM, LeCann NC, Reid LD: Consumption of ethanol solution is potentiated by morphine and attenuated by naloxone persistently across repeated daily administrations. *Alcohol* 1986; 3: 39-54.

Jones MA, Spratto SR: Ethanol suppression of naloxone-induced withdrawal in morphine-dependent rats. *Life Sciences* 1977; 20: 1549-1556.

Marlatt GA, Gordon JR: *Relapse Prevention*. New York, Guilford Press, 1985.

McLellan AT, Luborsky L, Woody GE, O'Brien CP: An improved diagnotic evalutation instrument for substance abuse patients: The Addiction Severity Index. *J Nerv Ment Dis* 1980; 168: 26-33.

Meyer RE: Prospects for a rational pharmacotherapy of alcoholism. *J Clin Psychiatry* 1989; 50: 403-412.

Middaugh LD, Read E, Boggan WO: Effects of naloxone on ethanol induced alterations of locomoter activity in C57BL/6 mice. *Pharmacology Biochemistry & Behavior* 1978; 11: 157-160.

Pfohl DN, Allen JI, Atkinson RL, Knopman DS, Malcolm RJ, Mitchell JE, Morley JE: Naltrexone hydrochloride (Trexan): A review of serum transaminase at high dosage, in Harris LS (ed): *Proceedings of the 47th annual scientific meeting, The Committee on Problems of Drug Dependence, Inc.* (National Institute on Drug Abuse Research Monograph 67) Rockville, M.D., National Institute on Drug Abuse, Office of Science, 1986, pp 66-72.

Reid LD, Hunter GA: Morphine and naloxone modulate intake of ethanol. *Alcohol* 1984; 1: 33-37.

Samson HH, Doyle TF: Oral ethanol self-administration in the rat: Effect of naloxone. *Pharmacology Biochemistry & Behavior* 1985; 22: 91-99.

Spitzer RL, Williams JBW: Structured Clinical Interview for DSM-III-R, patient version, 7/85. Biometric Research Department, New York State Pychiatric Institute, 722 West 168th Street, New York, NY 10032.

Volpicelli JR, Davis MA, Olgin JE: Naltrexone blocks the post shock increase of ethanol consumption. *Life Sciences* 1986; 38: 841-847.

Volpicelli JR, O'Brien CP, Alterman AI, Hayashida M: Naltrexone and the treatment of alcohol dependence: Initial observations, in Reid LB (ed): *Opioids, Bulimia, Alcohol Abuse and Alcoholism.* New York, Springer-Verlag, 1990, pp 195-214.

Part IV
The Role of Other Neurotransmitters in Regulating Alcohol Intake

14
Neurotransmitter Systems Regulating Alcohol Intake
Z. Amit and B.R. Smith

1 Neurobiology of alcohol's effects on Behavior: One vs multiple systems.

The ingestion of alcohol by most organisms including humans results in profound effects on a variety of behaviors. For example, alcohol induces narcosis and related changes in righting reflex, affects body temperature, locomotor activity, startle response, as well as several other behaviors. Perhaps, the most important impact alcohol has on behavior is related to the ingestion of alcohol itself. The ingestion of alcohol among humans, but also other species, results in the increase in the probability and frequency of future bouts of alcohol intake (10, 58, 93). This property of alcohol places it in the same category as other substances of abuse (e.g., opiates, cocaine). This by virtue of the fact that it is presumed that all of these substances are endowed with positive reinforcing properties which underlie the development of dependence on them. The search for the neurobiological substrates of alcohol's effects on behavior in general and its positive reinforcing effects in particular now span several decades (e.g., 25, 51). In view of the diversity and heterogeneity of alcohol's effects on behavior one would have presumed that the search would be broad in nature and that its focus would be the identification of multidimensional neural system interacting in the mediation of alcohol effects. Nevertheless, it is not completely surprising that in reality, the search tended to focus on one transmitter system which presumably accounted for the entire variance of alcohol's behavioral effects. Thus, for example, earlier studies including those emanating from our own laboratory attempted to identify "the neurotransmitter system" implicated in mediating alcohol induced changes in behavior (e.g., 4, 29, 46, 64). In this vein, the direction research took in this area paralleled those prevailing in other areas of psychobiology where the search for "the substance of reward" was the rage for quite some time (68, 94).

2 The Attempt to Identify One Controlling Mechanism

The search for a single regulatory system mediating the voluntary intake of ethanol has followed several seemingly independent paths. The goal of each of these lines of research have been to determine the involvement of a particular neurotransmitter in regulating this behavior. Thus, despite an acute scarcity of theoretical underpinning to guide and provide direction for such a search, for over twenty years, investigators have tended to persist in focussing their attention on a search for a single mechanism. In retrospect, it has become quite clear that this search was aided by nothing more substantial then the prevailing Zeitgeist. Nevertheless, as often happens in such cases, a large body of useful data did emerge. A brief description of these independent research lines follows.

2.1 Catecholamines

In the early 60's the pioneering work of Stein (88) and others (30) implicated brain catecholamines in the mediation of motivated behavior. In line with this body of data, investigators in the late 60's and early 70's, began to explore the possible role of the catecholamines (CA) in regulating ethanol intake. Several studies had demonstrated that changes to central CA activity could result in alterations in the effects of ethanol. It was demonstrated that electrical stimulation of the lateral hypothalamus produced an increase in voluntary ethanol consumption in laboratory rats and that the observed increased preference for ethanol persisted for some time following termination of the stimulation (3, 9, 10, 12). The proposal that the catecholamines were involved in the mediation of ethanol induced behaviors was reinforced by the identification of major CA pathways traversing the lateral hypothalamus (92). Indeed, the impact of Ungerstedt's chemical histofluorescence work on motivated research in general and drug and alcohol research in particular cannot be overemphasized.

The results of more pharmacologically related studies using the CA synthesis inhibitor, α-methyltyrosine (AMT), also suggested CA involvement. It was shown that treatment with AMT produced a transient attenuation of consumption of ethanol (65). In addition, it was found to interfere with the reacquisition of intragastric ethanol self-administration in rats (23). It was also shown that the use of this agent could suppress alcohol-induced euphoria in human subjects (2).

Several studies have examined the effects of physical destruction of CA pathways on ethanol intake in rats. Electrolytic lesions within the lateral hypothalamus (8) and direct central infusion of the catecholamine specific neurotoxin, 6-hydroxydopamine (6-OHDA) have been shown to attenuate ethanol intake (16, 64, 74). These findings lent support to the notion of CA involvement in the regulation of ethanol consumption. Perhaps unfortunately, at least it was felt so at the time, they did not provide any data regarding the relative importance of norepinephrine (NE) or dopamine (DA) in the mediation of the psychopharmacological effects of ingested ethanol.

2.1.1 Dopamine and/or Norepinehrine

In an attempt to isolate the respective roles for NE and DA in the psychopharmacology of ethanol, a series of studies were conducted using selective destruction of NE and DA pathways via the usage of neurotoxins. Brown and Amit (16) reported decreased ethanol intake in rats when both NE and DA were destroyed following 6-OHDA infusion but failed to see any change in consumption when NE neurons were protected by pretreatment with desmethylimipramine. These results were supported by other reports demonstrating that lesions of NE pathways and not DA neurons produced alterations in voluntary ethanol consumption (19, 44, 45, 46, 55).

Despite the apparent consistencies of these results, there have been several studies which have reported contradictory data or a lack of effect. Kiianmaa et al. (46) and Kiianmaa (44) demonstrated transitory increases in ethanol intake following 6-OHDA lesions of NE pathways which was in contrast to the observed decreases described above following this manipulation (16, 19, 55). In addition, the use of specific NE neurotoxins such as 6-hydroxydopa (74) and DSP-4 (21, 34) failed to alter ethanol intake. In an attempt to resolve this inconsistency, It was suggested (16) that NE systems are only marginally impaired following extensive depletions by neurotoxins as the remaining NE neurons are capable of compensation through various processes such as increased release, synthesis and turnover, as well as increased sensitivity of receptors (1, 98, 99). Given this, it would seem that the specific methodology used when neurotoxins were applied would be expected to have, on its own, a great impact on the nature of the alterations seen on ethanol related behavior, independent of its specific effects on neural tissue. However, despite the inconsistencies in this area of research, one common finding could be gleaned from this work; the specific destruction of DA neurons alone regularly failed to alter ethanol intake.

An alternative approach to the question of DA and/or NE involvement in ethanol intake was developed through the utilization of enzyme inhibitors and receptor blockers. The depletion of NE by dopamine-ß-hydroxylase (DBH) inhibitors FLA-63 and FLA-57 have been shown to attenuate voluntary ethanol consumption in rats (4, 7, 17). These authors suggested that the decrease in consumption was a result of an attenuation of the reinforcing properties of ethanol brought about via the depletion of NE (4, 7). Consistent with this suggestion, rats given the DBH inhibitor U14-624 failed to reacquire a response contingency for intragastric infusions of ethanol, whereas, haloperidol, a specific DA receptor blocker, was ineffective (23). FLA-57 was also shown to attenuate ethanol intragastric self-administration behavior and block the development of a secondary reinforcer to signalled ethanol infusions (24).

It was stated earlier, that destruction of DA neurons alone consistently failed to produce any alterations in ethanol drinking behavior. Similar findings using DA receptor manipulations have also generally failed to produce any alterations in ethanol intake. The use of the

DA antagonist pimozide resulted in no change in ethanol consumption using both a 24-hour drinking paradigm (18) and a 1-hour drinking paradigm (61). There are, however, some studies which have reported a decrease in operant responding for access to an ethanol solution following pimozide and haloperidol treatment (69, 70). However, it is of the utmost importance to note that these agents have been repeatedly shown to reduce fluid intake through mechanisms which may be unrelated to manipulation of the reinforcing properties of the appetitive stimulus (e.g., 54, 87, 91). A recent report by Linseman (54) indicated that those alterations in ethanol intake observed following treatment with various DA receptor manipulators were accompanied by similar alterations in water intake. It was concluded that dopamine may not play as critical a role in mediating the reinforcing properties of ethanol as it may do in relation to other psychoactive drugs (54). In addition to these studies, the administration of a DA reuptake inhibitor, nomifensine, also failed to alter voluntary ethanol consumption (20). Lastly, it has been shown that chronic low-level administration of amphetamine increased ethanol consumption (72) and that the increased intake was mediated by central NE (52).

These findings suggested that the reinforcing properties of ethanol may be mediated through the activity of central NE pathways. However, recent data has called into some question the specificity of NE manipulations such as FLA-57. It has been suggested that the mechanism whereby FLA-57 results in an attenuation of ethanol consumption may not be exclusively through a disruption of the reinforcing properties of ethanol but rather, at least in part, through an aversive mechanism (6, 83). It has also been suggested that FLA-57 may alter fluid intakes in general, and that its effects on ethanol drinking while robust, may be the result of a partial and/or indirect involvement of NE (21).

It would appear from the preceding section that the bulk of the research supports the notion that the integrity of central NE systems is essential for the regulation of ethanol consumption. The research regarding DA seems to be less convincing as there is a relative paucity of positive data (compared to that examining NE) relating DA's involvement in mediating ethanol intake. However, despite twenty years of research it is still unclear as to what role NE systems may play and whether Da pathways play a role altogether.

2.2 Serotonin

In recent years, there has been great interest in the possible use of serotonin (5-HT) uptake blockers as a potential pharmacological treatment for alcoholism. The interest in 5-HT interactions with ethanol, however, is not new and dates back to the late 1960's when Myers and Veale (65) first reported that the 5-HT synthesis inhibitor ρ-chlorophenylalanine (PCPA) reduced voluntary ethanol consumption in rats. Other attempts to lower central 5-HT content with the neurotoxin 5,6-dihydroxytryptamine (5,6-DHT) were found, in a seemingly contradictory fashion, to increase ethanol intake (41, 59) or to have no effect (43). However, there have been several reports in the literature that treatment with 5-HT uptake blockers consistently reduced voluntary ethanol consumption in rats (31, 33, 49, 77, 78). These results which were in contradiction to some of the studies discussed above (e.g., 41, 59) were, however in line with earlier studies which employed agents that increased 5-HT neurotransmission. Tryptophan and the 5-HT agonist quipazine was shown to reduce ethanol intake in rats given ethanol as their only source of fluid (95). Administration of 5-HT itself, as well as the precursor 5-HTP were also shown to decrease ethanol consumption (29, 40, 63, 96). The mechanism underlying the observed decrease in ethanol intake was proposed to be the result of an attenuation of the reinforcing properties of ethanol (77, 78). However, other investigators suggested that the increased availability of 5-HT reacted with ethanol to produce a profound conditioned taste aversion (97) and that this conditioned aversion may be the mechanism by which ethanol intake was reduced.

In the past several years this laboratory has published the results of several studies using the 5-HT uptake blocker, zimeldine, in rats voluntarily ingesting ethanol. These studies consistently demonstrated that zimeldine treatment produced a significant reduction in ethanol intake (35, 77, 78). Other similar acting compounds (e.g., fluoxetine, citalopram, fluvoxamine, sertraline) have also been tested yielding essentially the same results (22, 33, 36, 49, 62, 76, 95). In addition, there have been several reports showing that treatment with serotonin uptake inhibitors decreased ethanol consumption in human social drinkers (5, 66, 67).

The pharmacological mechanisms through which these drugs affect ethanol consumption are as yet unclear. For example, prior depletion of central 5-HT by the neurotoxin ρ-chloramphetamine failed to alter the actions of zimeldine despite substantial reductions in whole brain 5-HT levels (11, 35). It has been reported that a variety of NE and 5-HT receptor antagonists failed to block the inhibitory effects of fluoxetine and fluvoxamine on ethanol intake (62). In addition, the use of phenoxybenzamine (alpha-NE receptor antagonist), propranolol (beta-NE receptor antagonist), cinanserin (5-HT receptor antagonist) and methergoline with or without xylamidine tosylate (combined central and peripheral 5-HT receptor antagonists) all failed to attenuate the fluid suppressant effects of zimeldine (32). The inability to block, attenuate or even change the effects of 5-HT uptake inhibitors, while in itself an extremely puzzling phenomenon, leaves unanswered the important questions of pharmacological specificity as well as receptor specificity. Altogether, it is entirely possible that these 5-HT uptake inhibitors exert their influence on ethanol intake through indirect non-serotonergic mechanisms.

There is also increasing evidence that the effects of 5-HT uptake blockade may not reflect a specific interactions with ethanol. It has been reported that treatment with sertraline reduced saccharin consumption and preference (33) and was also shown to have a potent anorexic effect in which food intake was reduced by more than 50% following drug treatment (36). It has also been demonstrated that zimeldine significantly reduced the consumption of saccharin as well as dextrose solutions (35). It has been repeatedly shown that 5-HT uptake blockers and 5-HT agonists effect a number of consummatory behaviors. For example, they were shown to reduce the ingestion of a sucrose-morphine ingestion (75), consumption of sucrose, saccharin and sweet milk solutions (60) and well as food intake (37). It would appear likely that the primary actions of 5-HT uptake blockers may consist of a global effect on feeding with the reduction in ethanol consumption a secondary consequence of this suppression. However, even this explanation is problematic in view of the fact that 5-HT uptake inhibitors were reported to have an effect on taste factors independent of the caloric value of the food (32). When this body of data is evaluated as a whole it appears that serotonin is involved in the regulation of ethanol intake in a non-specific way involving a complex effect on food, taste and satiety processes. The future of this avenue of research with regards to the development of a pharmacological treatment for alcohol intake based on 5-HT manipulations would appear to rest on additional investigations of this transmitter system's involvement in the regulation of general consummatory behaviors.

2.1.3 Gamma-Aminobutyric Acid

For much of the past twenty years, research on the role of central neurotransmitter systems in the regulation of ethanol intake has focused on the CAs and 5-HT. This has coincided with the enormous attention placed on the mediation of these systems of motivated behavior. More recently, however, there has been increasing interest in the possible role of the inhibitory neurotransmitter gamma-aminobutyric acid in regulating behavior. As more information has been gathered on the functional significance of GABA in the central nervous system, attention has been placed on the possible involvement of GABA mechanisms in the mediation of some of the psychopharmacological properties of ethanol. Chronic exposure to ethanol has been shown to decrease GABA transmission which has been implicated in the mediation of the ethanol withdrawal syndrome (42, 48). However, acute exposure to ethanol results in a facilitation of GABA transmission (42, 48). GABAergic involvement in ethanol intoxication has been demonstrated in a number of behavior paradigms including locomotor activity (13, 53), sleep time in mice (53) and the tilt plane using rats (38). In addition, it has been suggested that GABAergic mechanisms may play an important role in the development of ethanol-induced conditioned taste aversion (86).

Some researchers have also examined the possible interaction between GABA and voluntary intake of ethanol in laboratory animals. Boismare et al. (14) showed that the administration of a GABA agonist, calcium acetyl-homotaurine reduced voluntary ethanol consumption in rats and that pretreatment with bicuculline, a GABA antagonist, blocked this decrease. As well, the administration of gamma-butyrolactone (a GABA agonist) to laboratory rats with a high preference for ethanol was reported to attenuate voluntary ethanol intake (27). It was shown that the propensity to self-select ethanol by rats was related to their respective sensitivity to the inhibitory effects of a GABA agonist (84). These experiments seem to suggest that GABA may play an important, yet, mostly inhibitory role in the control of voluntary ethanol intake in laboratory rats.

In an attempt to explore the possible role of GABAergic mechanisms in the mediation of voluntary ethanol intake it was shown that the administration of a GABA agonist can enhance the acquisition of voluntary ethanol consumption in laboratory rats (85). It was also shown by the same investigators that treatment with THIP (GABA-A agonist) induced a significant increase in the amount of ethanol consumed as well as the preference for ethanol. Partially similar effects were observed following the administration of baclofen (GABA-B agonist), suggesting, on first inspection, that the augmentation effects of GABA agonists may not be receptor specific. However, the increased preference for ethanol seen with THIP treatment was not duplicated with baclofen administration. In fact, baclofen treatment resulted in a significant increase in total fluid intake strongly suggesting that the increased ethanol consumption may be related more to a generalized increase in the intake of fluids rather than a specific interaction of GABA-B receptor activation and ethanol. Importantly, and in contrast, there was no total fluid effect with THIP treatment. Animals demonstrating an increase in the self-selection of ethanol compensated for this increased fluid intake by lowering their water consumption, hence, resulting in a corresponding elevation in ethanol preference. Taken together, these findings appear to suggest that GABAergic mechanisms may play an important role in the acquisition of voluntary ethanol consumption and, more specifically, this effect may be mediated through the GABA-A receptor (85).

Recent studies have suggested two different pharmacological and functional sites on GABA neurons. Hill and Bowery (39) identified two different sub-populations of GABAergic receptors, GABA-A and GABA-B. The well-established GABA-A receptor is a complex entity with, at least, three binding sites that form a complex and interact with a common chloride ionophore (79). It has also been shown that a bicuculline-insensitive GABA-B receptor can be identified on nerve terminals (15, 73). There is now increasing evidence to suggest that these two receptor sub-populations differ not only at the cellular level, but that they also have different functions within the CNS (for review: 56).

Previous research from this laboratory reported that picrotoxin administration attenuated an ethanol-induced conditioned taste aversion (86). Picrotoxin is believed to block chloride influx at the chloride ion channel (82) and it is the GABA-A receptor which is thought to be associated with this chloride ionophore (56). In addition, picrotoxin has been shown to attenuate ethanol-induced physical intoxication (38, 53). These findings suggest that GABAergic processes may play a mediational role in ethanol-induced intoxication and that these psychopharmacological effects may serve as important stimulus cues during the acquisition of ethanol intake.

This notion may also account for the apparent discrepancy of the findings examining the role of GABA in acquisition of ethanol intake with previous results which have reported decreased ethanol consumption following the administration of GABA agonists (14, 27). These latter studies examined the effect of this manipulation on the maintenance of ethanol intake with animals already experienced with the effects of ingested ethanol. An augmentation of ethanol's stimulus cues through GABA facilitation would be expected to have different behavioral consequences in ethanol-naive versus ethanol-experienced animals. It is important to note the in the entire body of literature examining the effects of manipulation of neural systems on ethanol intake, very few studies report enhanced intake. While reports of decreased ethanol ingestion following such manipulations abound (e.g., 4, 14, 23, 24, 27, 32), only a handful of noncontroversial studies reported elevated levels of drinking following any kind of neural manipulation (9, 41, 52, 72).

In comparison to research examining NE and/or DA and 5-HT involvement in ethanol's behavioral effects, the investigation of GABAergic involvement is still in its infancy. Extensive research is needed to determine its role in the mediation of ethanol-induced intoxication and, more importantly, the relevance of this GABA mediated behavioral consequence of ethanol exposure in the regulation of ethanol consumption.

III. Unitary or Interactional Mechanisms

The preceding text has provided a concise review of the main thrusts of psychopharmacological research aimed at identifying a mechanism regulating the voluntary self-selection of ethanol. Each of these lines of investigation have concentrated on the possible role of a single system or mechanism. However, as the knowledge of the functioning of the central nervous system becomes increasingly more sophisticated and complex, there is likely to be an attempt to integrate each of these independent lines of research into some form of interactional scheme. This is particularly true for the psychopharmacological effects of ethanol. The most salient feature of the research described above is the fact that the data most clearly demonstrates and supports a role, among all the possible putative candidates, for NE and GABA. Since the ingestion of ethanol is in its essence, a consummatory response, it is also likely that the 5-HT system forms part of some complex, yet non-specific, interaction in this regard. In addition, the extensive data describing a fundamental role for DA in motivated behavior in general, still, cannot be ignored when the specific case of the mediation of ethanol intake is considered. With regard to this last point, it is important to note that while the research on central mechanisms of ethanol self-administration has not provided support for a role of DA in the regulation of ethanol intake, this assertion is not intended to suggest that DA may not play some significant functional role in other ethanol effects, particularly those related to motor activity (47).

Over the past two decades, a body of data emerged which clearly implicated several neural systems in the mediation of ethanol intake in different ways and different levels of specificity. This fact by itself provides a convincing argument that it is unlikely that one single neuronal system would be identified as the primary-unitary system underlying ethanol's effects on behavior in general and ethanol intake in particular. What is far more likely is the emergence of a body of data pointing at a complex central multi-system interaction in the mediation of ethanol's behavioral effects. This notion that control of ethanol's behavioral effects is exerted through an interaction of several neuronal systems is also a logical extension of the fact that ethanol exerts such a varied and heterogeneous impact on behavior.

IV. An interaction of multiple systems underlying ethanol's effects.

Examples of the kind of multi-system neuronal interactions which may be of significance to ethanol consumption may be summarized as follows. GABA has been demonstrated to interact with cerebral and hippocampal NE systems (89). Several GABA agonists have been reported to enhance noradrenergic transmission (26, 28) and specific activation of GABA-A receptors with THIP was shown to increase the turnover of NE in brain as measured by the production of MHPG, a product of NE degradation (90). There is also considerable evidence that 5-HT and NE systems have close anatomical (50, 71) and biochemical (57) relationships suggesting that 5-HT neurons may modulate NE neuronal activity. The evidence concerning the role of serotonin in the regulation of ethanol intake, while probably non-specific, is nevertheless most likely exerted through an interaction with NE (76, 80) and possibly also DA.

The emergent accumulation of data suggesting the interaction of several neuronal system in the mediation of ethanol's effects is clearly in line with current notions on neuronal substrates of motivated behavior. In this sense, the parallel between research on the neurobiological substrates of ethanol intake in particular and motivated behavior in general is complete both temporally and conceptually. Most researchers in the area of the neurobiology of motivation tend to look for increasingly more complex interactions mediating a variety of motivated behavior (81).

In conclusion, it appears that the search for an effective pharmacological treatment of alcoholism will have to focus, in the future, on a treatment approach that will involve a complex array of agents which on the basis of currently available data will involve, as a minimum, GABAergic and noradrenergic mechanisms.

6. References

1. Acheson AL, Zigmond MJ, Stricker EM (1980) Compensatory increase in tyrosine hydroxylase activity in rat brain after intraventricular injections of 6-hydroxy-dopamine. Science 207:537-540.
2. Ahlenius S, Carlsson A, Engel J, Svensson TH, Sodersten P (1973) Antagonism by alpha methyltyrosine of the ethanol-induced stimulation and euphoria in man. Clin Pharmacol Ther 14:586-591.
3. Amir S, Stern MH (1978) Electrical stimulation and lesions of the medial forebrain bundle of the rat: Changes in voluntary ethanol consumption and brain aldehyde dehydrogenase activity. Psychopharmacol 57:167-174.
4. Amit Z, Brown ZW, Levitan DE, Ögren S-O (1977) Noradrenergic mediation of the positive reinforcing properties of ethanol: I. Suppression of ethanol consumption in laboratory rats following dopamine-ß-hydroxlase inhibition. Arch Int Pharmacodyn Ther 223:65-75.
5. Amit Z, Brown ZW, Sutherland EA, Rockman GE, Gill K, Selvaggi N (1985) Reduction in alcohol intake in humans as a function of treatment with zimeldine: Implications for treatment. In Naranjo CA, Sellers EM (eds) Research Advances in New Psychopharmacological Treatments for Alcoholism. Excerpta Medica: Amsterdam, pp 189-198.
6. Amit Z, Gill K, Ng Cheong Ton JM (1990) Attenuation of volunatry ethanol consumption by dopamine-ß-hydroxylase inhibition (FLA-57): Mediated by changes in aversion, reinforcement or both. Alcohol, submitted
7. Amit Z, Levitan DE, Lindros KO (1976) Suppression of ethanol intake following administration of dopamine-beta-hydroxylase inhibitors in rats. Arch Int Pharmacodyn Ther 223:114-119.

8. Amit Z, Meade RG, Levitan DE, Singer J (1976) The effects of dorsal and ventral hypothalamic lesions on voluntary ethanol consumption in rats. Quart J Stud Alcohol 37:1188-1196.

9. Amit Z, Stern MH (1971) A further investigation of alcohol preference in the laboratory rat induced by hypothalamic stimulation. Psychopharmacol 21:317-327.

10. Amit Z, Stern MH, Wise RA (1970) Alcohol preference in the laboratory rat induced by hypothalamic stimulation. Psychopharmacol 17:367-377.

11. Amit Z, Sutherland EA, Gill K, Ögren S-O (1984) Zimeldine: A review of its effects on ethanol consumption. Neurosci Biobehav Rev 8:35-54.

12. Atrens DM, Marfaing-Jallat P, Le Magnen J (1983) Ethanol preference following hypothalamic stimulation: Relation to stimulation parameters and energy balance. Pharmacol Biochem Behav 19:571-575.

13. Biswas B, Carlsson A (1978) Effect of intraperitoneally administered GABA on the locomotor activity of mice. Psychopharmacol 59:91-94.

14. Boismare F, Daoust M, Moore N, Saligaut C. Lhuintre JP, Chretien P, Durlach J (1984) A homotaurine derivative reduces the voluntary intake of ethanol by rats: are cerebral GABA receptors involved? Pharmacol Biochem Behav 21:787-789.

15. Bowery NG, Doble A, Hill DR, Hudson AL, Shaw J, Turnbull MJ (1980) ß-Chlorophenyl GABA (baclofen) is a selective ligand for a novel GABA receptor on nerve terminals. Brain Res Bull 5 (Suppl 2):497-502.

16. Brown ZW, Amit Z (1977) The effects of selective catecholamine depletions by 6-hydroxydopamine on ethanol preference in rats. Neurosci Lett 5:333-336.

17. Brown ZW, Amit Z, Levitan DE, Ögren S-O, Sutherland EA (1977) Noradrenergic mediation of the reinforcing properties of ethanol: II. Extinction of ethanol-drinking behavior in laboratory rats by inhibition of dopamine-beta-hydroxylase inhibition. Implications for treatment procedures in human alcoholics. Arch Int Pharmacodyn Ther 230:76-82.

18. Brown ZW, Gill K, Abitbol M, Amit Z (1982) Lack of effect of dopamine receptor blockade on voluntary ethanol consumption in rats. Behav Neural Biol 36:291-294.

19. Corcoran ME, Lewis J, Fibiger HC (1983) Forebrain noradrenaline and oral self-administration of ethanol by rats. Behav Brain Res 8:1-21.

20. Daoust M, Moore N, Saligaut C, Lhuintre JP, Chretien P, Boismare F (1986) Striatal dopamine does not appear involved in voluntary intake of ethanol by rats. Alcohol 3:15-17.

21. Daoust M, Protais P, Ladure P (1990) Noradrenergic system: Effect of DSP4 and FLA-57 on ethanol intake in ethanol preferring rats. Pharmacol Biochem Behav 36:133-137.

22. Daoust M, Saligaut C, Chadelaud M, Chretien P, Moore N, Boismare F (1984) Attenuation by anti-depressant drugs of alcohol intake in rats. Alcohol 1:379-383.

23. Davis WM, Smith SG, Werner TE (1978) Noradrenergic role in the self-administration of ethanol. Pharmacol Biochem Behav 9:369-374.

24. Davis WM, Werner TE, Smith SG (1979) Reinforcement with intragastric infusions of ethanol: Blocking effect of FLA-57. Pharmacol Biochem Behav 11:545-548.

25. Deneau D, Yanagita T, Seevers MH (1969) Self-administration of psychoactive substances by the monkey. Psychopharmacol 16:30-48.

26. Dennis T, Curet O, Nishikawa T, Scatton B (1985) Further evidence for, and nature of, the facilitatory GABAergic influence on central noradrenergic transmission. Naunyn-Schmiedeberg's Arch Pharmacol 331:225-234.

27. Fadda F, Argiolas A, Melis MR, De Montis G, Gessa GL (1983) Suppression of voluntary ethanol consumption in rats by gamma-butyrolactone. Life Sci 32:1471-1477.

28. Fung SC, Fillenz M (1985) Studies on the mechanism of modulation of 3H)noradrenaline release from rat hippocampal synaptosomes by GABA and benzodiazepine receptors. Neurochem Int 7:95-101.

29. Geller I (1973) Effects of para-chlorophenylalanine and 5-hydroxytryptophan on alcohol intake in the rat. Pharmacol Biochem Behav 1:361-365.

30. German DC, Bowden DM (1974) Catecholamine systems as the neural substrate for intracranial self-stimulation: A hypothesis. Brain Res 73:381-419.

31. Gill K, Amit Z (1987) Effects of serotonin uptake blocade on food, water and ethanol consumption in rats. Alcohol Clin Exp Res 11:444-449.

32. Gill K, Amit Z (1989) Serotonin uptake blockers and voluntary alcohol consumption. A review of recent studies. In Galanter M (ed) Recent Developments in Alcoholism, Vol 7. Plenum Press: New York, pp 225-248.

33. Gill K, Amit Z, Koe BK (1988) Treatment with sertraline, a new serotonin uptake inhibitor, reduces voluntary ethanol consumption in rats. Alcohol 5:349-354.

34. Gill K, Amit Z, Ögren S-O (1984) Selective depletion of norepinephrine in brain by N-2-chloroethyl-N-ethyl-2-bromobenzylamine fails to alter the voluntary consumption of ethanol in rats. Neuropharmacol 23:1379-1383.

35. Gill K, Amit Z, Ögren S-O (1985) The effects of zimeldine on voluntary ethanol consumption: Studies on the mechanism of action. Alcohol 2:343-347.

36. Gill K, Filion Y, Amit Z (1988) A further examination of the effects of sertraline on voluntary ethanol consumption. Alcohol 5:355-358.

37. Goudie AJ, Thornton EW, Wheeler TJ (1976) Effects of Lilly 110140, a specific inhibitor of 5-hydroxytryptamine uptake, on food intake and on 5-hydroxytryptophan-induced anorexia: Evidence for serotonergic inhibition of feeding. J Pharm Pharmacol 28:318-320.

38. Hakkinen HM, Kulonen E (1976) Ethanol intoxication and gamma-aminobutyric acid. J Neurochem 27:631-633.

39. Hill DR, Bowery NG (1981) 3-H-baclofen and H-GABA bind to bicuculline-insensitive GABA-B sites in the rat brain. Nature 290:149-152.

40. Hill SY (1974) Intraventricular injection of 5-hydroxytryptamine and alcohol consumption in rats. Biol Psychiat 8:151-158.

41. Ho AKS, Tsai CS, Chen R, Begleiter H, Kissin B (1974) Experimental studies on alcoholism. I. Increase in alcohol preference by 5,6-dihydroxytryptamine and brain acetylcholine. Psychopharmacol 40:101-107.

42. Hunt WA (1983) The effect of ethanol on GABAergic transmission. Neurosci Biobehav Rev 7:87-95.

43. Kiianmaa K (1976) Alcohol intake in the rat after lowering brain 5-hydroxytryptamine content by electrolytic midbrain raphe lesions, 5,6-dihydroxytryptamine or p-chlorophenylalanine. Med Biol 54:203-209.

44. Kiianmaa K (1980) Alcohol intake and ethanol intoxication in the rat: Effect of 6-OHDA-induced lesions on the ascending noradrenaline pathways. Eur J Pharmacol 64:9-19.

45. Kiianmaa K, Andersson K, Fuxe K (1979) On the role of ascending dopamine systems in control of voluntary ethanol intake and ethanol intoxication. Pharmacol Biochem Behav 10:603-608.

46. Kiianmaa K, Fuxe K, Jonsson G, Ahtee L (1975) Evidence for the involvement of central NA neurones in alcohol intake: Increased alcohol consumption after degeneration of the NA pathways to the cortex. Neurosci Lett 1:41-45.

47. Koechling UM, Smith BR, Amit Z (1990) Differential effects of catecholamine antagonists c ethanol induced excitation in mice. Psychopharmacol in press.

48. Kulonen E (1983) Ethanol and GABA. Med Biol 61:147-167.

49. Le Bourhis B, Uzan A, Aufrere G, LeFur G (1981) Effects of Indalpin, a specific 5-HT uptake inhibitor, on the ethanol behavioral dependence and on the voluntary ethanol consumption in rats. Ann Pharmaceut Fran 39:11-20.

50. Leger L, Descarries L (1978) Serotonin nerve terminals in the locus coeruleus of adult rat: A radioautographic study. Brain Res 145:1-13.

51. Lester D (1966) Self-selection of alcohol by animals, human variation and the etiology of alcoholism: A critical review. Quart J Stud Alcohol 28:395-438.

52. Levy AD, Ellison G (1985) Amphetamine-induced enhancement of ethanol consumption: Role of central catecholamines. Psychopharmacol 86:233-236.

53. Liljequist S, Engel J (1982) Effects of GABAergic agonists and antagonists on various ethanol-induced behavioral changes. Psychopharmacol 78:71-75.

54. Linseman MA (1990) Effects of dopaminergic agents on alcohol consumption by rats in a limited access paradigm. Psychopharmacol 100:195-200.

55. Mason ST, Corcoran ME, Fibiger HC (1979) Noradrenaline and ethanol intake in the rat. Neurosci Lett 12:137-142.

56. Matsumoto RR (1989) GABA receptors: are cellular differences reflected in function? Brain Res Rev 14:203-225.

57. McRae-Degueurce A, Dennis T, Leger L, Scatton B (1985) Regulation of noradrenergic neuronal activity in the rat locus coeruleus by serotonergic afferents. Physiol Psychol 13: 188-196.

58. Meisch RA (1977) Ethanol self-administration: Infrahuman studies. In Thompson T, Dews PB (eds) Advances in Behavioral Pharmacology, Vol 1. Academic Press: New York, pp 35-84.

59. Melchior C, Myers RD (1976) Genetic differences in ethanol drinking of the rat following injection of 6-OHDA, 5,6-DHT or 5,7-DHT into the cerebral ventricles. Pharmacol Biochem Behav 5:63-72.

60. Montgomery AMJ, Burton MJ (1986) Effects of peripheral 5-HT on consumption of flavoured solutions. Psychopharmacol 88:262-266.

61. Mudar PJ, LeCann NC, Czirr SA, Hubbell CL, Reid LD (1986) Methadone, pentobarbital, pimozide and ethanol-intake. Alcohol 3:303-308.

62. Murphy JM, Waller MB, Gatto CJ, McBride WJ, Lumeng L, Li T-K (1985) Monoamine uptake inhibitors attenuate ethanol intake in alcohol-preferring (P) rats. Alcohol 2:349-352.

63. Myers RD, Martin GE (1973) The role of cerebral serotonin in the ethanol preference of animals. Ann NY Acad Sci 215:135-144.

64. Myers RD, Melchior CL (1975) Alcohol drinking in the rat after destruction of serotonergic and catecholaminergic neurons in the brain. Res Comm Chem Pathol Pharmacol 10:363-378.

65. Myers RD, Veale WL (1968) Alcohol preference in the rat: Reduction following depeletion of brain serotonin. Science 160:1469-1471.

66. Naranjo CA, Sellers EM, Roach CA, Woodley DV, Sanchez-Craig M, Sykora K (1984) Zimelidine induced variations in ethanol intake in non-depressed heavy drinkers. Clin Pharmacol Ther 35:374-381.

67. Naranjo CA, Sellers EM, Sullivan JT, Woodley DV, Kadlec K, Sykora K (1987) The serotonin uptake inhibitor citalopram attenuates ethanol intake. Clin Pharmacol Ther 41:266-274.

68. Olds ME, Fobes JL (1981) The central basis of motivation: Intracranial self-stimulation studies. Ann Rev Psychol 32:523-574.

69. Pfeffer AO, Samson HH (1986) Effect of pimozide on home cage ethanol drinking in the rat: Dependence on drinking session length. Drug Alcohol Depend 17:47-55.

70. Pfeffer AO, Samson HH (1988) Haloperidol and apomorphine effects on ethanol reinforcement in free feeding rats. Pharmacol Biochem Behav 29:343-350.

71. Pickel VM, Joh TH, Reis DJ (1977) A serotonergic innervation of noradrenergic neurons in nucleus locus coeruleus: Demonstration by immunocytochemical localization of the transmitter specific enzymes tyrosine and tryptophan hydroxylase. Brain Res 131:197-214.

72. Potthoff AD, Ellison G (1982) Low-level continuous amphetamine selectively increases alcohol consumption. Psychopharmacol 77:242-245.

73. Reimann W (1983) Inhibition by GABA, baclofen and gabapentin of dopamine release from rabbit caudate nucleus: Are there common or different sites of action? Eur J Pharmacol 94:341-344.

74. Richardson JS, Novakovski DM (1978) Brain monoamines and free choice ethanol consumption in rats. Drug Alcohol Depend 3:253-264.

75. Rockman GE, Amit Z, Bourque C, Brown Z, Ögren S-O (1080) Reduction of voluntary morphine consumption following treatment with zimelidine. Arch Int Pharmacodyn Ther 244:123-129.

76. Rockman GE, Amit Z, Brown Z, Bourque C, Ögren S-O (1982) An investigation of the mechanism of action of 5-hydroxytryptamine in the suppression of ethanol intake. Neuropharmacol 21:341-347.

77. Rockman GE, Amit Z, Carr G, Brown Z, Ögren S-O (1979) Attenuation of ethanol intake by 5-hydroxytryptamine uptake blockade in laboratory rats. I. Involvement of brain 5-hydroxytryptamine in the mediation of the positive reinforcing properties of ethanol. Arch Int Pharmacodyn Ther 241:245-259.

78. Rockman GE, Amit Z, Carr G, Ögren S-O (1979) Attenuation of ethanol intake by 5-hydroxytryptamine uptake blockade in laboratory rats. II. Possible interaction with brain norepinephrine. Arch Int Pharmacodyn Ther 241:260-265.

79. Schofield PR, Darlison MG, Fujita N, Burt DR, Stephenson FA, Rodriguez H, Rhee LM, Ramachandran J, Reale V, Glencorse TA, Seeburg PH, Barnard EA (1987) Sequence and functional expression of the GABA-A receptor shows a ligand-gated receptor super-family. Nature 328:221-227.

80. Shaskan GE, Snyder SH (1970) Kinetics of serotonin accumulation into slices from rat brain: Relationship to catecholamine uptake. J Pharmacol Exp Ther 175:404-418.

81. Shizgal P, Murray B (1989) Neuronal basis of intracranial self-stimulation. In Liebman JM, Cooper SJ (eds) The Neuropharmacological Basis of Reward. Clarendon Press: Oxford, pp 106-163.

82. Simmonds M (1982) Classification of some GABA antagonists with regard to site of action and potency in slices of rat cuneate nucleus. Eur J Pharmacol 80:347-358.

83. Sirota P, Boland FG (1987) A role for taste aversion learning in FLA-57 induced reductions of voluntary alcohol intake. Alcohol 4:21-24.

84. Smith BR, Amit Z (1985) The role of gamma-aminobutyric acid (GABA) in the regulation of ethanol and acetaldehyde self-administration. Prog Neuro-Psychopharmacol Biol Psychiat 9:759-763.

85. Smith BR, Robidoux J, Amit Z (1990) GABAergic involvement in the acquisition of voluntary ethanol intake in laboratory rats. Alcohol Clin Exp Res, submitted.

86. Smith BR, Segal RB, Amit Z (1989) Administration of a GABA antagonist selectively attenuates an ethanol-induced conditioned taste aversion. Pharmacol Biochem Behav 33:269-271.

87. Spivak K, Amit Z (1986) The effects of pimozide on drinking behavior in the rat: An investigation using the conditioned taste aversion paradigm. Pharmacol Biochem Behav 24:1527-1531.

88. Stein L (1969) Chemistry of purposive behavior. In Tapp JT (ed) Reinforcement and Behavior. Academic Press: New York, pp 328-355.

89. Suzdak PD, Gianutsos G (1985) Parallel changes in the sensitivity of gamma-aminobutyric acid and noradrenergic receptors following chronic administration of antidepressant and GABAergic drugs. A possible role in affective disorders. Neuropharmacol 24:217-222.

90. Suzdak PD, Gianutsos G (1985) Differential coupling of GABA-A and GABA-B receptors to the noradrenergic system. J Neur Trans 62:77-89.

91. Tombaugh TN, Tombaugh J, Anisman H (1979) Effects of dopamine receptor blockade on alimentary behaviors: Home cage food consumption, magazine training, operant acquisition and performance. Psychopharmacol 66:219-225.

92. Ungerstedt U (1971) Stereotaxic mapping of the monoamine pathways in the rat brain. Acta Physiol Scand 367:1-48.

93. Wise RA (1973) Voluntary ethanol intake in rats following exposure to ethanol on various schedules. Psychopharmacol 29:203-210.

94. Wise RA (1980) Action of drugs of abuse on brain reward systems. Pharmacol Biochem Behav 13(Suppl. 1):213-223.

95. Zabik JE, Binkerd K, Roache JD (1985) Serotonin and ethanol aversion in the rat. In Naranjo CA, Sellers EM (eds) Research Advances in New Psychopharmacological Treatments for Alcoholism. Excerpta Medica: Amsterdam, pp 87-101.

96. Zabik JE, Liao S, Jeffreys M, Maickel RP (1978) The effects of DL-5-hydroxytryptophan on ethanol consumption by rats. Res Comm Chem Pathol Pharmacol 20:69-78.

97. Zabik JE, Roache JD (1983) 5-Hydroxytryptophan-induced conditioned taste aversion to ethanol in the rat. Pharmacol Biochem Behav 18:785-790.

98. Zigmond MJ, Acheson AL, Chiodo LA, Stricker EM (1981) Increased norepinephrine turnover and increased firing rate in residual neurons after NE-depleting lesions. Soc Neurosci Abstr 7:456.

99. Zigmond MJ, Stricker EM (1973) Recovery of feeding and drinking by rats after intraventricular 6-hydroxydopamine or lateral hypothalamic lesions. Science 182:717-720.

15

Agents Which Modify Channels as Potential Treatments in Alcohol Withdrawal

J.M. Littleton and O. Bouchenafa

Introduction

The genesis of alcohol physical dependence is usually viewed as a consequence of adaptive mechanisms within the central nervous system. In this scheme alcohol produces inhibitory effects on neurones by some mechanism and this evokes an opposing adaptation in these neurones. Removal of alcohol once neurones have adapted in this way exposes this adaptation which causes the hyperexcitability of the alcohol withdrawal syndrome.

In the clinical setting the alcohol withdrawal syndrome still represents a serious challenge. It is usually treated with sedative/tranquillizers which effectively suppress the signs of withdrawal. This treatment is unsatisfactory not least because it runs the risk of introducing another potentially dependence-producing drug into the clinical picture. It would be a more satisfactory approach, both theoretically and practically, if the withdrawal syndrome could be treated in some way which attacked the actual process of physical dependence rather than simply substituting one sedative for another.

In this paper we will consider the possible mechanisms which lead to the acute actions of ethanol and potential adaptations in the CNS to these actions. We will concentrate on the role of neuronal calcium flux in both the acute effects of ethanol and the adaptive response which these evoke. We will then describe experiments in cell cultures and animal models which show that drugs which modify calcium channel activity in vitro and in vivo are effective in reducing the severity of ethanol withdrawal seizures. The reasons for our concentration on the role of calcium are given below.

Background

There is a great deal of evidence that ethanol acutely can inhibit the depolarisation-induced entry of calcium into neurones (see below). Since calcium entry is crucial for the activation of neurones this effect could underlie the inhibitory effects of ethanol on neuronal excitability. We originally suggested in 1983 that adaptation to this acute effect of ethanol on calcium entry may be of importance in determining physical dependence on the drug(1). We suggested that the inhibitory effects of ethanol could be overcome by adaptive changes within nerves which increased their "calcium sensitivity" in some way(1). While ethanol is present in the brain this mechanism can contribute to drug tolerance whereas, on the removal of ethanol, it should lead to neuronal hyperexcitability and could therefore cause the ethanol withdrawal syndrome.

Acute effects of ethanol

Ethanol can reduce depolarisation-induced calcium entry into neurones in a variety of ways both direct and indirect. The drug probably has a direct effect on calcium flux through voltage-operated calcium channel (VOCC) proteins(2) by a non-specific effect within the membrane bilayer. A rather more selective effect on calcium entry through receptor-operated calcium channels (ROCC) is suggested by the inhibitory effect of ethanol on NMDA receptor activity while it has little effect on other receptors for glutamate(3).

These direct effects of ethanol on calcium flux may be relatively insignificant when compared with indirect effects. For example ethanol has been shown to have markedly potentiating effects on GABA receptor function leading to a potentiation of the effects of GABA on $GABA_A$ receptors(4). This effect of ethanol would be expected to inhibit the effect of depolarising influences on neurones and therefore to reduce calcium flux in the neurones carrying $GABA_A$ receptors.

In relation to which of these several effects, if any, is most closely related to sedative/tranquillizing effects of ethanol in the intact animal most evidence favours the effect on $GABA_A$ receptors. The most direct evidence comes from experiments using the imidazo diazepine RO 15-4513. This compound is able to inhibit the effects of ethanol on GABA-stimulated chloride flux in vitro(4), and can also overcome sedative/tranquillizing effects of ethanol at low doses in vivo(4).

Potential adaptive mechanisms

Clearly all these different effects of ethanol might well evoke different adaptive responses in neurones. However it is equally possible that a single adaptive strategy based on calcium flux could occur.

Given the probable importance of GABA in the actions of ethanol there has been a great deal of interest in the possibility of alterations in GABA receptor proteins playing some role in adaptation to ethanol. Despite this interest no consistent changes have emerged. In contrast there is recent evidence(5) that adaptive alterations (increases) in MK 801 binding sites, representing NMDA receptor proteins occur in animals after chronic ethanol treatment. These changes represent a potential response opposing the effects of ethanol on calcium flux since the NMDA receptor is a receptor-operated calcium channel.

We have been more interested in the possibility that changes may take place in voltage -operated calcium channels (VOCCs) to oppose the acute effect of ethanol. In this scheme the acute effect of the drug would be expected to evoke an increase in VOCCs which would confer a generalised hyperexcitability on neurones which had adapted in this way. This would oppose the inhibitory action of ethanol on cell excitability, causing tolerance, but it could also lead to increased excitation on removal of the drug. This hyperexcitability could cause the ethanol withdrawal syndrome.

These concepts are very simple and although they were originally developed from experiments in intact animals it would be much easier to investigate these possibilities in a simple system. Both my own group and that of Dr Ivan Diamond in San Fracisco have utilised cell cultures of adrenal origin to study the adaptive processes to ethanol involving calcium flux.

Cell culture models of ethanol dependence

Cells obtained from either bovine adrenals or a rat pheochromocytoma cell line (PC12 cells) resemble undifferentiated neurones and can be kept in primary culture for up to 3 weeks. They are easy to separate and to maintain in culture. Also they express a wide variety of receptor and ion channel proteins. In many respects they are ideal for studies on the cellular basis of drug tolerance and dependence.

Adrenal cells growing in culture release Catecholamines in response to depolarising stimuli as a result of calcium entry through different types of VOCCs. A major route of calcium entry linked to Catecholamine (CA) release is the Dihydropyridine (DHP) calcium channel antagonist-sensitive VOCC. Bovine adrenal chromaffin cells, which we have used extensively, release GABA as well as CAs. The GABA acts back on the cells which have just released it to inhibit further release of GABA and CAs by a $GABA_A$ receptor-mediated effect(6).

Ethanol is strongly inhibitory to CA release from these cells and this inhibition is sensitive to nanomolar concentrations of the imidazo diazepine RO 15-4513 suggesting that the effect of ethanol is largely a consequence of potentiation of released GABA(6).

In addition to their possessing DHP-sensitive VOCCs and $GABA_A$ receptors we have recently found that BACCs in culture also express NMDA receptors(7). The NMDA receptors can be activated by glutamate or NMDA to cause release of CAs from BACCs. Under concentrations of magnesium ions in the physiological range these NMDA receptors are inactive. The magnesium block can however be relieved by depolarisation.

Activation by the selective agonist, homocysteic acid , and inhibition by the selective antagonists amino phosphonovalerate and MK 801 confirm the response as NMDA receptor-mediated. In relation to this paper we have recently found that the compound acetyl homotaurine (calcium acamprosate or AOTAL) is a potent inhibitor of responses induced by NMDA receptor stimulation in bovine adrenal cells.

Chronic exposure to ethanol of Adrenal cells in culture.

When either PC12 cells or BACCs are exposed to ethanol for several days in culture the inhibitory effects of ethanol are lost(8,9). In addition removal of ethanol after this time is associated with a hyperexcitability in the cells which is manifest by enhanced release of CAs to some depolarising stimuli. These changes are what would be predicted in a cellular model of ethanol tolerance and dependence. The hyperexcitability in "withdrawal" could clearly be a consequence of increased numbers of VOCC proteins.

The VOCC proteins can be labelled using tritiated DHP calcium channel antagonist drugs. This technique of course labels only the VOCC sub-group which is sensitive to the DHP drugs but this is currently the only type susceptible to study in this way.

Both in PC12 cells(8) and in bovine adrenal cells(10) exposure to ethanol for a period of 6 days caused a very marked increase in the numbers of binding sites for [3H]DHPs. The increase reached a plateau after 4-6 days at between 175-350% of the control numbers of binding sites. Various techniques including calcium flux studies(11) and biochemical consequences of calcium entry(12) demonstrate that the increase in DHP binding sites probably represents an increase in functional VOCC proteins. This change could therefore be an adaptive response to ethanol opposing its inhibitory effects and conferring hyperexcitability on removal of the drug.

If this alteration in VOCC number is truly an adaptive response to the acute inhibitory effect of ethanol then prevention of this acute effect should remove the need for the adaptive response. The imidazo diazepine RO 15-4513 almost completely prevents the acute inhibitory effect of ethanol on BACCs in culture. Growth of these cells in medium containing ethanol and RO 15-4513 prevented the increase in DHP binding sites observed previously(4).

This result suggests strongly that the increase in DHP binding sites induced by growth in ethanol is an adaptive response to the effect of ethanol on $GABA_A$ receptors. Subsequently we have shown that benzodiazepine tranquillizers can have a similar effect when present in the culture medium for several days and that this effect is blocked by benzodiazepine receptor antagonists(13).

The increase in DHP-sensitive VOCCs which is caused by growth of these cells in ethanol can be prevented by inhibitors of protein synthesis (cycloheximide, anisomycin) or mRNA (lomofungin)(10). It is likely therefore that gene transcription is involved in the response.

Similar experiments utilising different inhihibitors suggests a complex series of signals link membrane calcium flux to intracellular second messengers and activation of protein kinases which eventually control expression of the VOCC gene(14). Ethanol and virtually any drug which inhibits electrical activity in these cells activates this pathway leading to an increase in the synthesis and insertion of calcium channel proteins in the neuronal membrane. This then opposes the inhibitory effect of the drug.

In relation to its potential role in ethanol dependence one of the crucial questions is "What functional change would an increase in this sub-type of VOCC have in the intact CNS?". Only if this question is answerable does this finding become verifiable in the intact animal.

Functional role of DHP-sensitive calcium channels

The DHP-sensitive VOCCs on mature neurones in the CNS do not appear to have much influence on neurotransmitter release. They may be primarily important on nerve cell bodies rather than nerve terminals. At this site VOCCs would be expected to play a role in the spread of excitatory depolarising influences over the neuronal membrane.

One potentially very important consequence of an increased number of these VOCCs would be removal of the "depolarisation-dependent" block by magnesium ions of the NMDA receptors on cell bodies and dendrites. This would confer dramatic hyperexcitability on affected neurones and would be a convincing potential explanation of the withdrawal syndrome in the intact animal.

Experiments on BACCs in culture support this possibility. The excitatory effects of glutamate are increased dramatically in cells removed from ethanol after several days(7). The increased response shows all the characteristics of an NMDA receptor-mediated response potentiated as a result of an increased susceptibility to depolarisation of the cell membrane(7).

Experiments on intact animals

Clearly these results in cell cultures have relevance to ethanol dependence only if they can be shown in intact, ethanol dependent animals. The increase in DHP binding sites has been shown in the cerebral cortices of rats exposed to ethanol for a period of 8-10 days by inhalation. The increase in DHP binding sites was almost exactly 50% and the animals showed evidence of a withdrawal syndrome when ethanol was removed(15). Brain slice preparations from these animals showed biochemical evidence of functional changes compatible with an increase in VOCC proteins(15).

These functional changes have been explored further by the researh group of my colleague Dr Hilary Little. Using the Hippocampal slice preparation from ethanol-dependent rodents she has been able to show evidence of hyperexcitability electrophyiologically(16). This in vitro counterpart of the ethanol withdrawal syndrome appears to be a consequence of increased responses to excitatory amino-acids as a result of increased DHP-sensitve VOCC activity(17).

Further evidence that this increase in DHP-sensitive VOCCs is related to the ethanol withdrawal syndrome comes from experiments which we have recently completed with Dr John Crabbe. Mice have been selectively bred for 26 generations for the severity of their withdrawal syndrome from alcohol. Since this is the only criterion used, very few trait-irrelevant genetic characteristics should have been co-selected. The withdrawal seizure prone (WSP) line show a 130% increase in their DHP binding sites in brain after chronic exposure to ethanol whereas the withdrawal seizure resistant (WSR) line show only a 25% increase(18). Clearly this suggests that the increase in DHP-sensitive VOCCs in brain is causally related to the genetic variability in the severity of the ethanol withdrawal syndrome.

Drug effects on ethanol withdrawal seizures

In addition to this genetic evidence there is considerable pharmacological evidence that DHP drugs can modify the ethanol withdrawal syndrome in intact animals. Not only can DHP calcium channel antagonists block the withdrawal syndrome, but the syndrome can be mimicked by DHP activators of the VOCCs(19). A puzzling finding is that chronic treatment with DHP calcium channel activators and inhibitors both appear to block the development of dependence(17), and (in cell cultures) prevent the increase in DHP binding sites associated with the prolonged presence of ethano(16).

Recently we have obtained evidence that inhibitors of NMDA receptors are also good inhibitors of alcohol withdrawal seizures. The NMDA receptor antagonist MK 801 can inhibit withdrawal seizures as can the compound calcium acamprosate (acetyl homotaurine). In experiments in cell cultures the latter drug is as effective as MK 801 on NMDA responses but it is less potent in vivo(20).

Implications for drug dependence

The evidence presented here suggests a very simple mechanism which could account for many of the changes which accompany ethanol physical dependence. The adaptive changes in response to ethanol which we have described here could also be of importance in other general-depressant drug dependency.

Any drug which inhibits the electrical excitability of a nerve for a prolonged period may evoke an increase in the genetic expression of calcium channel proteins. These oppose the inhibitory effects of the drug by making the neurone more susceptible to depolarising influences. This adaptive response can therefore provide a mechanism for tolerance.

If the adaptive mechanism just described persists after the drug has been removed from the brain (which we believe it does) then hyperexcitability in affected nerves will result. If these affected nerves are in pathways which are important in movement or autonomic control then the hyperexcitability will be expressed as a physical withdrawal syndrome. If it occurs in pathways with more subtle effects then either psychological changes will result or the withdrawal excitability may be completely "hidden".

Implications for therapy

One of the most important aspects of this hypothesis is that it holds out the hope of being able to control depressant drug withdrawal without simply substituting one drug of dependence with another.

The DHP calcium channel antagonists are not ideal because they have been developed for selectivity on the cardiovascular system rather than the CNS. As a result they may have severe cardiovascular side effects if used at the high doses needed to suppress ethanol withdrawal signs. The development of new CNS selective calcium channel antagonists, or the combination of DHP calcium channel antagonists in low doses with other drugs may provide a solution to these problems.

NMDA receptor antagonists too may have an important role to play if side effects can be controlled. Although inhibitors of

NMDA receptors should not have any important peripheral effects they are known to cause phencyclidine-like dissociative anesthesia and hallucinations. It is quite possible however that these side effects are restricted to the compounds which act by blocking the NMDA receptor calcium channel.

Calcium acamprosate (acetyl homotaurine) does not appear to act in this way (its structure is completely different and it does not influence MK 801 binding to preparations of brain membranes). In addition no evidence of CNS side effects have emerged in the considerable clinical experience with this drug. There is evidence that calcium acamprosate is an effective drug in limiting alcohol intake both in experimental animals(21) and in alcoholic patients(22). This drug may prove very valuable in the treatment of alcohol withdrawal states.

REFERENCES

1 Lynch M A & Littleton J M Possible association of alcohol tolerance with increased synaptic calcium sensitivity. Nature 303: 175-176, 1983.

2 Harris R A & Hood W F Inhibition of synaptosomal calcium uptake by ethanol. J. Pharmacol. Exp. Ther. 213: 562-568, 1980

3 Lovinger D M , White G & Weight F F Ethanol inhibits the NMDA activated ion current in hippocampal neurones. Science 243: 1721-1724, 1989.

4 Suzdak P D, Glowa J R, Crawley J N, Schwartz R D, Skolnick P & Paul S M. A selective imidazodiazepine antagonist of ethanol in the rat. Science 234: 1243-1247, 1986.

5 Hoffman P L, Rabe C S, Valverius P, Grant K A, Gulya K, Crabbe J C & Tabakoff B. The NMDA receptor is implicated in the acute effects of ethanol and ethanol withdrawal. International Society for Biomedical Research on Alcohol, Toronto 1990.

6 Brennan C H, Lewis A & Littleton J M. Membrane receptors involved in up-regulation of calcium channels in bovine adrenal chromaffin cells chronically exposed to ethanol. Neuropharmacol. 28; 1303-1307, 1989.

7 Cwynarski K, Bouchenafa O, Brennan C H & Littleton J M. Bovine adrenal cells grown in culture medium containing ethanol show hyperexcitability to glutamate. Alcohol & Alcoholism 24: 370, 1989.

8 Messing R O, Carpenter C L, Diamond I & Greenberg D A. Ethanol regulates calcium channels in clonal cells. Proc. Natl. Acad. Sci.83: 6213-6215, 1986.

9 Harper J C & Littleton J M. Development of tolerance to ethanol in cultured adrenal chromaffin cells. Alcoholism, Clin. Exp. Res. (in press).

10 Harper J C, Brennan C H & Littleton J M. Genetic up-regulation of calcium channels in a cell culture model of ethanol dependence. Neuropharmacol. 28: 1299-1302, 1989.

11 Greenberg D A, Carpenter C L & Messing R O. Ethanol-induced component of 45 Ca2+ uptake in PC 12 cells is sensitive to Ca2+ channel modulating drugs. Brain Res. 410: 143-146, 1987.

12 Brennan C H. The role of dihydropyridine-sensitive calcium channels in alterations of cell excitability associated with ethanol dependence. University of London Ph.D. thesis 1990.

13 Brennan C H & Littleton J M. Chronic exposure to anxiolytic drugs working by different mechanisms causes up-regulation of dihydropyridine binding sites on cultured bovine adrenal chromaffin cells. Neuropharmacol.(in press).

14 Brennan C H & Littleton J M. Second messenger systems involved in genetic regulation of Ca2+ channels in adrenal chromaffin cells. Neuropharmacol. (in press).

15 Dolin S J, Little H J, Hudspith M J, Pagonis C & Littleton J Increased dihydropyridine-sensitive calcium channels in rat brain may underlie ethanol physical dependence. Neuropharmacol.26: 275-280, 1987.

16 Little H J, Whittington M A, Dolin S J, Patch T L, Siarey R J & Ripley T. Evidence that neuronal calcium channels are involved in ethanol dependence. Brain Res. (in press).

17 Whittington M & Little H J. Nitrendipine prevents the ethanol withdrawal syndrome when administered chronically with ethanol prior to withdrawal. Br. J. Pharmacol. 94: 385P,1988.

18 Brennan C H, Crabbe J & Littleton J M. Genetic regulation of dihydropyridine sensitive calcium channels in brain may determine susceptibility to ethanol physical dependence. Neuropharmacol (in press).

19 Littleton J M Little H J, Dolin S J, Patch T & Whittington M A. Dihydropyridine calcium channel antagonists in ethanol withdrawal;effects of BAY K8644, stereospecificity and brain concentrations. Psychopharmacologia (in press).

20 Bouchenafa O, Cwynarski K & Littleton J M. Interactions between excitatory amino acids and AOTAL in a cell culture model of ethanol dependence. ISBRA meeting ,Toronto 1990.

21 Littleton J M, Dunnage J & Pagonis C. Alcohol dependence and modulation of calcium channels. In "Biomedical and Social aspects of Alcohol and Alcoholism" Eds Kuriyama K, Takada A & Ishii H. Elsevier Amsterdam 1988.

22 L'huintre J P, Daoust M, Moore N, Chretien P, Saligaut C, Tran G, Boismare F & Hillemand B. Ability of calcium bis acetyl homotaurine, a GABA agonist, to prevent relapse in weaned alcoholics. Lancet I, 8436: 1014-1016, 1985.

16

Management of Alcohol Consumption with Angiotensin Converting Enzyme Inhibitors: A Review of the Animal Findings

L.A. Grupp, G. Spinosa, and T. Lingham

The prevalence of alcoholism throughout the world is a significant problem in contemporary society. However, few if any demonstrably effective drug treatments have been developed and efforts to encourage the reduction in excessive intake have therefore been addressed at the sociological, political and educational levels. The present paper reviews our animal work showing that the angiotensin converting enzyme (ACE) inhibitors produce a significant, and reliable reduction in alcohol intake. Using either the two-bottle 24 hr choice procedure or the bout-producing limited access procedure we have seen that a variety of different ACE inhibitors including Captopril, Abutapril and the pro-drug formulations Enalapril and Benzapril can reduce alcohol intake in normotensive animals by as much as 50%. Animals with elevated renin levels (Two-Kidney,One-Clip hypertensive) show a faster onset of this effect, while animals with suppressed renin levels (Dahl Salt Sensitive hypertensive) do not appear to respond to ACE inhibitor treatment, suggesting that the initial level of activity in the renin-angiotensin system may be an important determinant of the speed and ability of ACE inhibition to attenuate alcohol intake. This effect does not appear to be related to an ACE inhibitor-induced reduction in blood pressure, increased thirst or altered pharmacokinetics. Taken together, these findings suggest that ACE inhibitors may be useful in the treatment of human alcohol abuse.

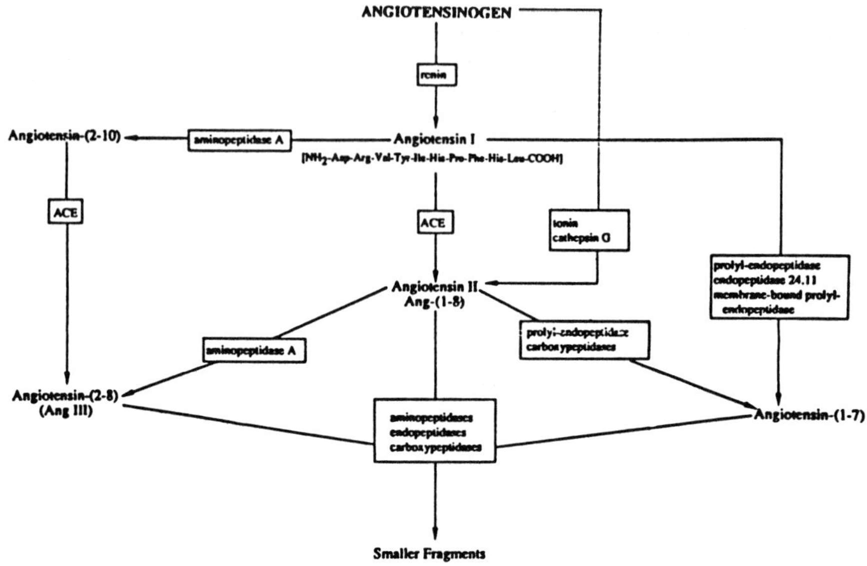

FIGURE 1. Schematic illustration of the pathways for the formation of angiotensin peptides. (From Ferrario et al. Hypertension 15 (Suppl 1): I13-I19, 1990.

THE RENIN-ANGIOTENSIN SYSTEM

The renin-angiotensin (R-A) system is involved in the endocrine control of blood pressure and fluid/electrolyte balance. The pathway for the formation and metabolism of Angiotensin II (ANG II), the biologically active element of the system is illustrated in Figure 1. Renin, a specific acid protease, cleaves the plasma protein angiotensinogen, which is formed in the liver, to produce the inactive decapeptide Angiotensin I (ANG I). Angiotensin converting enzyme splits off two amino acids from ANG I to form the octapeptide ANG II which is a potent pressor and dipsogenic agent. ANG II is then degraded by the aminopeptidases and carboxipeptidases to angiotensin III (ANG III), and other smaller fragments . In addition, aminopeptidase A can convert ANG I into a nonapeptide (DES ASP^1 Angiotensin I) which is then itself degraded by angiotensin converting enzyme into ANG III. Thus the development of agents which could prevent the formation of ANG II would have obvious utility in the treatment of hypertension. Ferreira (1965) was the first to describe a mixture of peptides found in the venom of the Brazilian arrowhead viper, Bothrops jararaca, which could enhance bradykinin effects. When it was subsequently demonstrated that one of these peptides could also inhibit the conversion of ANG I to ANG II (Bakhle 1968, Ferreira et al 1970), the search for a long lasting orally active form eventually resulted in the development of Captopril (Ondetti et al 1977). Inhibition of ANG II formation by active-site directed inhibitors such as Captopril or the pro-drug, Enalapril, has turned out to be a very effective therapeutic means to reduce blood pressure and treat congestive heart failure and is an important and increasingly popular approach to cardiovascular therapy.

Our interest in examining the effect of ACE inhibitors on alcohol intake came directly out of our previous work which demonstrated the direct involvement of the R-A system in modulating alcohol consumption (Grupp 1987, Stewart et al 1988). In particular we found that when activity in the R-A system was enhanced either by drugs, diet, or surgical intervention, alcohol consumption was severely curtailed and conversely that manipulations which lowered the level of R-A activity led to an increase in alcohol drinking. In this context we decided to assess the effect of the ACE inhibitors on alcohol intake with the expectation that since these drugs lower activity in the R-A system, they might increase alcohol intake. In fact what we found in a series of experiments and replications is that these drugs reduced alcohol consumption (Spinosa et al 1988, Lingham et al 1990). In what follows I shall review the results of these experiments and offer some possible explanations for this finding.

ACE INHIBITORS REDUCE ALCOHOL CONSUMPTION

Figure 2 illustrates the first experiment done with Captopril. In this experiment, two groups of rats, one with renin-dependent (i.e., high renin) hypertension, the other normotensive, were offered alcohol using the two bottle 24 hr choice procedure where food, water and a 4% w/v alcohol solution were continuously available. Renin-dependent hypertension or Two-Kidney, One-Clip (2-K,1-C) hypertension is produced by applying a silver clip to one renal artery and leaving the contralateral kidney intact (Goldblatt et al 1934). After a baseline period, Captopril was administered intraperitoneally twice daily for a total daily dose of 50 mg/kg for 11 days and then in a dose of 100 mg/kg for a further 11 days. Captopril reduced alcohol intake in both the normotensive and hypertensive rats. Blood pressure measured before and after Captopril treatment (Figure 3) was significantly reduced in both hypertensive and normotensive rats and the reduction in blood pressure in the normotensive rats to 100 mmHg which is low end of the normal range indicates that this reduction was not so great as to render these rats hypotensive.

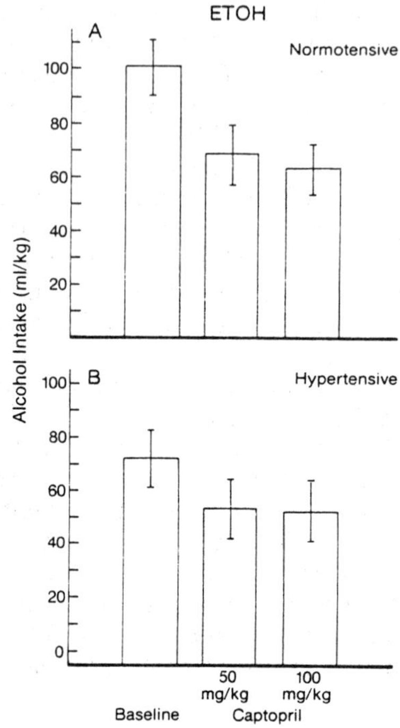

FIGURE 2. Average 24-hr alcohol intake in a group of normotensive and a group of 2-K,1-C hypertensive rats prior to (Baseline) and following the administration of two different doses of captopril. The drug was administered by the intraperitoneal route.

THE EFFECT OF ACE INHIBITORS ON ALCOHOL INTAKE IS NOT DEPENDENT ON A REDUCTION IN BLOOD PRESSURE

Is a reduction in blood pressure a necessary condition for the ACE inhibitors to reduce alcohol intake. To assess this, two groups of renin-dependent hypertensive rats were chronically treated with 1 mg/kg of Enalapril for 14 days during which they were offered limited access (1 hr) to 3% w/v alcohol. Water was continuously available but food was not present during this 1 hr period. Figure 4 shows that this dose of Enalapril was not sufficient to produce a significant change in blood pressure. However as is clearly shown

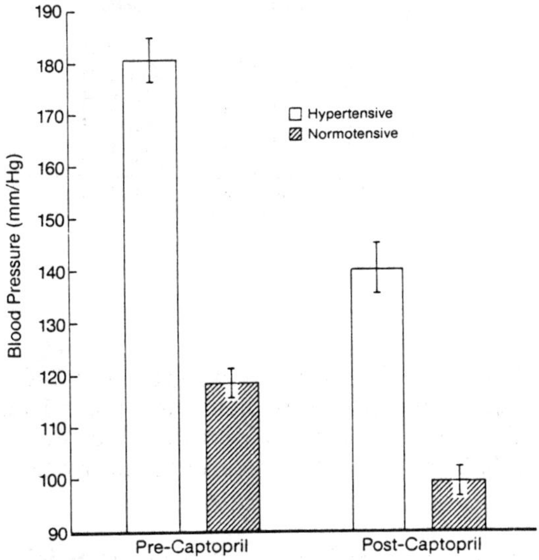

FIGURE 3. Mean blood pressure prior in the 2-K,1-C hypertensive rats and the normotensive rats before and after daily treatment with 100 mg/kg captopril. The drug was administered by the intraperitoneal route.

in Figure 5, this same dose of Enalapril produced a greater than 50% reduction in the consumption of alcohol. These findings suggest that the reduction in alcohol consumption is independent of any concomitant reduction in blood pressure.

BASAL RENIN LEVELS AND THE TIME COURSE OF THE ACE INHIBITOR EFFECT ON ALCOHOL INTAKE

In order to examine the time course of the reduction in alcohol intake mediated by the ACE inhibitors, 4 groups of normotensive animals were offered alcohol (6% w/v) using the limited access procedure and then treated for a further two weeks with either 5,10,20 mg/kg Abutapril or the saline vehicle. Figure 6A illustrates that Abutapril did not appear to influence alcohol consumption during the first week of treatment, but did produce a dose-dependent reduction in alcohol intake during the second week. In contrast, water intake was significantly elevated during both weeks of treatment (Figure 6B) suggesting that the reduction in alcohol intake during week two is not secondary to an increase in water intake. The prompt and

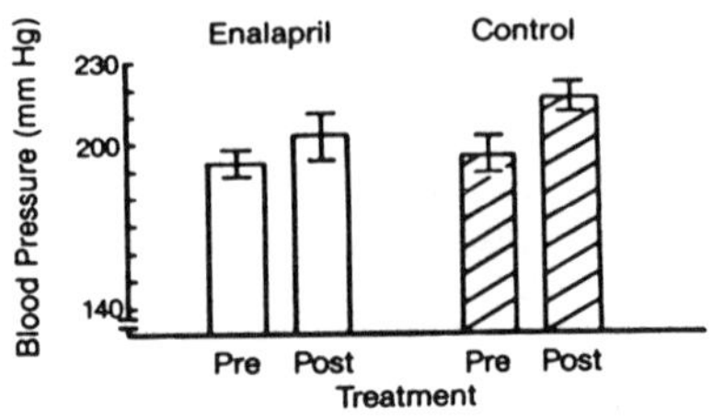

FIGURE 4. Mean blood pressure in two groups of 2-K,1-C hypertensive rats before and after treatment with either 1 mg/kg of enalapril or the saline vehicle (control). The drug and vehicle were administered by the intraperitoneal route.

sustained increase in water intake following ACE inhibitor treatment is a well-documented finding and has been linked to an increase in central R-A system activity (Schiffrin and Genest 1982, Rowland and Fregly 1988). The proposed mechanism of this increase in water consumption and its possible relationship to the reduced alcohol intake will be discussed below.

Alcohol abuse in humans is often accompanied by significant changes in cardiovascular function, the most notable of which is hypertension (Saunders et al 1981, Friedman et al 1983, Potter et al 1984). In this context, we attempted to examine the time course of the effect of ACE inhibitors on alcohol consumption in animals with two different forms of hypertension : a) the renin-dependent renovascular form as modelled by the Two-Kidney, One-Clip (2-K,1-C) high renin rat and b) the renin-independent form as modelled by the low renin genetically selected Dahl Salt Sensitive rat (Dahl 1961). The 2-K,1-C rats became hypertensive 3 weeks following application of a 0.2 mm solid silver clip. Systolic blood pressure was then measured and only those rats with pressures above 160 mmHg were used. The Dahl Salt sensitive rats were fed an 8% salt supplemented diet and as they became hyperetensive over a 3 week period, the salt concentration was reduced and then eliminated. As with the 2-K,1-C rats only those rats with pressures above 160 mmHg were used. The Dahl Salt sensitive rats start with low renin levels prior to the feeding of a salt supplemented diet (Iwai et al 1973, Rapp et al 1980).

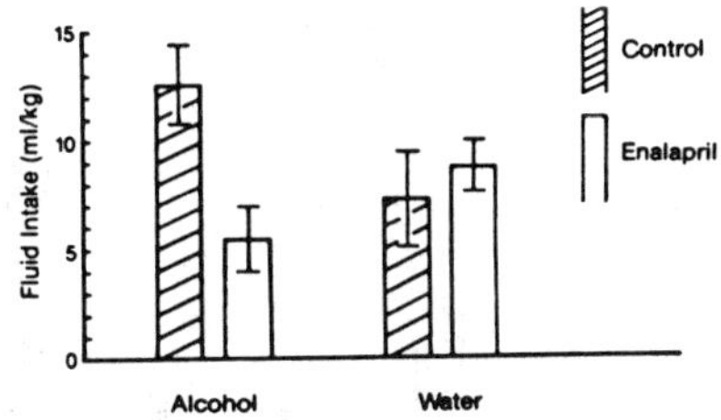

FIGURE 5. Average alcohol and water intake in the two groups of 2-K,1-C hypertensive rats which received either the saline vehicle or 1 mg/kg enalapril. The drug and vehicle were administered by the intraperitoneal route.

Figure 7 illustrates the alcohol intake in the high renin rats before Abutapril treatment (i.e. Baseline) and over the course of the two week Abutapril treatment period. The same 20 mg/kg dose which in normotensive rats was able to reduce alcohol consumption during the second week of treatment appeared to have a quicker onset of action in that it already reduced alcohol intake during the first week of treatment and continued to do so during the second week as well. Figure 8 illustrates the alcohol intake in the low renin rats before Abutapril treatment (i.e. Baseline and Saline injections) and over the course of the two week Abutapril treatment period. In contrast to the effects seen in both the normotensive and high renin rats, the same 20 mg/kg dose failed to alter alcohol consumption over the two week treatment period in these low renin rats. Taken together, these findings suggest that the basal level of renin activity is an important determinant of the effect of the ACE inhibitors on alcohol intake. Thus, when renin levels were normal or elevated as in the case of normotensive or 2-K,1-C hypertensive rats, respectively, 20 mg/kg of Abutapril produced a strong reduction in alcohol intake. Furthermore, the 2-K,1-C animals with the elevated renin levels were more responsive to the ACE inhibitor-induced decrease in alcohol intake as shown by the more rapid onset of the reduction in intake during the first week of Abutapril treatment. However, in the case of the Dahl Salt Sensitive rats with low renin levels, this same dose of Abutapril failed to have any impact on alcohol intake. Abutapril reduced blood pressure in both the 2-K,1-C rats (from 200 mmHg to 143 mmHg) and the Dahl Salt Sensitive rats (from 212 mmHg to 150 mmHg) but attenuated alcohol intake only in the 2-K,1-C rats again indicating that the effect of the ACE inhibitor on alcohol intake is

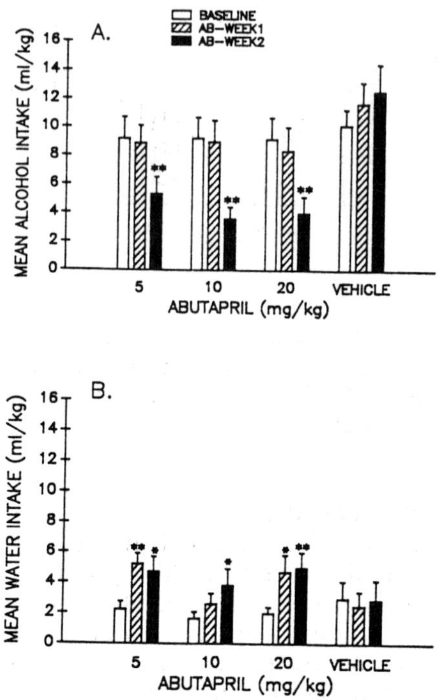

FIGURE 6. Mean alcohol intake (A) and water intake (B) in a saline vehicle group and in three groups receiving different doses of abutapril during baseline (i.e. no treatments) and during the subsequent two weeks of treatment (AB-WEEK1, AB-WEEK2) . All animals were normotensive. The drug and vehicle were administered by the intraperitoneal route.

not conditional upon a change in blood pressure. Taken together, these findings indicate that the effect of ACE inhibitors on alcohol intake may in part be dependent on the basal levels of renin at the time of ACE inhibitor administration.

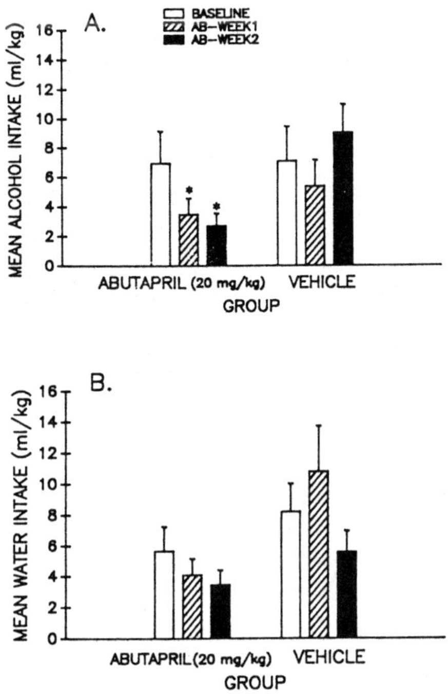

FIGURE 7. Mean alcohol intake (A) and water intake (B) in a saline vehicle group and in a group receiving 20 mg/kg of abutapril during baseline (i.e. no drug) and during the subsequent two weeks of treatment (AB-WEEK1, AB-WEEK2) . All animals were 2-K,1-C renin-dependent hypertensive rats. The drug and vehicle were administered by the intraperitoneal route.

POSSIBLE MECHANISMS OF THE EFFECT OF ACE INHIBITORS ON ALCOHOL INTAKE

The replicability of the reduction in alcohol intake by the ACE inhibitors indicates that this effect is a reliable one. By what mechanism(s) could the ACE inhibitors reduce alcohol intake? It is possible that the ACE inhibitors act on alcohol consumption through mechanisms other than the R-A system. For example, ACE inhibitors are also kininase and enkephalinase inhibitors thereby raising kinin and enkephalin levels (Williams and Hollenberg 1977, Norman et al 1985, Blum et al 1987). Captopril can also raise prostaglandin

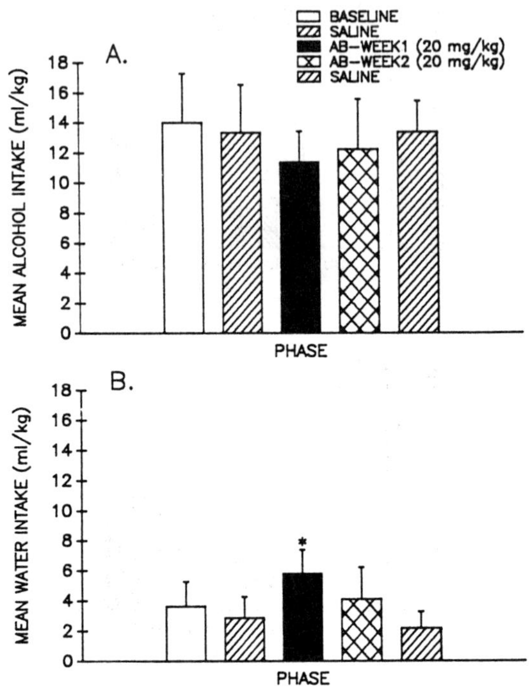

FIGURE 8. Mean alcohol intake (A) and water intake (B) in a group of low renin Dahl Salt sensitive hypertensive rats. The experiment consisted of a baseline phase (i.e. no drug) followed by a phase with daily saline injections followed by two weeks of daily drug treatment (AB-WEEK1, AB-WEEK2) with 20 mg/kg abutapril followed by a final saline injection phase. The drug and vehicle were administered by the intraperitoneal route.

levels (Abe et al 1980). It is possible that alcohol consumption may, in part, be suppressed by these or as yet unidentified extra-R-A system effects of ACE inhibitors. The ACE inhibitors, however, could actually reduce alcohol intake via the R-A system in the following way. ACE inhibitors increase renin and ANG I levels in the periphery because the decrease in ANG II synthesis they produce removes the feedback inhibition on renin release (Schiffrin and Genest 1982, Brunner et al 1987, DiNicolantonio 1984). Elevated concentrations of ANG I in the plasma could gain access to sites in the central nervous system not accessible to the ACE inhibitors themselves, there to be converted to ANG II and thereby produce a reduction in alcohol intake. Support for the suggestion that ACE inhibitors may raise central ANG II levels comes from the finding that the increase in water intake produced by peripherally administered Captopril could be blocked by the concomitant central administration of Captopril (Schiffrin and Genest 1982, DiNicolantonio 1984). It is therefore possible that as a consequence of lowering peripheral ANG II, the ACE inhibitors may also produce an elevation in central ANG II levels which mediate the reduction in alcohol consumption. Alternatively, ANG I might be converted in the periphery to the naturally occurring ANG I fragment Des Asp^1ANG I because ACE inhibitors do not inhibit the aminopeptidase A which converts ANG I to this fragment. If Des Asp^1ANG I is active and can reduce alcohol intake, it may mediate some of the effects of the ACE inhibitors on alcohol intake.

If elevated levels of renin and consequently the angiotensins are an important part of the effect of the ACE inhibitors on alcohol intake, we hypothesize that the process they participate in may be one related to satiety (Grupp 1987, Grupp et al 1988). This process would monitor levels of activity in the R-A system and send a "stop" signal to halt alcohol consumption once the level of activity is sufficiently elevated to enter a satiety range. Thus, any manipulation which would alter basal levels of R-A activity would have the potential to increase intake if the basal level were to be shifted away from the satiety range or to decrease intake if basal level were to be moved closer to the putative satiety range. Thus, the failure of the Dahl salt sensitive rats to respond to ACE inhibitor treatment would be related to their low levels of basal R-A activity which would therfore require a greater degree of change in the R-A activity in order to achieve satiety. On the other hand, the increased responsiveness in the 2-K,1-C hypertensive rats would be related to their elevated levels of R-A activity which would consequently require a smaller degree of change in R-A system activity in order to achieve satiety. This could translate into a more rapid onset of effect as observed in the present experiments.

In summary, the basal level of activity in the R-A system appears to be an important setting condition in determining the ability of the ACE inhibitors to reduce alcohol intake in laboratory animals. Pretreatment screening of plasma renin levels may be a useful and convenient way of selecting those patients who might benefit most from this treatment.

REFERENCES

Abe K, Itoh T, Satoh M, Haruyama T, Imai Y, Goto T, Satoh K, Otsuka Y, Yoshinaga K: Indomethacin inhibits enhanced renin release following captopril, SQ 14225, administration. Life Sci 26: 561-565, 1980.

Bakhle YS Conversion of angiotensin I to angiotensin II by cell-free extracts of dog lung. Nature 220: 919-921, 1968.

Blum K, Briggs AH, Trachtenberg MC, Delallo L, Wallace JE: Enkephalinase inhibition: Regulation of ethanol intake in genetically predisposed mice. Alcohol 4:449-456, 1987.

Brunner HR, Waeber B, Nussberger J: Pharmacology of converting enzyme inhibitors. Clin Exp Hypertension A9(2&3): 257-288, 1987.

Dahl LK: Effects of chronic excess salt feeding. Induction of self sustaining hypertension in rats. J. Exp. Med. 114:231-236, 1961.

DiNicolantonio R: Angiotensin converting enzyme blockade and thirst. Clin. Exp. Hyperten A6: 2025-2029, 1984.

Ferreira SH: A bradykinin-potentiating factor (BPF) present in the venom of Bothrops jararaca. Br J Pharm 24: 163-169, 1965.

Ferreira SH Greene LJ Alabaster VA Bakhle YS: Activity of various fractions of bradykinin potentiating factor against angiotensin I converting enzyme . Nature 225: 379-380,1970.

Friedman GD, Klatsky AL, Siegelaub AB: Alcohol intake and hypertension. Annals Int Med 98: 846-849, 1983.

Goldblatt H, Lynch J, Hanzal RF, Summerville WW:
Studies on experimental hypertension. The production of persistent elevation of the systolic blood pressure by means of renal ischemia. J. Exp. Med. 59: 347-360, 1934.

Grupp LA: Alcohol satiety, hypertension and the renin-angiotensin system. Medical Hypotheses 24: 11-19, 1987.

Grupp LA, Perlanski E, Leenen FHH, Stewart RB: Voluntary alcohol intake is attenuated in Two-Kidney,One-Clip but not in One-Kidney, One-Clip Goldblatt hypertensive rats. Alcohol 5: 173-179, 1988.

Iwai J, Dahl LK, Knudsen KD: Genetic influences on the renin-angiotensin system. Low renin activities in hypertension prone rats. Circ. Res. 32: 678-684, 1973.

Lingham TL, Perlanski E, Grupp LA: Angiotensin converting enzyme inhibitors reduce alcohol consumption: Some possible mechanisms and important conditions for their therapeutic use. Alcoholism: Clin Exp Res 14: 92-99, 1990.

Norman JA, Autry WL, Barbaz BS: Angiotensin converting enzyme inhibitors potentiate the analgesic activity of [Met]-Enkephalin-Arg^{6}-Phe^{7} by inhibiting its degradation in mouse brain. Mol. Pharmacol. 28: 521-526, 1985.

Ondetti MA Rubin B Cushman DW Design of specific inhibitors of angiotensin converting enzyme: A new class of orally active antihypertensive agents Science 196: 441-444, 1977.

Potter JF,Bannan LT Beevers DG: Alcohol and hypertension. Br J Addict 79: 365-372, 1984.

Rapp JR, McPartland RP, Sustarsic DL: A qualitative difference in plasma renin activity in Dahl rats susceptible or resistant to salt-induced hypertension. Biochem Genet 18: 1087-1096, 1980.

Rowland NE. Fregly MJ: Sodium appetite: Species and strain differences and role of renin-angiotensin-aldosterone system. Appetite 11: 143-178, 1988.

Saunders JB, Beevers DG, Paton A: Alcohol induced hypertension. Lancet 2: 653-656, 1981.

Schiffrin EL, Genest J: Mechanism of captopril-induced drinking. Am. J. Physiol. 242: R136-R140, 1982.

Spinosa G, Perlanski E, Stewart RB, Grupp LA: Angiotensin converting enzyme inhibitors: Animal experiments suggest a new pharmacological treatment for alcohol abuse in man. Alcoholism: Clin Exp Res 12: 65-70, 1988.

Stewart RB, Perlanski E, Grupp LA: Ethanol as a reinforcer for rats: Factors of facilitation and constraint. Alcoholism: Clin Exp Res 12: 599-608, 1988.

Williams GH, Hollenberg NK: Accentuated vascular and endocrine response to SQ 20881 in hypertension. N Engl J Med 297: 184-188, 1977.

ACKNOWLEDGEMENTS

The authors would like to thank Ms Susan Loh for preparation of the typescript. This work was supported by the Addiction Research Foundation of Ontario and Ciba-Geigy Canada Ltd.

17

Enalapril Does not Decrease Alcohol Intake in Normotensive Alcoholics

C.A. Naranjo, K.E. Bremner, P. Sanhueza, and E.M. Sellers

1. ABSTRACT

Some studies in rats have found that angiotensin converting enzyme (ACE) inhibitors, e.g., enalapril (E), decrease alcohol intake. Therefore, we tested E in normotensive moderately dependent drinkers, (36 male, 6 female), aged 24 to 65 years, consuming 8.2+2.3 ($\bar{x}$+S.D.) standard alcoholic drinks per day. They were randomized to receive E 10 mg/day (n=20) or E 20 mg/day (n=22) and placebo (P) for 4 weeks each in a double-blind, crossover study. Patients monitored their alcohol intake, but received no other treatment. E 10 mg/day and P decreased mean daily drinks ($\bar{x}$+SEM) from baseline (8.1+0.5) to 7.5+0.5 and 7.2+0.5, respectively, (both $p<0.05$). The effects of E 10 mg/day and P did not differ. Decreases from baseline were also observed with E 20 mg/day (from 8.3+0.5 to 6.8+0.6, $p<0.01$) and its P (to 7.2+0.4, $p<0.01$), but the effects of E 20 mg/day and P did not differ. Responses varied: 14 (64%) of E 20 mg/day patients decreased their alcohol intake by 21% (range=1.6% to 78.3%) compared with P. Plasma renin activity increased from P with E 10 and E 20 mg/day (both $p<0.05$). Blood pressure decreased within the normotensive range, except for one patient who discontinued the study because of hypotension after 5 days of E 10 mg. Otherwise, side effects were few and mild. No variables correlated with changes in alcohol intake. Our findings suggest that enalapril may not be a potential treatment for alcoholism.

2. INTRODUCTION

Effective pharmacological treatments for alcoholism are yet to be developed, but studies with animals have identified several drugs which decrease alcohol consumption. For example, serotonin uptake inhibitors decreased ethanol intake in rats in a dose-dependent manner (Lawrin *et al*, 1986; Naranjo *et al*, 1986). These drugs have also been shown to decrease ethanol intake in humans with moderate alcohol dependence (Naranjo *et al*, 1984, 1987, 1989, 1990, 1991a). Some recent studies

---

Parts of this manuscript have been published in abstracts and other articles by the authors.

suggest that angiotensin converting enzyme inhibitors, such as enalapril and captopril, decrease ethanol intake in normotensive and hypertensive rats (Grupp, 1987; Grupp *et al*, 1991), but others detected only some effect (Brands *et al*, 1991). However, because of the potential clinical importance of angiotensin converting enzyme inhibitors, we tested the efficacy and safety of enalapril in decreasing alcohol intake in normotensive moderately dependent alcoholics.

3. METHODS

3.1 Study Design and Procedures

The randomized, double-blind, crossover trial consisted of an initial assessment, a two-week baseline period (pre-randomization), 4 weeks of enalapril 10 mg/day, enalapril 20 mg/day, or placebo, a two-week washout period (no drug treatment), and 4 weeks of the alternate treatment (placebo or one dose of enalapril) (Figure 1). At the initial

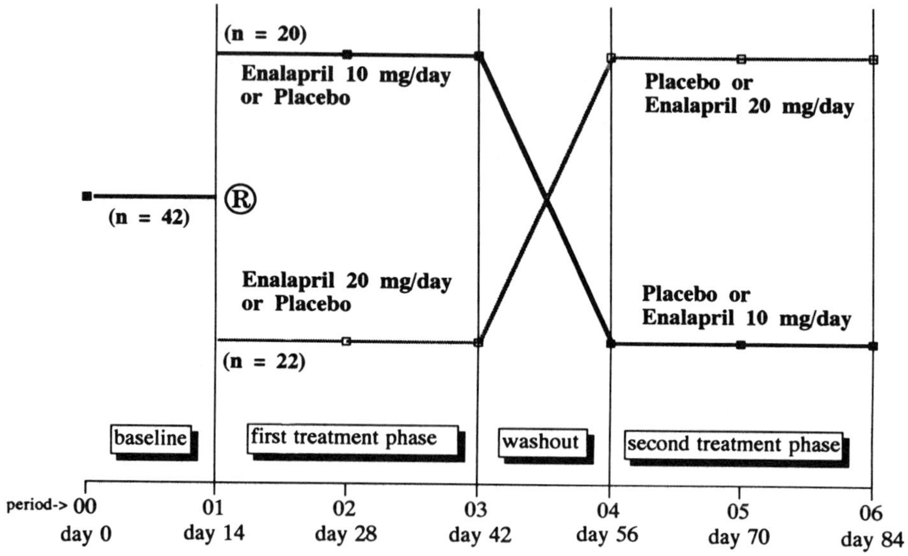

Fig. 1. Study Design

assessment, patients were screened for psychiatric and medical disorders, social stability and alcohol dependence and problems as in our previous studies (Naranjo *et al*, 1984, 1987, 1989, 1990, 1991a). Patients met DSM-III-R criteria for mild to moderate alcohol dependence (American Psychiatric Association, 1987).

During the first two weeks of the study (baseline) patients recorded their daily alcohol consumption (one standard drink = 13.6 g ethanol) on a self-monitoring form and took daily evening (10:00 p.m.) urine samples which were analyzed for ethanol and riboflavin concentrations. Those who complied with these procedures and reported at least 28 standard drinks and 4 drinking days per week were randomized to one of the enalapril/placebo treatment groups. In order to minimize the occurrence of side effects, the dose of each medication was gradually increased over one week. By day 7, patients were taking enalapril 10 mg/day, 20 mg/day, or placebo in two equal doses at 8:00 a.m. and 8:00 p.m. daily. To confirm compliance a separate riboflavin (20 mg) tablet was taken with the evening medication. After washout, the dose of each medication was again gradually increased. Daily throughout the study, patients recorded their alcohol intake, times of medication and took evening urine samples. They returned every 2 weeks for a physical examination and assessment of anxiety and depression. Also, following 15 minutes of rest in a recumbent position, blood samples were drawn for laboratory tests (hematology and liver and renal function) and for assay of enalapril concentration and plasma renin activity, details of which are described elsewhere (Naranjo *et al*, 1991b). A urine sample was taken to screen for drugs of abuse, and adverse events (using an open-ended questionnaire and a symptom checklist) were assessed. Patients monitored their daily alcohol intake and attended the biweekly assessments but did not receive any other pharmacologic or formal psychosocial treatment during the study.

3.2 Data Analysis

Alcohol intake (mean daily drinks, percent of days abstinent and drinks per drinking day), levels of serum gamma-glutamyl transpeptidase, which are related to alcohol intake (Orrego *et al*, 1985), blood pressure and plasma renin activity were assessed. Differences between each dose of enalapril and the respective placebo were determined with repeated measures analysis of covariance tests using baseline values as covariates. Also, treatment and baseline measures were compared with repeated measures analysis of variance. Since interindividual variations in clinical response were observed, Pearson correlations were used to relate decrease in alcohol intake with patient characteristics and other variables.

The daily self-reports of alcohol consumption were validated by correlation with the ethanol concentration in the daily urine samples. The frequencies of reported adverse events during enalapril and placebo were compared with McNemar's tests.

4. RESULTS

The complete results of the study are presented in detail elsewhere (Naranjo *et al*, 1991b). The most important findings are briefly discussed here.

4.1 Patients and Compliance

The 42 patients who completed the study were physically healthy, intelligent, socially stable, and had no evidence of clinical depression or anxiety. They met DSM-III-R criteria for mild to moderate alcohol dependence (American Psychiatric Association, 1987), and had been drinking at least 28 drinks per week for an average of 13 years. They were normotensive and their plasma renin activity levels were within the normal range for individuals on a normal diet (i.e., not low-sodium) (Tietz, 1986). There were no significant differences between those who received enalapril 10 mg/day ($n=20$) and those who received enalapril 20 mg/day ($n=22$) (ANOVAs, all $p>0.05$).

All measures of compliance confirmed adherence to the study protocol and the medication schedule, as well as complete and accurate monitoring of alcohol intake (Naranjo et al 1991b).

4.2 Plasma Renin Acitivity and Blood Pressure

Both doses of enalapril increased plasma renin activity compared to placebo (both $p<0.01$). The average increases of 1.6 ng/L/sec after enalapril 10 mg/day (Table 1) and 2.5 ng/L/sec after enalapril 20 mg/day (Table 2) were within the normal range for patients on a normal diet (Davies *et al*, 1984).

Table 1: Effects ($\bar{x}$+SEM) of enalapril 10 mg/day (n=20)

	Baseline	Enalapril	Placebo	p[1]
Plasma renin activity (ng/L/sec)	0.32+0.04	1.89+0.3	0.32+0.04	<.001
Systolic blood pressure (mmHg)	124.2+2.5	118.4+2.4	124.4+3.3	n.s.
Diastolic blood pressure (mmHg)	80.3+2.0	71.8+1.7	78.1+1.8	.005
Mean daily drinks	8.1+0.5	7.5+0.5	7.2+0.5	n.s.
% decrease from baseline		7.8+3.1	11.9+3.7	n.s.
Abstinent days (%)	2.3+1.1	3.8+1.7	7.2+2.2	n.s.
Drinks per drinking day	8.3+0.5	7.8+0.5	7.7+0.5	n.s.
Serum gamma-glutamyl transpeptidase (IU/L)	52.6+9.9	44.5+7.4	47.5+8.6	n.s.

[1]enalapril vs placebo in repeated measures analysis of variance tests with 1, n-1 degrees of freedom

Blood pressure slightly decreased with enalapril treatment but all 42 patients remained normotensive. The average decreases in systolic and diastolic blood pressures, from placebo, were 6.0 and 8.5 mmHg after 28 days of enalapril 10 mg/day treatment (Table 1), and 7.7 and 5.0 mmHg after enalapril 20 mg/day treatment (Table 2). One patient dropped out of the study because of lowered blood pressure and lightheadedness, as described in the Adverse Events Section.

4.3 Alcohol Intake

In repeated measures analysis of covariance tests using baseline values as covariates, neither dose of enalapril significantly changed any of the measures of alcohol intake compared with its placebo (Tables 1 and 2). However, both enalapril 10 mg/day and its placebo reduced mean daily drinks compared with baseline (both $p<0.05$), (Table 1). Enalapril 20 mg/day and its placebo also reduced alcohol intake from baseline (both

Table 2: Effects ($\bar{x}$+SEM) of enalapril 20 mg/day (n=22)

	Baseline	Enalapril	Placebo	p[1]
Plasma renin activity (ng/L/sec)	0.28+0.05	2.75+0.8	0.39+0.07	<.01
Systolic blood pressure (mmHg)	124.3+2.8	116.6+2.5	122.3+2.5	<.05
Diastolic blood pressure (mmHg)	79.1+2.3	74.2+2.2	77.7+2.2	n.s.
Mean daily drinks	8.3+0.5	6.8+0.6	7.2+0.4	n.s.
% decrease from baseline		20.0+4.1	11.0+3.5	n.s.
Abstinent days (%)	5.2+1.9	8.6+3.8	3.9+1.9	n.s.
Drinks per drinking day	8.8+0.6	7.3+0.5	7.5+0.4	n.s.
Serum gamma-glutamyl transpeptidase (IU/L)	51.1+8.0	47.2+7.0	47.4+7.6	n.s.

[1]enalapril vs placebo in repeated measures analysis of variance tests with 1, n-1 degrees of freedom

$p<0.01$), (Table 2). However, the decrease from baseline with enalapril 20 mg/day (1.5 drinks per day) was significantly greater than with enalapril 10 mg/day (0.6 drinks per day) ($p<0.05$). Order of treatment (enalapril or placebo first) had no significant effect on alcohol intake.

Only 13 (65%) of the patients who received enalapril 10 mg/day and 10 (45%) of those who received enalapril 20 mg/day had any abstinent days during the 12 weeks of the study. Percent of days abstinent did not change with enalapril 10 mg/day or 20 mg/day treatments compared with their placebos or baselines (all $p>0.05$), (Tables 1 and 2).

Drinks per drinking day were not different during enalapril 10 mg/day and its placebo ($p>0.05$). The change from baseline to enalapril was also not significant, but placebo decreased drinks per drinking day from baseline ($p<0.05$) (Table 1). Drinks per drinking day during enalapril 20 mg/day decreased from baseline ($p<0.01$), but not compared with placebo ($p>0.05$). The baseline to placebo decrease was also significant ($p=0.001$), (Table 2).

Serum gamma-glutamyl transpeptidase (SGGTP) levels decreased significantly from baseline to the end of enalapril 10 mg/day treatment ($p<0.05$), (Table 1), and from baseline to the end of enalapril 20 mg/day treatment ($p<0.05$), (Table 2), and non-significantly with their placebos. Enalapril did not decrease SGGTP concentrations compared with placebo. These variations parallel those for reported drinks. There was a significant correlation between changes (enalapril 20 mg/day vs placebo) in alcohol intake and SGGTP ($r=0.41$, p(1-tail)<0.05).

The response to enalapril varied. Fourteen (64%) of the patients who received enalapril 20 mg/day decreased their alcohol intake compared with placebo by an average of 21% (range=1.6 to 78.3%). Response to enalapril 10 or 20 mg/day did not correlate with any patient characteristic, plasma renin activity, blood pressure, or enalapril concentration (Pearson correlations, all $p>0.05$).

A power analysis indicated that if enalapril 20 mg/day were capable of decreasing alcohol intake by 1.1 drink per day compared with placebo (a change similar to that detected with other agents, e.g., serotonin uptake inhibitors (Naranjo *et al* 1984, 1987, 1989, 1990, 1991a), we should have been able to detect it in 22 patients with 80% power at $\alpha = 0.05$. Thus, the inability to detect an overall effect is not due to a type 2 error (i.e. lack of power).

4.4 Attitudinal Responses to Alcohol

Desire, interest, craving and liking for alcohol were indicated on a 5-point scale (from 0=not at all, to 4=an awful lot) at each biweekly visit. Neither dose of enalapril had significant effects compared with placebo. Desire, interest and liking for alcohol decreased from baseline during both enalapril and placebo treatment periods for the patients in both dosage groups (all $p<0.05$). "Craving" showed no change.

4.5 Adverse Events

Three patients dropped out of the study because of symptoms possibly associated with enalapril. One patient experienced lightheadedness and decreased blood pressure (from 130/80 to 100/40 mmHg) after 5 days of treatment with enalapril 10 mg/day, one reported gastrointestinal symptoms after 7 days of enalapril 10 mg/day, and the other experienced gastrointestinal symptoms one day after discontinuing enalapril 20 mg/day. All three had complied with the titration procedure.

For the 42 patients who completed the study, adverse events were few and mild (e.g. headache, fatigue, anxiety during both enalapril and placebo). No symptom was reported more frequently during enalapril than placebo (McNemar's tests, all $p>0.05$).

5. DISCUSSION

This study indicates that enalapril 10 mg/day and 20 mg/day had no significant overall effect on alcohol consumption in normotensive, moderately alcohol-dependent patients. However, enalapril 20 mg/day did reduce alcohol consumption in 14 (64%) of 22 patients by an average of 21% (range from 1.6% to 78.3%) compared with placebo. The inability to detect a statistically significant effect of a clinically important magnitude was not due to insufficient sample size. In addition, we detected no variation in liking or desire for alcohol. Other drugs (e.g., serotonin uptake inhibitors) which reduced alcohol intake also reduced desire to drink (Naranjo *et al*, 1989, 1990, 1991a).

This study did not confirm the effects of enalapril detected in some studies in rats. However, some recent animal studies indicate that response to angiotensin converting enzyme inhibitors may be dependent upon basal plasma renin activity (Grupp *et al*, 1991). When genetically-bred salt-sensitive rats with low basal plasma renin activity were made hypersensitive with a salt-supplemented diet, they did not reduce their alcohol intake when administered the angiotensin converting enzyme inhibitor, abutapril. When Wistar rats, which have elevated basal plasma renin activity, were made hypertensive with the two-kidney, one-clip method, they did decrease their alcohol intake when administered abutapril (Lingham *et al*, 1990). In the present clinical trial with enalapril, patient selection, for health and safety reasons, ensured that all were normotensive and had normal plasma renin activity. This may explain our inability to detect any relationships between drinking, response to enalapril, blood pressure and plasma renin activity. No other patient characteristic could be identified as a predictor of response. As would be expected with an angiotensin converting enzyme inhibitor, plasma renin activity increased and blood pressure decreased during enalapril treatment. Except for one patient who had to discontinue because of lowered blood pressure, all patients remained normotensive. Otherwise, adverse side effects were few and mild and could not account for the variation in response.

In some studies in rats, enalapril slightly decreased alcohol intake (Brands *et al*, 1991; Hubbell *et al*, 1990), perhaps due to non-specific malaise (Hubbell *et al*, 1990) or inhibition of acetaldehyde dehydrogenase (Guivernau *et al*, 1990). The results of our study illustrate the difficulties and vagaries of extrapolating from animals to humans. The predictive values of most animal models remain untested (Naranjo *et al*, 1991c). Therefore, it is necessary to test the effects of medications in humans to determine their potential clinical value.

Higher doses of enalapril may have produced a clinically important decrease in alcohol intake. However, the frequency and severity of side effects might increase, making this impractical even in hypertensive alcoholics. Therefore, angiotensin converting enzyme inhibitors do not seem to be promising agents for treating alcoholics.

6. ACKNOWLEDGEMENTS

We thank the staff of the Clinical Research Unit, Addiction Research Foundation, Toronto, Ontario, Canada, for their help in conducting the study and Merck Frosst Canada, Dorval, Quebec, Canada, for providing enalapril.

7. REFERENCES

American Psychiatric Association (1987). DSM-III-R Diagnostic and Statistical Manual of Mental Disorders (Third Edition-Revised), Washington D.C.

Brands, B., C.A. Naranjo, R. Collis, and E.M. Sellers (1991). Effects of angiotensin converting enzyme inhibitors on free choice ethanol consumption by rats. In: *Novel Pharmacological Interventions for Alcoholism* (C.A. Naranjo, E.M. Sellers eds.), Springer-Verlag New York Publishers, New York .

Davies, R.D., H.J. Gomez, J.D. Irvin, and J.F. Walker (1984). An overview of the clinical pharmacology of enalapril. *Br. J. Clin. Pharmacol.*, 18 (supplement 2), 215-229.

Grupp, L.A. (1987). Alcohol satiety, hypertension and the renin-angiotensin system. *Medical Hypotheses*, 24, 11-19.

Grupp, L.A., G. Spinosa, and T. Lingham (1991). Management of alcohol consumption with angiotensin converting enzyme inhibitors: a review of the animal findings. In: *Novel Pharmacological Interventions for Alcoholism* (C.A. Naranjo, E.M. Sellers eds.), Springer-Verlag New York Publishers, New York.

Guivernau, M., M.E. Quintanilla, and L. Tampier (1990). Effect of dipyridamole and captopril on prostacyclin production and ALDH activity (abstract). *Alcohol Clin. Exper. Res.*, 14, 295.

Hubbell, C.L., G.A. Chrisbacher, E.J. Bilsky and L.D. Reid (1991). Angiotensin converting enzyme inhibitors and intake of an alcoholic beverage. *Abstracts, Symposium on Novel Pharmacological Interventions for Alcoholism*, Toronto, Canada. June 16-17, 1990 [abstract #39].

Lawrin, M.O., C.A. Naranjo and E.M. Sellers (1986). Identification and testing of new drugs for modulating alcohol consumption. *Psychopharmacol. Bull.*, 22, 1020-1025.

Lingham, T., E. Perlanski, L.A. Grupp (1990). Angiotensin converting enzyme inhibitors reduce alcohol consumption: some possible mechanisms and important conditions for its therapeutic use. *Alcohol Clin. Exp. Res.*, 14, 92-99.

Naranjo, C.A., E.M. Sellers, and M.O. Lawrin (1986). Modulation of ethanol intake by serotonin uptake inhibitors. *J. Clin. Psychiatry*, 47(4), 16-22.

Naranjo, C.A., E.M. Sellers, C.A. Roach, D.V. Woodley, M. Sanchez-Craig, and K. Sykora (1984). Zimelidine-induced variations in alcohol intake by non-depressed heavy drinkers. *Clin. Pharmacol. Ther.*, 35, 374-381.

Naranjo, C.A., E.M. Sellers, J.T. Sullivan, D.V. Woodley, K. Kadlec, and K. Sykora (1987). The serotonin uptake inhibitor citalopram attenuates ethanol intake. *Clin. Pharmacol. Ther.*, 41, 266-274.

Naranjo, C.A., J.T. Sullivan, K.E. Kadlec, D.V. Woodley-Remus, G. Kennedy, and E.M. Sellers (1989). Differential effects of viqualine on alcohol intake and other consummatory behaviours. *Clin. Pharmacol. Ther.*, 46, 301-309.

Naranjo, C.A., K.E. Kadlec and C.X. Poulos (1991a). Citalopram decreases the desire for alcohol. In: *Novel Pharmacological Interventions for Alcoholism* (C.A. Naranjo, E.M. Sellers eds.), Springer-Verlag New York Publishers, New York.

Naranjo, C.A., K.E. Kadlec, P. Sanhueza, D. Woodley-Remus, and E.M. Sellers (1990). Fluoxetine differentially alters alcohol intake and other consummatory behaviours in problem drinkers. *Clin. Pharmacol. Ther.*, 47, 490-498.

Naranjo, C.A., K.E. Kadlec, P. Sanhueza, D. Woodley-Remus and E.M. Sellers (1991b). Enalapril effects on alcohol intake and other consummatory behaviors in alcoholics. *Clin. Pharmacol. Ther.*, 50, 96-106.

Naranjo, C.A., Kadlec, K.E. and C.X. Poulos (1991c). A human model for testing drug-induced concomitant variations in alcohol consumption and desire to drink. In: *Novel Pharmacological Interventions for Alcoholism* (C.A. Naranjo, E.M. Sellers eds.), Springer-Verlag New York Publishers, New York.

Orrego, H., J.E. Blake, and Y. Israel (1985). Relationship between gamma-glutamyl transpeptidase and mean urinary alcohol levels in alcoholics while drinking and after alcohol withdrawal. *Alcohol Clin. Exper. Res.*, 9, 10-13.

Tietz, N.W. (ed) (1986). *Textbook of Clinical Chemistry*. WB Saunders, Philadelphia.

Poster Papers: General Methodologic Issues

Rational vs. reflexive alcohol drinking

J. D. Sinclair[1] and R. Thomas[2]

[1]Research Laboratories of Alko Ltd., Helsinki, SF-00101 Finland, and [2]South Glamorgan Health Authority, Whitchurch Hospital, Cardiff, UK CF4 7XB

Most people assume they choose their behavior rationally, selecting the response they expect will bring them the most pleasure and the least pain. Opposed to this "Theory of Rational Behavior" (TRB), S-R Learning Theory (LT) stipulates that behavior is emitted reflexively by stimuli triggering the response to which they have the strongest connections, and that these connections are subsequently reinforced or weakened.

The area of alcoholism and drug abuse offers an unusual opportunity to evaluate these two theories because it is one of the few in which they make quite different predictions. The results in turn suggest how treatments could be improved.

According to TRB (but not LT), people choose their responses not only on the basis of personal experience but also from what they have heard, read, or seen happen to others, and such secondary information should help alcoholics and drug addicts to abstain. TRB also predicts alcohol or drug abuse would stop if the consequences were made sufficiently painful. According to LT such punishment of reinforced responses produces only attempts to "escape from the field".

The euphoria from alcohol is so small that TRB must postulate that another factor is the major reason for alcoholics taking alcohol: the avoidance of withdrawal reactions. The desire for alcohol thus should increase as physical dependence develops and decrease as dependence disappears, and forced abstinence should be an effective treatment. LT predicts the opposite: since the propensity for making a response increases during a period when the response cannot be made, forced abstinence will not cure alcoholism but instead will increase the alcohol craving.

LT (but not TRB) predicts that changing the stimuli from those in which alcohol or drug taking responses were learned will reduce the chances of relapse. LT also predicts that extinction of these responses should be an effective adjunct to treatment. TRB does not recognize the existence of extinction.

As reviewed elsewhere (Sinclair, 1990a), the evidence supports LT rather than TRB. Secondary information is ineffective: alcoholics and addicts usually are well aware already of the consequences of continued abuse, and the disorders are still found in medical doctors and others who are extremely knowledgeable about the likely effects. Punishment usually does lead to various forms of escaping from the field, such as discontinuing disulfiram use. Loss of physical dependence does not stop a patient from being an alcoholic, or drug addict; forced abstinence would be a useful treatment only if it could be maintained indefinitely and otherwises increases craving. Major environmental or stimulus changes are good predictors of successful treatments, as in the notable example of the treatment of heroin addiction in returning Vietnam veterans. Extinction is a real process: it can weaken the alcohol-drinking response of rats (Sinclair, 1990b), and there is clinical evidence that it is useful in the treatment of opiate addiction (Renault, 1980).

Perhaps all behavior is reflexive -- there is no choice or freewill, and we are all automatons merely reeling off sequences of responses. A more conservative interpretation is that alcohol drinking and drug taking are learned responses that become progressively stronger as positive reinforcement accumulates, and like bicycle riding, become more automatic as the learning proceeds. These responses in alcoholics and drug addicts are so well learned that they are no longer subject to rational choices and can only be modified by methods that alter reflexive actions, such as stimulus change, extinction, cue exposure, and the learning of alternative responses. Treatments involving rational behavioral choices may, however, be effective once the reflexive component has been weakened.

References

Sinclair, J D (1990a) Alcoholism treatment: Misdirection by the common-sense theory of rational behavior. Proceedings of the 34th International Institute on the Prevention and Treatment of Alcoholism, Pontalult-Combault, France, May 31-June 9, 1989 (in press).

Sinclair, J D (1990b) Drugs to decrease alcohol drinking. Annals of Medicine Proceedings of the Alcohol and Brain Symposium, Helsinki, Finland, Jan. 10-11, 1990 (in press).

Renault P F (1980) Treatment of heroin-dependent persons with antagonists: Current status. In: Willett RE,Barnett G (eds) Naltrexone: Research Monograph 28, Washington,D.C., Nat Inst Drug Abuse, 1980, pp 11-22.

RATS' INTAKES OF DIFFERENT ALCOHOLIC BEVERAGES

Michael L. Nichols, John D. Delconte, Kenneth D. Wild,
Christopher L. Hubbell and Larry D. Reid

A major issue associated with rats' intake of alcoholic beverages is the palatability of the presented ethanol solution (ES). It is well-known that rats prefer sweet solutions and aver bitter ones. Furthermore, rats perceive an ES of only ethanol (E) in water as bitter [1,2]. Consequently, rats do not avidly take solutions of only E and water.

Given rats' differential reactivity to various kinds of ESs, the question remains, what is the optimal solution to use. If, for example, only E in water is presented, then rats must overcome a barrier (bitterness) to take large amounts of E. Also, any manipulations enhancing or reducing reactivity to aversive stimulation might have a dramatic effect on rats' intakes. If, for another example, rats are presented a sweet ES, their intake may be for the sweetness rather than for E. Any manipulation changing intake of a sweet ES might also be due to changing reactivities to taste rather than reactivity to E.

Despite the saliency of the issue of what kind of an ES to use in studies of rats' intake of alcohol, there has been little systematic study of this issue. Here, we present some relevant data.

METHOD

Male, Sprague-Dawley rats (Taconic Farms, Germantown, NY) were maintained on a daily regimen involving 22 hr of water-deprivation followed by a 2-hr opportunity to take an ES and water. The ESs varied in flavor and concentrations of E. All ESs were prepared by mixing weighed amounts of pure E, flavoring and, most of the time, tap water. Beer was made by mixing pure E into a commercially available, nonalcoholic malt beverage that had been allowed to go "flat" overnight. Each day, rats' body weights and intakes of fluids were tabulated. The data associated with rats' intake of E are presented in terms of g/kg (g of pure E taken per kg of body weight).

The data of Figure 1 involved rats who had an opportunity to take a sweetened ES for, at least, 20 days. Then some had the ES changed. Intakes were observed until they became stable. Each index of intake involves mean g/kg across, at least, 3 days and for, at least, 8 rats. Figure 2 summarizes the 1st month of opportunity to take ES, in terms of g/kg, i.e., the data represent the initial history of taking 6 different kinds of ES.

RESULTS

Figure 1 presents mean g/kg intakes of rats given the opportunity to take various kinds of ESs. Notice the relatively low intake of rats given only E in water. When rats are offered a flavored ES, they take about 2.5 g/kg. Rats limit their intakes of E regardless of how sweet the ES. The amount of ES taken is considerably less than the amount of sweet solution they would take with no E. Without a barrier of bitterness, rats' intakes of ES rise to a level in which they show signs of intoxication (reduced righting reflexes) and then they stop drinking.

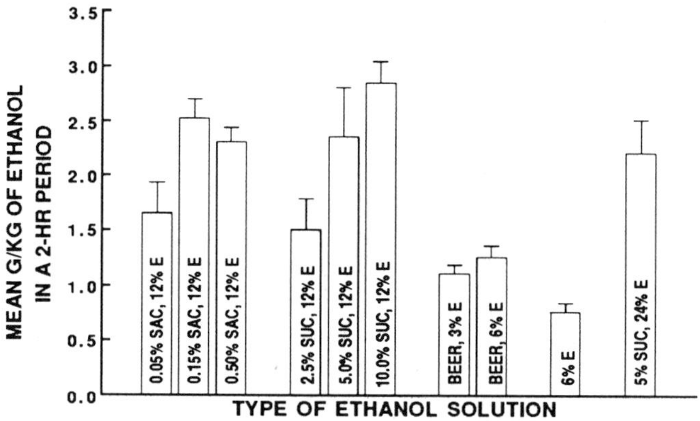

FIGURE 1. Summarized are mean intakes of ethanol (E), in terms of g/kg by rats offered a variety of alcoholic beverages. SAC = saccharin. SUC = sucrose. BEER = nonalcoholic malt beverage. Percentages are in terms of weight of flavoring or E to the total weight of the alcoholic beverage (e.g., each 100 g of the 5.0% SUC,12% E solution contained 5 g of SUC, 12 g of pure E and 83 g of tap water. Solutions of BEER were made by mixing E into the nonalcoholic malt beverage. These data were taken from a number of experiments. Error bars represent standard errors of the means.

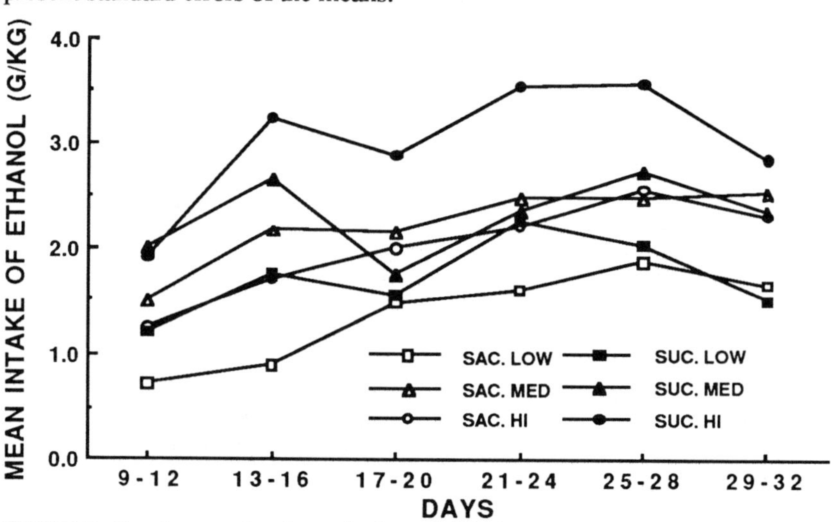

FIGURE 2. Rats' mean intakes of ethanol (E), in terms of g/kg are summarized. Each of the alcoholic beverages contained 12% E. The alcoholic beverages contained 0.05% (LOW), 0.15% (MED) or 0.50% (HI) saccharin (SAC.), or 2.5% (LOW), 5.0% (MED) or 10.0% (HI) sucrose (SUC.). An ANOVA of these data leads to the conclusion that there are no reliable differences associated with the factor of SAC versus SUC. In general, there are no reliable differences in intake among the four sweetest beverages and these intakes differ from the two less sweet solutions.

Notice, in Figure 2, that the highest concentration of sucrose ES lead to higher levels of intake than the next highest concentration, but the level decreased toward the end of the period of measurement. Data not presented indicates that the high level of intake with the 10% sucrose solution is peculiar to this group of rats.

DISCUSSION

One could reasonably choose to ignore the whole issue of flavoring of alcoholic beverages in studies of rats' intake of E by providing alcoholic beverages of the type taken by people. If a manipulation modified rats' intakes of these kinds of beverages, then presumably such a manipulation would similarly modify people's intake. Our data, for example, indicate that rats do, indeed, take meaningful amounts of E when presented beer (Fig. 1). Rats also take sweet ESs, which are also taken by people.

If the goal is to assess a drug's effect on opportunistic intake of E, rather than assess a drug's effects on intake that is held in check by an aversive barrier of taste, then presenting a beverage of only E in water is inappropriate. Even in confirmed alcoholics, minimal barriers to drinking (such as the requirement to press a lever to get alcohol) will reduce intakes [3]. Indeed, alcoholics' drinking is opportunistic, i.e., they drink excessively when it is easy to do so. Consequently, it may be desirable to study rats' drinking when it is not constrained by barriers. Indeed, it seems desirable to assess drugs' effects on intake of E when that intake is highly probable, sustained, and goaded by a number of factors. Presumably, a drug that would curb that kind of intake is more apt to curb an alcoholic's intake.

If a goal is to minimize the intrusiveness of palatability, then it might not be wise to use a beverage of only E in water. This idea seems to be at variance with others' conceptualizations of the problem (e.g., [4]). Not flavoring an alcoholic beverage, however, does not resolve the issue of palatability. In fact, because bitterness is so salient to rats, using a nonflavored ES makes the issue of palatability very salient.

If an unflavored ES is not optimal, what kinds of standards can be used to choose an optimal ES? The beverage should have a sufficiently high concentration of E that rats can take meaningful levels of E across a short period of time without reaching the holding capacity of their gut. An ES of only 3% E may not be, by this criterion, concentrated enough. The ES should not be so concentrated that rats' cannot meaningfully modulate their intake. Also, we need to be able to measure the intake in large enough units so that error of measurement does not become a factor. Concentrations of 6 or 12% seem to meet these standards.

There may be a way to rationally determine the kind of flavoring to use to minimize the intrusiveness of palatability. Notice in Fig. 1 that a number of ESs lead to an intake of about 2.25 g/kg of E despite considerable variation in concentrations of sweetener and E. When using our general procedures, this is the g/kg that our rats typically take after about 21 days of daily opportunity to take ES. These observations lead to the suggestion that palatability is not salient when it can be shown that intakes of E, in terms of g/kg, do not shift radically when there are some changes in flavoring or concentration of E.

When only E in water is the beverage presented, a change in concentration of E results in dramatic changes in g/kg. When concentration of E is modified in a sweet solution from 6 to 24%, rats' intakes of E tend, in our daily regimen, to be about 2.25 g/kg. By using the specified criteria, sweetening an ES may minimize the intrusiveness of palatability.

An optimal ES to use, then, may be one that the concentration of flavoring can be changed across a relatively broad range (all other variables remaining constant) without changing rats' intake of E in terms of g/kg. Also, the optimal ES to use is one in which changes in concentrations of E lead to changes in intake of amount of fluid, but not in terms of g/kg of E. Taste may not be the salient factor, but rather avidity for E is the factor, when there can be changes in concentrations of flavoring and/or E with a kind of ES, but intake of E remains rather constant in terms of g/kg.

Adding sucrose to an ES also adds calories to the solution. The data with saccharin leads to the suggestion that this might be an unnecessary complication.

The effects of palatability can be mitigated by flavoring the ES with an acceptable taste. That introduces another problem, of course. A manipulation may change the rats' reactivity to the flavoring rather than reactivity to E. That problem is, however, extant with procedures using only E in water as well (e.g., a manipulation may accentuate aversiveness). There is just no way to avoid having palatability as a factor when measuring rats' intake of alcoholic beverages, one can only mitigate the saliency of the factor.

There is a way of knowing whether or not a manipulation is peculiar to any given flavor. Try the manipulation in question across a variety of flavors. If the manipulation affects intake of different flavored ESs similarly, then it is reasonable to conclude that the resultant effect is not a product of palatability of a particular flavor.

There are ways of interpreting changes in rats' intake of ES rather than those focusing on E's reinforcing (or addictive, or incentive, or appetitive) effects. A decrease in intake of ES is particularly difficult to understand. Making rats sick, for example, will lead to a decrease in intake. When a manipulation concurrently reduces intake of water as well as intake of ES, it is reasonable to conclude that the manipulation might be debilitating. In brief, the concurrent intake of water provides a nonalcohol related behavior to observe, and the data concerning that behavior helps to understand changes in intake of ES.

A way to assess the possibility that sickness is causing decreased E intake is to give the manipulation day after day while monitoring indices such as body weight and intake of water as well as intake of ES. Consequently, it is usually necessary, before a strong conclusion is reached about how a manipulation affects E's reinforcing value, to do tests across a number of daily sessions.

Providing rats deprived of water a daily (but rather brief, say, 2 hr) opportunity to take a sweetened ES (having a considerable concentration of E, say, 12%) and water engenders, across days, considerable intake of E. This intake of E is motivated by a number of setting conditions which additively increase intake of E (e.g., the deprivation schedule, the flavor of the ES, days of opportunity to drink, and daytime presentation [5]). Consequently, this motivated propensity to take E is one metric to use to assess the effects of drugs and germane hypotheses.

REFERENCES

1. Kiefer, S.W., & Dopp, J.M. Behavioral Neuroscience 103:1318-1326; 1989.
2. Kiefer, S.W., et al. Alcohol 7:115-120; 1990.
3 Mello, N.K. In: Kissin, B., & Begleiter, H. (Eds.), The Biology of Alcoholism: Vol. 2. Physiology and Behavior. New York: Plenum Press, 1972.
4. Dole, V.P. Alcoholism: Clinical and Experimental Research 10:361-363; 1986.
5. Hubbell, C.L., & Reid, L.D. In: Reid, L.D. (Ed.), Opioids, Bulimia, and Alcohol Abuse & Alcoholism. New York: Springer-Verlag, pp. 145-174, 1990.

ACKNOWLEDGEMENTS

This research was supported, in part, by a grant from NIDA (DA04440). M.L. Nichols was supported by funds made available from the Ewing Marion Kauffman Foundation. We thank Yizhao Hui for help with the data collection. K.D. Wild is now with the Department of Pharmacology, University of Arizona.

DRUG-INDUCED SPECIFIC AND NONSPECIFIC CHANGES IN VOLUNTARY ETHANOL INTAKE BY RATS

J. Mardones, R. Alvarado, S. Contreras and N. Segovia-Riquelme

1. ABSTRACT

Drug-induced changes in the voluntary intake of ethanol by experimental animals are known to be influenced by the appetite for calories and for water. Thus, at least a part of these changes can be considered nonspecific for ethanol. It is convenient to know which part of the effect is not due to the caloric value or the water of ethanol solution, since it can be considered as a specific change. We have proposed a method for recognizing such specific effect by simultaneously measuring the changes in the consumption of ethanol solution, water and solid food, and by analyzing data in a particular way, the rationale of which was also discused (ALCOHOL 5: 15-19, 1988). We have applied this method to the effects of some drugs acting on CNS in rats genetically low (UChA) and high (UChB) ethanol consumer. The results show that Disulfiram, Cyanamide, Pyrazole, Clofibrate, 5-HTP, PCPA, Sulpiride, Sch 23390, Metamphetamine, MDMA, Clonidine, AMPT, Benserazide Carbidopa, Diazepam, Caffeine, Aminophylline and Oxyphenonium decrease specifically ethanol intake in UChB rats; while Haloperidol, Chlorpromazine, Sulpiride, Diazepam, Atropine and Trihexyphenidyl, increase it in UChA rats. Other drugs did not show specific effect in rats of any of the strains. These results are useful for recognizing the kind of neurons playing a role in the mechanisms of appetite for and satiety with ethanol, and also as an aid in the choice of drugs to be tested in the treatment of alcoholism.

2. INTRODUCTION

It has been known for years that laboratory rats (1) and mice (2) exhibit appetite for and satiation with ethanol solutions, that the daily amount they consumed is determined genetically (3,4), and that this can bc quantitatively modified by nutrimental and pharmacological actions, as well as by lesion or stimulation of determined zones of the central nervous system (Rev in 5,6). These facts imply the presence of neurophysiological mechanisms involved in the expression of such behavior.

Useful tools for the study of this matter are the drugs of known action on determined central synapses, especially when they are given to laboratory animals genetically low or high ethanol consumers. For this purpose some strains of rats, such as ANA and A (7), NP and P (8), and UChA and UChB (3,9), and of mice, DBA and C57B1 (10) are available among others. A considerable difficulty for the interpretation of the results obtained by experimental actions on voluntary ethanol intake of rodents, arises from the fact that the amount of ethanol solution they consume appears to be determined not only by the specific search of this substance, but also by the ingestive drive, and by the appetite for and satiation with calories and/or water.

We have proposed a method (11) for recognizing specific changes of ethanol intake (supposedly occurring in the search for its pharmacological effects) as different from those secondary to effects on appetite or satiation of calories or water, or on ingestive drive. We have applied this method to the analysis of the effects of CNS acting drugs on ethanol intake in rats of our two strains UChA and UChb.

The present paper summarizes the results reported in recent studies (11-14), and some others to be published in detail, as well as the recalculation of data of experiments we have already published (15-22).

3. MATERIALS AND METHODS

3.1 Experimental Procedure

The experiments were performed on adult rats of both sexes of UChA and UChB strains. Animals of 2 to 3 months, weighing 200 to 250 grams the males and 150 to 200 grams the females, were housed in individual cages. Each animal had access to distilled water and 10% v/v ethanol solution offered in graduate bottles, and was fed ad libitum on a balanced diet. The consumption of water and ethanol solution was measured daily. After at least one month under these conditions, rats exhibiting regular intake of ethanol solution were selected for the experiment. During pretreatment (baseline), treatment and postreatment periods of 3 or 4 days in consecutive weeks, the measurement of food consumption was added to the procedure. The means of the daily consumption of water, ethanol solution and solid food during these periods were expressed in terms of 100 g of body weight. The drugs were administered daily in the doses and by route stated in Tables, during the treatment period.

3.2 Data Analysis and Definitions

The data were analyzed according to the method proposed in a previous paper (11), where the rationale, the performance, the symbols and the formulas have been detailed. An effect in the consumption of ethanol solution induced by a drug is considered specific when the following differences are of the same sign (plus or minus and significantly different to zero): a) the consumption of ethanol during the treatment period minus that during the pretreatment one (Δ_0E), b) this difference depurated from either the effects in the consumption of calories (Δ_1E), or of total water (Δ_2E) and of both calories and total water (Δ_3E), c) the ratio [consumption of ethanol solution: consumption of food] during the treatment period minus that during the pretreatment one (ΔCR) and d) the ratio [consumption of ethanol solution: consumption of total fluid] during the treatment period minus that of the pretreatment one (ΔVR). When the signs of all these differences are positive and significantly different to zero, meaning that the action of the drug is consistent with a lowering of the threshold of internal marks inducing appetite for ethanol, or with a rising of the threshold of the internal marks inducing satiation with it, the criteria accept that the drug effect is specific for ethanol consumption. Obviously, when the sign of all these difference is negative, the interpretation of the results is the contrary. The changes in the consumption of ethanol are considered secondary to alteration of the ingestive drive when the difference of the consumption of ethanol (Δ_0E) is of the same sign as that of the consumption of both solid food (ΔF) and total water (ΔTW), and any of the other conditions for accepting a specific effect is not fulfilled. When a coincidence in the sign of Δ_0E and ΔF, but not with that of ΔTW is observed, the change of ethanol solution intake is considered consequence of action on the mechanisms of appetite for or satiety with calories. By the same way, when the sign of Δ_0E is the same of ΔTW, but not that of ΔF, the change of the consumption of ethanol solution is considered consequence of action on the mechanisms of appetite for or satiation with water.

3.3 Statistical Analysis

Since only the signs of the differences are considered in the criteria, one tailed Student's t test is used for estimating the significance of all the changes, for $p<.05$. When no significant sex influence is observed in any of the signs of the differences employed in the criteria, data of male and female groups were pooled, in the same way, when consecutive doses did not produce significant differences in the signs of any of the differences employed in the criteria, the data of respective dose groups were pooled.

4. RESULTS AND DISCUSSION

The results obtained in rats genetically low ethanol consumer (UChA) are summarized in Table 1. A specific increase in the consumption of ethanol appeared to be produced by atropine, low doses of chlorpromazine, haloperidol, low doses of sulpiride and diazepam. These results suggest that neurones with muscarinic receptor and with D2 receptor are playing a role in the neurophysiological mechanisms responsible for the satiation with ethanol present in the rats of this strain, and that diazepine-sensitive-GABA receptor neurons can block this mechanism. A lowering of ethanol intake secondary to a decrease of ingestive drive, appeared to be produced by zimelidine, fluvoxamine, citalopram and p-chlorophenylalanine (PCPA). Since the three first mentioned drugs are known to block the synaptic serotonin uptake, this results suggests that the decrease of ethanol intake induced by these drugs, reported by different authors (rev in 13), may be the consequence of an effect of serotonergic drugs on the ingestive drive. The effect of PCPA seems to be induced by a yet unknown mechanism, different of the blocking of serotonin, synthesis (14). Caffeine appeared to lower the ethanol solution intake of UChA rats as a consequence of a decrease in the thirst, or an increase of the satiation with water. Other tested drugs did not show any significant effect in the ethanol intake of rats of this strain.

The effects of drugs on ethanol intake by genetically high consumer rats (UChB) are summarized in Table 2. None of the tested drugs induced an increase on the consumption of ethanol. In contrast, many of them decreased it in a specific manner. Obviously this decrease could be the consequence of a stimulation of satiety with ethanol mechanisms or by an inhibition of the appetite for it. The results of the application of the method of data analysis cannot decide about this alternative.

The drug blocking the ethanol metabolism in any of the steps, namely disulfiram, cyanamid and pyrazole, induced a specific decrease of ethanol consumption, presumably by activation of the sensor of the ethanol satiation mechanism.

Atropine and trihexyphenydil-anticholinergic drugs which cross the blood-brain-barrier decreased ethanol intake, but they did not accomplish the requirements for a specific action on it, because this decrease was not maintained when depurated from the effect of appetite for food and water (Δ3E). In contrast, oxyphenonium, a drug which does not enter in CNS induced a specific decrease in ethanol intake. When these facts are considered together with the specific increase of ethanol intake induced by atropine in UChA rats it suggests that the cholinergic synapses in the satiation mechanisms are located in CNS while cholinergic synapses not protected by the blood brain barrier may play a role in the appetite for alcohol.

The specific decrease of ethanol intake induced by high doses of sulpiride and by Sch 23390 suggests that the activity of both D1 and D2 neurones is necessary for the expression of the high ethanol intake observed in UChB rats. The unspecific decreases of ethanol intake induced by high doses of chlorpromazine and by haloperidol, considered together with the effects induced by these drug in UChA rats suggests that it can be the result of simultaneous blocking of the appetite and satiation mechanisms. In the same way, the nonspecific decrease of ethanol consumption induced by the dopaminergic agonists apomorphine, amantadine and bromocriptine in UChB rats, and the absence of effect of these drugs in UChA rats can be explained.

The specific decrease of ethanol intake induced by metamphetamine and metilendioxymetamphetamine (MDMA)-agonists of both dopaminergic and noradrenergic synapses - different of that induced by dopaminergic agonist, together with the specific effect of clonidine and the unspecific decrease induced by phenoxibenzamine, suggest that alpha-adrenergic neurones are playing a role in the appetite for ethanol. On the other hand, the specific decrease induced by propranolol suggests that beta-adrenergic neurones may play a role in the satiation mechanism.

The effects of serotonin uptake blockers and of 5-hydroxytryptophan and of PCPA have been recently discussed (13,14).

The effects of benserazide and carbidopa deserve further studies. The inhibition of aldehydehydrogenase by serazide, recently reported (23), could explain its specific decrease of ethanol intake. We are not aware of a similar effect of carbidopa. The effects of caffeine also deserve further studies. The role played by its activity on phosphodiesterase and in adenosine receptors in the action on ethanol intake need to be clarified.

The specific decrease of ethanol intake induced by diazepam suggests that benzodiazepine-sensitive-GABAergic neurones may inhibit the neurophysiological mechanisms of ethanol appetite.

In summary, the present communication which is planned to be followed by detailed reports of the non published results and their discussions shows that our method (11) for recognizing specific from secondary actions of drugs on the voluntary consumption of alcohol seems to be a useful tool to orientate further research on the neurophysiological mechanism involved in appetite for and satiation with ethanol.

5. REFERENCES

1. Richter, C.P. and Campbell, K.H. (1940). Alcohol taste threshold and concentrations of solutions preferred by rats. *Science*, 91, 507-508.

2. Loiseleur, J. and Petit, M. (1947). L'ethylisme experimental de la souris (The experimental alcohlism of the mouse), *C.R. Soc. Biol.* (Paris), 141, 568-569.

3. Mardones, J., Segovia, N. and Hederra, A. (1953). Heredity of alcohol preference in rats: II. Coeficient of heredity. *Quart. J. Studies Alc.*, 14, 1-2.

4. McClearn, G.E. and Rodgers, D.A. (1961). Genetic factors in alcohol prefrence of laboratory mice. *J. Comp. Physiol. Psychol.*, 54, 116-119.

5. Segovia-Riquelme, N., Varela, A. and Mardones, J (1971). Appetite for alcohol. In: *Biological Basis of Alcoholism* (Y. Israel and J. Mardones eds.), New York Wiley-Interscience, 299-334.

6. Meisch, R.A. (1984). Alcohol self-adminstration by experiemntal animals. *Res. Adv. Alcohol Drug Problems*, 8, 23-45.

7. Eriksson, K. (1968). Genetic selection for voluntary alcohol consumption in the albino rats. *Science*, 159, 739-741.

8. Lumeng, L., Hawkins, T.D. and Li, T.-K (1977). In: *Alcohol and Aldehyde Metabolizing Systems* (J.R. Thurman, J.R. Williamson, H.R. Drott and R. Chance (eds.), New York Academic Press, Vol. 3, 537-544; quoted by Li, T.-K.

9. Lumeng, L., McBride, W.J. and Murphy, J.M.(1987). Rodent lines selected for factors affecting alcohol consumption. *Alc. Alcoholism*, Suppl 1, 91-96.

10. Mardones, J. and Segovia-Riquelme, N. (1983). Thirty two years of selection of rats by ethanol preference: UChA and UChB strains. *Neurobehav. Toxicol. Teratol.*, 6, 171-178.

11. McClearn, G.E. and Rodgers, D.A. (1959). Differences in alcohol preference among inbred strains of mice. *Quart. J. Studies Alc.*, 20, 691-695.

12. Mardones, J., Contreras, S. and Segovia-Riquelme, N.A. (1988). A method for recognizing specific effects on ethanol intake by experimental animals. *Alcohol*, 5, 15-19.

13. Contreras, S. and Mardones, J. (1988). Effects of pyrazole on the voluntary consumption of ethanol, water and solid food in UChA and UChB rats. *Alcohol*, 5, 367-369.

14. Alvarado, R., Contreras, S., Segovia-Riquelme, N. and Mardones, J. (1990). Effects of serotonin uptake blockers and of 5-hydroxytryptophan on the voluntary consumption of ethanol, water and solid food by UChA and UChB rats. *Alcohol*, 7, 315-319.

15. Contreras, S., Alvarado, R. and Mardones, J. (in press). Effecst of p-chlorophenylalanine on the voluntary consumption of ethanol, water and solid food by UChA and UChB rats. *Alcohol*.

16. Mardones, J. and Segovia-Riquelme, N. (1982). Effects of chlorpromazine on voluntary consumption of ethanol water and solid food in UChA rats. *IRCS Med. Sci.*, 10: 564.

17. Segovia-Riquelme, N. and Mardones, J. (1983). Effects of chlorpromazine on the voluntary consumption of ethanol, water and solid food in UChB rats. *IRCS Med. Sci.*, 11, 203-209.

18. Mardones, J. and Segovia Riquelme, N. (1982). Effects of haloperidol on voluntary consumption of ethanol, water and solid food in UChA rats. *IRCS Med. Sci.*, 10, 197-198.

19. Segovia-Riquelme, N. and Mardones, J. (1982). Effects of haloperidol on the voluntary consumption of ethanol, water and solid food in UChB rats. *IRCS Med. Sci.*, 10, 375-376.

20. Mardones, J., Segovia-Riquelme, N. and Contreras, S. (1984). Effects of sulpiride on the voluntary consumption of ethanol, water and solid food by UChA and UChB rats. *IRCS Med. Sci.*, 12, 600-601.

21. Mardones, J., Segovia-Riquelme, N. and Hederra, A. (1980). Effects of apomorphine on the voluntary consumption of ethanol total fluid and solid food by rats of the UChA and UChB strains. *IRCS Med. Sci.*, 8, 503-504.

22. Segovia-Riquelme, N. and Mardones, J. (1980). Effects of amantadine on the voluntary consumption of ethanol, water and solid food by UChB rats. *IRCS Med. Sci.*, 8, 505.

23. Segovia-Riquelme, N. and Mardones J. (1980). Effects of bromocriptine on the voluntary consumption of ethanol, total fluid and solid food by UChB rats. *IRCS Med. Sci.*, 8, 911.

24. Milano, F.J. and Myers, R.D. (1989). Inhibition of brain dopa-decarboxylase by RO 4-4602 infused ICV blocks ethanol drinking induced in rats by cyanamide. *Psychopharmacology*, 98, 1976-1982.

Table 1

Effects of drugs on the voluntary consumption of ethanol solution, total water, and solid food in UChaA rats

Drug	Route	Dose mg/kg	n	Δ_0E	Δ_1E	Δ_2E	Δ_3E	ΔF	ΔCR	ΔTW	ΔVR	Act	Ref
Disulfiram	PO	300	14	n.s.	n.s.	n.s.	n.s.	n.s.	n.s.	n.s.	n.s.	n.s.	11
Cyanamide	IP	25	13	n.s.	n.s.	n.s.	n.s.	n.s.	n.s.	n.s.	n.s.	n.s.	11
Pyrazole	IP	70	11	n.s.	n.s.	n.s.	n.s.	-	n.s.	-	n.s.	n.s.	12
Atropine	IP	1	24	+	+	+	+	-	+	n.s.	+	S+	np
Trihexyphenydil	IP	10-20	28	n.s.	+	+	+	-	+	-	+	n.s.	np
Oxyphenonium	IP	2.5-5	20	n.s.	+	+	+	-	+	-	+	n.s.	np
Chlorpromazine	IP	0.5-1	27	+	+	+	+	n.s.	+	-	+	S+	15
Chorpromazine	IP	4	21	n.s.	+	n.s.	+	-	+	-	n.s.	n.s.	15
Haloperidol	IP	0.5-1	32	+	+	+	+	-	+	-	+	S+	17
Sulpiride	IP	5	18	+	+	+	+	n.s.	+	n.s.	+	S+	19
Sulpiride	IP	20-40	21	n.s.	n.s.	n.s.	n.s.	-	n.s.	-	n.s.	n.s.	19
SCH 23390	IP	0.64-1.28	15	n.s.	n.s.	n.s.	n.s.	n.s.	n.s.	-	n.s.	n.s.	np
Apomorphine	IP	2-5.6	22	n.s.	n.s.	n.s.	n.s.	-	n.s.	-	n.s.	n.s.	20
Amantadine	IP	8	8	n.s.	n.s.	n.s.	n.s.	n.s.	n.s.	n.s.	n.s.	n.s.	np
Bromocriptine	IP	1-4	26	n.s.	n.s.	n.s.	n.s.	-	n.s.	-	n.s.	n.s.	np
Metamphetamine	IP	10	15	n.s.	+	n.s.	n.s.	-	+	+	n.s.	n.s.	np
MDMA	IP	10	18	n.s.	n.s.	n.s.	n.s.	-	n.s.	n.s.	n.s.	n.s.	np
Clonidine	IP	0.6-1.2	14	n.s.	n.s.	-	n.s.	-	n.s.	n.s.	-	n.s.	np
Phenoxybenzamine	IP	2	16	n.s.	n.s.	n.s.	n.s.	-	n.s.	-	n.s.	n.s.	np
Propranol	IP	1	17	n.s.	n.s.	n.s.	n.s.	n.s.	n.s.	n.s.	n.s.	n.s.	np
Zimeldine	IP	10-30	18	-	n.s.	n.s.	+	-	n.s.	n.s.	-	D-	13
Fluvoxamine	IP	30-40	15	-	n.s.	-	n.s.	-	n.s.	-	n.s.	D-	13
Citalopram	IP	30	7	-	n.s.	n.s.	n.s.	-	n.s.	-	-	D-	13
5-Hydroxytryptophan	IP	70	14	n.s.	n.s.	n.s.	n.s.	-	n.s.	+	n.s.	n.s.	13
Benserazide	IP	50	10	n.s.	n.s.	n.s.	n.s.	n.s.	n.s.	n.s.	-	n.s.	np
Caffeine	IP	8	15	-	-	n.s.	n.s.	n.s.	-	-	n.s.	W-	np
Diazepam	IP	0.5-4	67	+	+	+	+	n.s.	+	n.s.	+	S+	np

Significant changes ($p<0.05$, one tailed Student's t test): + = up; - = down; n.s. = nonsignificant. Type of action: Specific for ethanol = S; Secondary to: D = ingestive drive; F = calories; W = water. Reference: np = not published

Table 2

Effects of drugs on the voluntary consumption of ethanol solution, total water, and solid food in UChab rats

Drug	Route	Dose mg/kg	n	Δ_0E	Δ_1E	Δ_2E	Δ_3E	ΔF	ΔCR	ΔTW	ΔVR	Act	Ref
Disulfiram	PO	300	17	-	-	-	-	-	-	-	-	S-	11
Cyanamide	IP	25	17	-	-	-	-	+	-	n.s.	-	S-	11
Pyrazole	IP	70	12	-	-	-	-	n.s.	-	n.s.	-	S-	12
Atropine	IP	1	20	-	-	-	-	n.s.	-	-	-	D-	np
Trihexyphenydil	IP	10-20	30	-	n.s.	-	n.s.	-	n.s.	-	-	D-	np
Oxyphenonium	IP	2.5-5	20	-	-	-	-	-	-	-	-	S-	np
Chlorpromazine	IP	1	8	n.s.	n.s.	n.s.	+	-	n.s.	n.s.	n.s.	n.s.	16
Chorpromazine	IP	4-8	21	-	-	-	n.s.	n.s.	-	-	n.s.	W-	16
Haloperidol	IP	0.5-1	35	-	n.s.	n.s.	+	-	n.s.	-	+	D-	18
Sulpiride	IP	5	22	n.s.	n.s.	n.s.	n.s.	n.s.	n.s.	+	n.s.	n.s.	19
Sulpiride	IP	20-40	21	-	-	-	-	n.s.	-	n.s.	-	S-	19
SCH 23390	IP	0.64-1.28	17	-	-	-	-	n.s.	-	-	-	S-	np
Apomorphine	IP	2-8	36	-	n.s.	-	n.s.	-	n.s.	-	-	D-	21
Amantadine	IP	32-80	16	-	n.s.	n.s.	n.s.	-	n.s.	-	-	D-	21
Bromocriptine	IP	1-4	35	-	n.s.	-	n.s.	-	n.s.	n.s.	-	F-	22
Metamphetamine	IP	10	14	-	-	-	-	n.s.	-	n.s.	-	S-	np
MDMA	IP	10	19	-	-	-	-	n.s.	-	n.s.	-	S-	np
Clonidine	IP	0.6-1.2	24	-	-	-	-	-	-	n.s.	-	S-	np
Phenoxybenzamine	IP	2	14	-	n.s.	n.s.	n.s.	-	n.s.	n.s.	-	F-	np
Propranol	IP	0.5-1	30	-	-	-	-	n.s.	-	n.s.	-	S-	np
Zimeldine	IP	1-30	24	-	-	-	n.s.	-	-	-	-	D-	13
Fluvoxamine	IP	30-40	14	-	-	-	+	-	-	-	-	D-	13
Citalopram	IP	30	9	-	n.s.	-	+	-	n.s.	-	-	D-	13
5-Hydroxytryptophan	IP	70	18	-	-	-	-	n.s.	-	n.s.	-	S-	13
P-Chlorophenylalanine	IP	129	16	-	-	-	-	-	-	n.s.	-	S-	14
Benserazide	IP	50	10	-	-	-	-	n.s.	-	n.s.	-	S-	np
Carbidopa	IP	5-10	18	-	-	-	-	n.s.	-	-	-	S-	np
Caffeine	IP	8	16	-	-	-	-	n.s.	-	n.s.	-	S-	np
Diazepam	IP	1-2	17	-	-	-	-	+	-	n.s.	-	S-	np

Rationale for Alcoholism Treatment Based on Inhibition of Aldehyde Dehydrogenase

H.T. Nagasawa*†, C.-H. Kwon†, J.A. Elberling*, M.J.C. Lee†, E.G. DeMaster*, F.N. Shirota*, and D.J.W. Goon†.

It has been long recognized that certain individuals, particularly of Oriental origin, present a pronounced facial flush on consumption of only modest quantities of alcoholic beverages, thereby sustaining a natural aversion to alcohol (ethanol). These individuals lack a functional low Km hepatic mitochondrial aldehyde dehydrogenase (AlDH2) that metabolizes acetaldehyde, the first product of ethanol metabolism (1). This inborn trait observed in 40-50% of Orientals has been shown to be due to a genetic defect manifested by a point mutation on AlDH2, with the amino acid lysine replacing a glutamate residue near the C-terminal end of the enzyme (2). The consumption of ethanol by such individuals gives rise to elevated blood acetaldehyde levels and a flushing reaction reminiscent of the disulfiram-ethanol reaction (3), leading to alcohol avoidance.

Individuals with this polymorphic AlDH2 (flushers) are much less prone to alcoholism and have a correspondingly low incidence of alcoholic liver disease (4-6). Conversely, individuals with normal AlDH2 (nonflushers) have a higher rate of alcoholism and a higher incidence of alcoholic liver disease. These genetic-epidemiological data, therefore, provide a persuasive rationale for pharmacological intervention with agents specifically designed to inhibit AlDH2 - - the same enzyme that is deficient in 50% of Orientals - - for the treatment of alcoholism.

Accordingly, we have synthesized a series of rationally designed, second generation aldehyde dehydrogenase inhibitors that target AlDH2. They are based on the postulated molecular mechanism of AlDH2 inhibition by a variety of agents such as cyanamide (a fertilizer component), coprine (found in inky cap mushrooms), and chlorpropamide (a hypoglycemic drug), all of which are known to provoke a disulfiram-like flushing syndrome when consumed with alcohol. Prodrugs of cyanamide, hybrid molecules of coprine, and analogs of chlorpropamide that are even more effective inhibitors of AlDH2 than the parent drug from which they were derived are now available.

---

* Medical Research Laboratories, V.A. Medical Center, and
† University of Minnesota, Minneapolis, MN 55417.

Figure 1 depicts the derivatization of cyanamide with amino acids, peptides and fatty acids, thus providing rationally designed prodrugs of cyanamide whose bioactivation requires two sequential enzymatic steps before the inhibition of AlDH2 can take place (7,8). Thus, the action of an amidase, peptidase, or esterase on these cyanamide derivatives releases cyanamide itself, which is then further bioactivated by catalase to produce nitroxyl (9), the putative inhibitor of AlDH2.

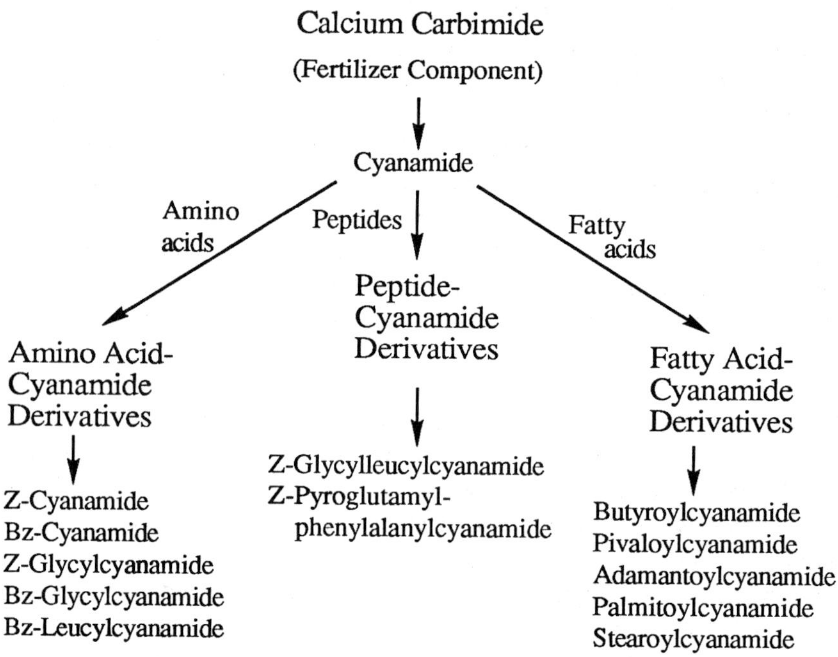

Figure 1. Rationally Designed Derivatives of Cyanamide

Coprine-pargyline hybrids where the toxic moiety (propargyl group) of pargyline has been replaced by the active moiety (cyclopropyl group) from coprine (10) are described in Figure 2. Here again, metabolism is required in order to release cyclopropanone, a known inhibitor of aldehyde dehydrogenase.

We have also shown that substitution at the N^1-position of the hypoglycemic drug, chloropropamide (CP), with various alkyl groups leads to a series of direct-acting inhibitors of AlDH2 (Figure 3) (11,12). These do not require prior metabolism for activity as in the case of CP itself; moreover, CP is rendered nonhypoglycemic by this molecular modification.

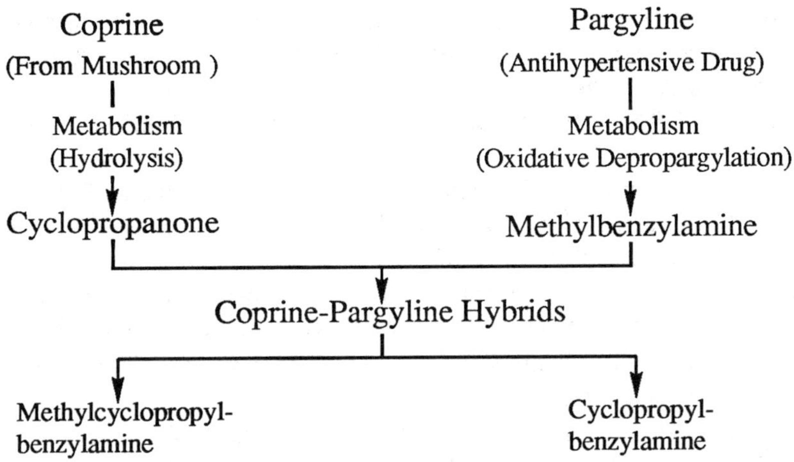

Figure 2. Coprine-Pargyline Hybrids

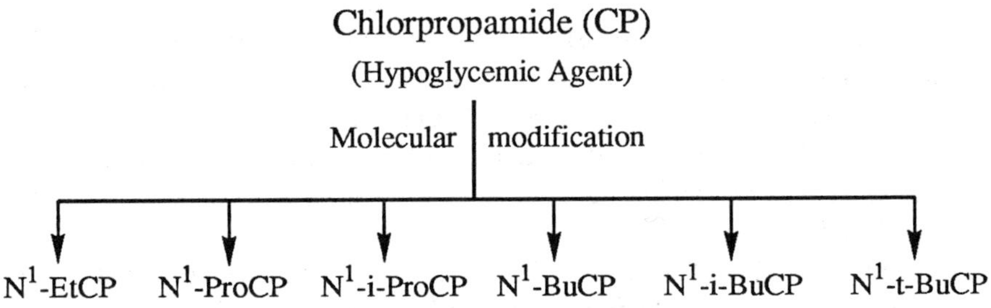

Figure 3. N^1-Alkyl-substituted Chlorpropamide Analogs

In summary, second generation enzyme inhibitors that block the action of AlDH2 have now been synthesized. The biological effects of these AlDH2 inhibitors mimic the alcohol flushing reaction observed in an ethnic group that naturally avoids alcohol due to a genetic defect on the same enzyme. The development of these agents for the treatment of alcoholism should, therefore, be seriously considered. (Supported by the Department of Veterans Affairs and by Grant 1R01-AA07317, ADAMHA.)

REFERENCES

1. Goedde HW, Agarwal DP: Acetaldehyde Metabolism: Genetic variation and physiological implications, in Goedde HW, Agarwal DP (eds): Alcoholism, Biomedical and Genetic Aspects, New York, Pergamon Press, 1989, pp 21-56.

2. Yoshida A, Huang I-Y, Ikawa M: Molecular abnormality of an inactive aldehyde dehydrogenase variant commonly found in Orientals. Proc Natl Acad Sci USA 81:258-261, 1984.

3. Kitson TM: The disulfiram-ethanol reaction: a review. J Stud Alc 38:96-113, 1977.

4. Harada S, Agarwal DP, Goedde HW, Takagi S, Ishikawa B: Possible protective role against alcoholism for aldehyde dehydrogenase isozyme deficiency in Japan. Lancet II:827, 1982.

5. Shibuya A, Yoshida A: Genotypes of alcohol-metabolizing enzymes in Japanese with alcoholic liver diseases: a strong association of the usual Caucasian-type aldehyde dehydrogenase gene ($ALDH_2^1$) with the disease. Am J Hum Genet 43:744-748, 1988.

6. Yoshihara H, Sato N, Kamada T, Abe H: Low Km AlDH isozyme and alcoholic liver injury. Pharmacol Biochem Behav 18(Suppl 1):425-428, 1983.

7. Nagasawa, HT, Kwon C-H, DeMaster EG, Shirota FN: Prodrugs of cyanamide as (long-acting) alcohol deterrent agents. Biochem Pharmacol 35:129-132, 1986.

8. Kwon C-H, Nagasawa HT, DeMaster E.G., Shirota FN: Acyl, N-protected α-aminoacyl, and peptidyl derivatives as prodrug forms of the alcohol deterrent agent cyanamide. J Med Chem 29:1922-1929, 1986.

9. Shirota FN, DeMaster EG, Nagasawa HT: Cyanide is a product of the catalase-mediated oxidation of the alcohol deterrent agent, cyanamide. Toxicol Lett 37:7-12, 1987.

10. Nagasawa HT, Elberling JA, DeMaster EG: Latent inhibitors of aldehyde dehydrogenase as alcohol deterrent agents. J Med Chem 27:1335-1339, 1984.

11 Nagasawa HT, Elberling JA, Shirota FN, DeMaster EG: A nonhypoglycemic chlorpropamide analog that inhibits aldehyde dehydrogenase. Alcoholism 12:563-565, 1988.

12. Nagasawa HT, Elberling JA, DeMaster EG, Shirota FN: N^1-Alkyl-substituted derivatives of chlorpropamide as inhibitors of aldehyde dehydrogenase. J Med Chem 32:1335-1340, 1989.

THE EFFECT OF LOW ALCOHOL BEVERAGES ON ALCOHOLISM LEVELS IN CANADA IN 1986

M. Adrian, P.M. Jull

A basic pharmacologic intervention in reducing alcoholism is to reduce the consumption of alcohol. Changes in public taste - preference for sweet flavours and low-calorie products - has led the alcohol industry to market 'coolers' and 'light' beers with a lower alcohol content than traditional beer, wine and spirits. The reduction in average per capita consumption of absolute alcohol resulting from the switch to low alcohol beverages was calculated by converting sales data for beer, wine, and spirit alcoholic beverages into absolute alcohol using a conversion factor based on the relative volume market share for 'light' beers and wine- and spirit-coolers relative to total alcoholic beverage sales, as reported by the Brewers' Association of Canada, the Canadian Wine Institute and the Association of Canadian Distillers (Table 1). The impact on total consumption is based on the percentage of all consumption due to each type of beverage alcohol, as well as the percentage market share of 'light' beer or 'coolers' as a proportion of all alcohol beverage sales. This results in reduced factors for converting alcoholic beverages into absolute alcohol (Table 2).

We found that because the relationship between per drinker consumption and the proportion of the population consuming alcohol at specified levels is non-linear, the drop in alcoholics exceeded the corresponding drop in alcohol consumption (Figure 1). It is expected that as market share of low alcohol beverages increases, continued decreases in both consumption and alcoholism levels will occur.

Table 1 – Market Share of Light Beer and Wine and Spirits Coolers, Canada and Provinces, 1986

Province	% Light Beer Relative to Total Beer Sales	% Wine Coolers Relative to Total Wine Sales	% Spirits Coolers Relative to Total Spirits Sales
Nfld.	5.1	3.9	0.4
P.E.I.	8.3	4.9	0.0
N.S.	6.8	11.8	4.8
N.B.	7.6	8.1	1.3
Que.	5.6	3.1	0.2
Ont.	14.7	5.9	2.5
Man.	24.6	9.6	2.2
Sask.	21.5	10.8	2.1
Alta.	18.2	17.1	2.3
B.C.	4.9	11.2	0.5
Yukon	0.0	3.5	0.0
N.W.T.	0.0	9.5	0.2
Canada	11.4	7.3	1.8

Table 2 – Conversion Factors From Beverage Alcohol to Absolute Alcohol, Canada and Provinces, 1986

	Beer	Wine	Spirits
Old Conversion Factors (%)			
Canada	5.00	13.00	40.00
New Conversion Factors (%)			
Nfld.	4.95	12.67	39.86
P.E.I.	4.92	12.58	40.00
N.S.	4.93	12.00	38.32
N.B.	4.92	12.31	39.55
Que.	4.94	12.74	39.93
Ont.	4.85	12.50	39.13
Man.	4.75	12.18	39.23
Sask.	4.79	12.08	39.27
Alta.	4.82	11.55	39.20
B.C.	4.95	12.05	39.83
Yukon	5.00	12.70	40.00
N.W.T.	5.00	12.19	39.93
Canada	4.89	12.38	39.37

Sources: Brewers Association of Canada, "Annual Statistical Bulletin 1988" (Ottawa: Brewers Association of Canada, 1989); Canadian Wine Institute, Canadian Wine Institute Annual Statistical Report 1986" (Mississauga: Canadian Wine Institute, 1987); Association of Canadian Distillers, "Annual Statistical Report 1988" (Ottawa: Association of Canadian

Figure 1
Alcohol Consumption & Alcoholism Levels
Canada, 1986

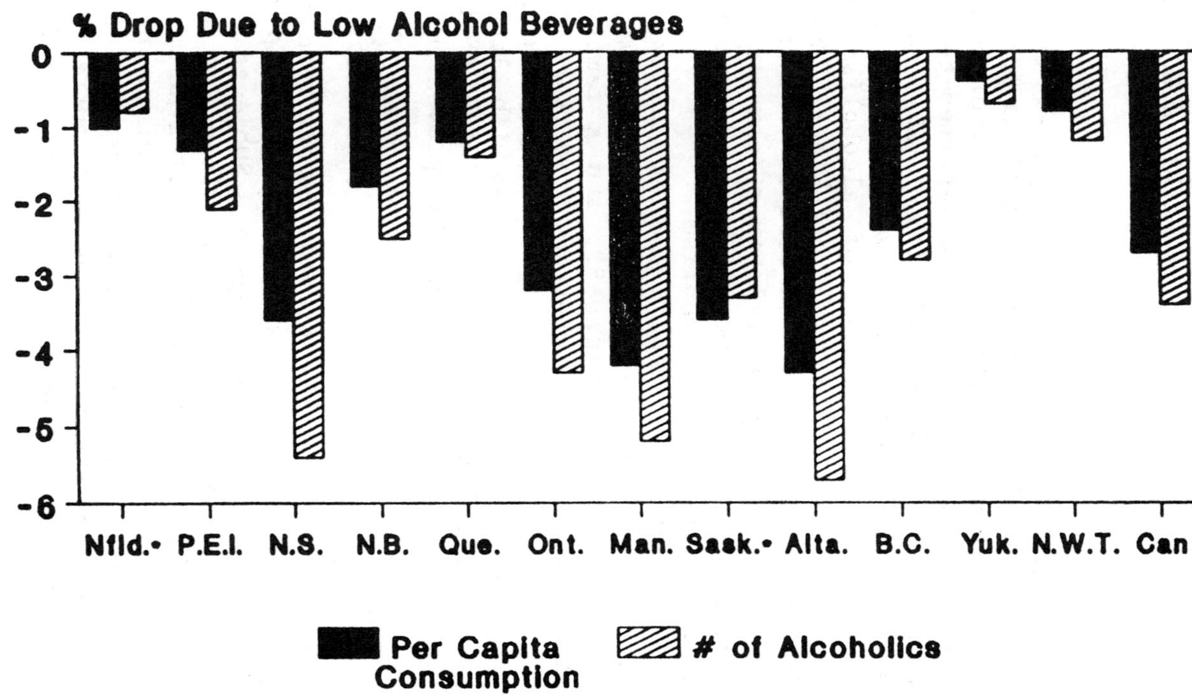

*Due to rounding, effects are masked.

ALCOHOLISM, ANTISOCIAL BEHAVIOR, AND FAMILY HISTORY: A SYNOPSIS

Collins E. Lewis, M.D., and Kathleen K. Bucholz, Ph.D.

INTRODUCTION

Investigators have long recognized the association between alcoholism and criminal behavior[1] and with the recent advent of standardized psychiatric diagnostic criteria, many studies[2] have reported that individuals with antisocial personality (ASP) have a higher prevalence of alcoholism than individuals without. A second robust correlate of alcoholism is a family history of problem drinking, and numerous investigations[3] have demonstrated that individuals who have close biological relatives (parents, siblings, or children) with problem drinking are themselves at an increased risk for alcoholism.

Research from selected samples (medical inpatients,[4] black urban men,[5] white men with unipolar depression)[6] indicates that gender, ASP, and a family history of problem drinking are important predictors of alcoholism. The purpose of this analysis is to determine whether these factors are also associated with alcoholism in the general population; and, if associated, whether they are useful as screening devices for prevention.

METHODS

The data used in the present report were collected as part of the St. Louis component of the Epidemiological Catchment Area (ECA) project. Subjects were selected from households and institutions by a multistage cluster-probability sampling strategy and interviewed by lay examiners with the NIMH Diagnostic Interview Schedule. This structured instrument elicited detailed information about lifetime and current psychiatric symptoms[7] and produced diagnoses based on DSM-III criteria.[8]

The St. Louis sample included 2572 subjects. For this analysis, the DSM III criteria for ASP were modified to exclude symptoms related to substance abuse and driving while intoxicated to avoid any spurious correlation between ASP and alcoholism. Subjects were diagnosed to have conduct disorder if they had three or more childhood symptoms of ASP, all of which began before the age of 15. Again, repeated intoxication and substance use were removed to avoid false associations. Stepwise logistic regression[9] was used to determine the contributions of gender, antisocial behavior and family history to having a lifetime DSM III diagnosis of alcohol abuse or dependence (alcoholism). The variables were dichotomous and represented the presence or absence of a clinical condition and male or female gender. Odds ratios[+] and confidence intervals were calculated from the logistic regression coefficients and their standard errors according to the methodology of Lemeshow and Hosmer.[10] We hypothesized that antisocial behavior, gender, and a family history of problem drinking would all be significantly associated with alcoholism.

RESULTS

Psychosocial data

39.2% of the sample were men, and 60.8%, women. Most of the subjects were in their early forties, had been married, and had a high school education. The majority of the respondents (55.7%) were employed at the time of the interview.

Whites comprised the largest ethnic group with 58.5%, and blacks, the second largest with 38.1%. Hispanics comprised 0.5% of the sample, and other ethnic groups including Asians, American Indians, and Pacific Islanders comprised the remaining 2.9%.

[+]The odds ratio is the odds of an event occurring given a set of independent variables divided by the odds of the event occurring given a different value on one of those variables. This measures the likelihood of an event given a change in a specific independent variable; hence, this illustrates the association of that event with the given variable.

TABLE 1

The Risk of Alcoholism Controlling for Gender, ASP, and Family History of Problem Drinking

Gender	ASP	FHx	Predicted Probability of Alcoholism ± SE
Male	no	no	0.1893 ± 0.0140
Male	no	yes	0.3622 ± 0.0350
Male	yes	no	0.5429 ± 0.0442
Male	yes	yes	0.7429 ± 0.0390
Female	no	no	0.0300 ± 0.0043
Female	no	yes	0.0700 ± 0.0110
Female	yes	no	0.2408 ± 0.0507
Female	yes	yes	0.4355 ± 0.0693

ASP - Antisocial Personality
FHx - Family history of problem drinking

FIGURE 1

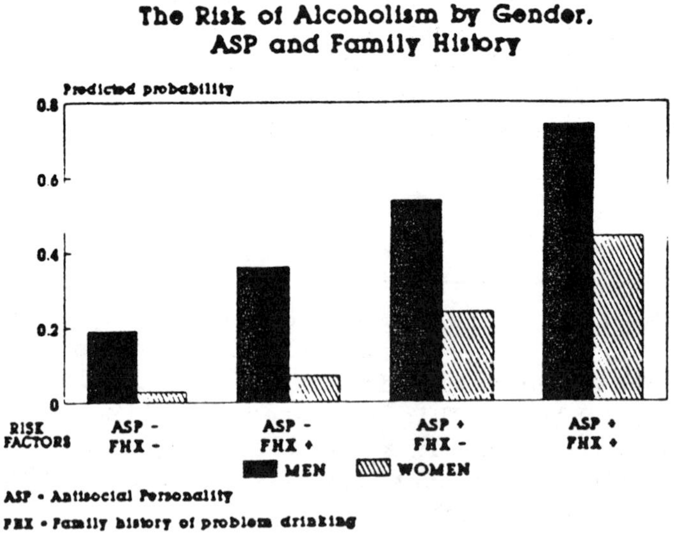

To determine the association of alcoholism with ASP, gender, and family history, we used stepwise logistic regression with a diagnosis of alcoholism (DSM-III alcohol abuse or dependence) as the dichotomous dependent variable and with ASP, gender, a family history of alcohol problems, drug problems, and antisocial problems as the five dichotomous independent variables. The results showed that gender, ASP, family history of alcohol problems, and the interaction of gender with ASP were all significantly related to alcoholism. The model goodness of fit was 5.845 with a "p" value of 0.119.

Being male, having ASP, and having a family history of problem drinking all increased the probability of developing alcoholism in the St. Louis sample. The interaction between gender and ASP indicated that alcoholism was more closely associated with ASP in women than in men. (Table 1 and Figure 1)

Alcoholism, conduct disorder, and family history

TABLE 2

The Risk of Alcoholism Controlling for Gender, Conduct Disorder, and Family History of Problem Drinking

Gender	Conduct Disorder	FHx	Predicted Probability of Alcoholism ± SE
Male	no	no	0.1914 ± 0.0146
Male	no	yes	0.3824 ± 0.0355
Male	yes	no	0.4136 ± 0.0358
Male	yes	yes	0.6485 ± 0.0410
Female	no	no	0.0266 ± 0.0041
Female	no	yes	0.0668 ± 0.0109
Female	yes	no	0.1684 ± 0.0320
Female	yes	yes	0.3463 ± 0.0532

FHx = Family history of problem drinking

FIGURE 2

The Risk of Alcoholism by Gender, Conduct Disorder and Family History

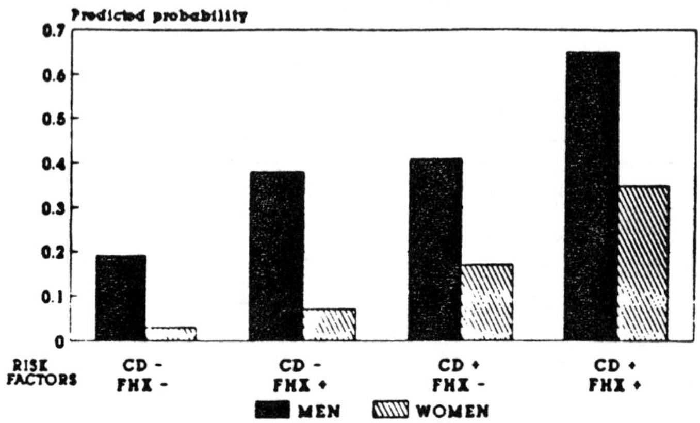

CD = Conduct Disorder

FHX = Family history of problem drinking

We repeated the analytic strategy substituting conduct disorder for antisocial personality, and the results were strikingly similar. Gender, conduct disorder, a family history of problem drinking, and the interaction of gender with conduct disorder were associated with alcoholism after all other variables had been taken into account. The goodness-of-fit chi square of the model with these four variables was 2.822 with a "p" value of 0.420 indicating an adequate fit.

Being male, having conduct disorder, and having a family history of alcohol problems all increased the probability of developing alcoholism in the St. Louis sample. The interaction between gender and conduct disorder indicated that alcoholism was more closely associated with conduct disorder in women than in men. (Table 2 and Figure 2)

Strengths of Association

Family history showed the weakest association with alcoholism with an odds ratio of 2.56 for both sexes;

ASP had a much stronger association with odds ratios of 5.09 for men and 10.24 for women. The interaction of ASP with gender was shown by the higher odds ratio for women than for men. The same pattern was noted for conduct disorder. Family history had a weaker association with alcoholism than conduct disorder. Family history had an odds ratio of 2.61 in both men and women, and conduct disorder had odds ratios of 2.98 and 7.40 in men and women respectively.

The chronology of antisocial behavior and alcohol abuse

In subjects with ASP, antisocial behavior began 11.0 ± 5.5 years ($t = 16.19$ with 65 df, $p < 0.0001$) before alcohol abuse in men and 12.1 ± 6.4 years ($t = 8.03$ with 17 df, $p < 0.0001$) before alcohol abuse in women. In subjects with conduct disorder, antisocial behavior began 11.9 ± 6.9 years ($t = 15.26$ with 77 df, $p < 0.0001$) before alcohol abuse in men and 11.9 ± 5.9 years ($t = 9.34$ with 20 df, $p < 0.0001$) before alcohol abuse in women with conduct disorder. Hence, antisocial behavior significantly preceded pathological drinking in both men and women with either ASP and alcoholism or conduct disorder and alcoholism.

Risk factors, epidemiology, and alcoholism

Gender, antisocial behavior, and a family history of problem drinking were three important antecedents of alcoholism. However, when either ASP or conduct disorder was combined with a positive family history of problem drinking and used as an overall predictor of alcoholism, the sensitivities and predictive values were quite low. Only 48.1% of all male alcoholics and 63.2% of all female alcoholics had either ASP or a positive family history or both. Similarly, only 51.5% of all male alcoholics and 67.1% of all female alcoholics had conduct disorder or a positive family history. Having either ASP or a positive family history predicted only 49.4% male and 13.6% female alcoholism, and having either conduct disorder or a positive family history predicted only 43.7% male and 12.9% female alcoholism.

DISCUSSION AND SUMMARY

These data confirm that serious early onset antisocial behavior, gender, and a family history of problem drinking all act as predispositions to alcoholism. Conduct disorder, antisocial personality, male gender, and a positive history of problem drinking in a close relative all increase the probability of alcoholism in the individual. Both conduct disorder and antisocial personality are more closely associated with alcoholism than a family history of problem drinking and both of these disorders interact with gender so that they are more closely associated with alcoholism in women than in men.

Although antisocial behavior and family history are two important predispositions to alcoholism, their use as screening devices for primary prevention only identifies about 51.5% of the men and 67.1% of women with alcoholism. Thus, these factors are somewhat inefficient screeners, but their utility lies in that they are readily identifiable in adolescents by teachers and parents.

A major question that remains is why some individuals with antisocial and familial risk factors do not develop alcoholism and why other individuals without these risk factors do. These issues cannot be answered directly by this data and pose the most challenging and difficult questions for future investigation.

Appreciation is expressed to Ms. Linda Heise for secretarial assistance, and Ms. Paula Stewart for graphical consultation.

REFERENCES

1. Schuckit MA. Alcoholism and sociopathy - diagnostic confusion. *Quarterly Journal of Studies on Alcohol*, 34:157-164, 1973.

2. Lewis CE. Alcoholism, antisocial personality, narcotic addiction: An integrative approach. *Psychiatric Developments*, 3:223-235, 1984.

3. Cotton, N. The familial incidence of alcoholism: A review. *Journal of Studies on Alcohol*, 40:89-116, 1979.

4. Lewis CE, Rice JP, Helzer JE. Psychiatric diagnostic interactions: alcoholism and antisocial personality. *Journal of Nervous and Mental Disease*, 171:105-113, 1985.

5. Lewis CE, Robins LN, Rice JP. Association of alcoholism with antisocial personality in urban men. *Journal of Nervous and Mental Disease*, 173:166-174, 1985.

6. Lewis CE, Rice JP, Andreasen N, et al. Clinical and familial correlates of alcoholism in men with unipolar major depression. *Alcoholism: Clinical and Experimental Research*, 10:657-662, 1986.

7. Robins LN, Helzer JE, Croughan JL. The National Institute of Mental Health Diagnostic Interview Schedule: its history, characteristics, and validity. *Archives of General Psychiatry*, 38:381-389, 1981.

8. American Psychiatric Association: Diagnostic and Statistical Manual of Mental Disorder, Third Edition, (1980) (American Psychiatric Assocation, Washington, D.C.).

9. Engelman, L. (1983) Stepwise Logistic Regression, in Dixon, W.J., Brown, M.B., Engelman, L. et al (Eds). BMDP Statistical Software, pp. 330-344 (Los Angeles, University of California Press).

10. Lemeshow S, Hosmer DW. Estimating odds ratios with categorically scaled covariates in multiple logistic regression analysis. *American Journal of Epidemiology*, 119:147-151, 1984.

PERCEPTION OF WHETHER DRUG OR PLACEBO HAS BEEN ADMINISTERED IS A DETERMINANT OF DRINKING REDUCTION

T. TONEATTO, E.M. SELLERS, L.C. SOBELL & M.B. SOBELL

In placebo-conducted clinical trials, a placebo is used to distinguish effects due to factors (i.e., expectancies, beliefs, motivation) other than the active treatment. The effects of subjects' perceptions of whether they are receiving drug or placebo are typically not assessed. This study evaluated the impact of such perceptions on the efficacy of an experimental drug to modify problem drinkers' alcohol consumption and on their reported urges to consume alcohol.

SUBJECTS

Subjects were 71 socially stable, male problem drinkers who responded to newspaper advertisements soliciting individuals who were interested in modifying their pattern of alcohol use. Subjects ranged in age from 19 to 65 years, had no concurrent medical or psychiatric problems requiring treatment, reported no excessive use of psychoactive drugs besides alcohol, had not received treatment for alcohol problems within the past year, and did not have DSM-III R (American Psychiatric Association, 1980) diagnoses of severe alcohol dependence.

PROCEDURE

During a two-week baseline phase, subjects completed daily self-monitoring forms assessing alcohol consumption. Twice daily, subjects also assessed their urge to drink alcohol, stress level, affect, and perceived effectiveness of alcohol to alter affective states. After completing the baseline phase, subjects were randomized, double-blindly, to one of two dosages of the experimental drug or to placebo. Subjects received drug or placebo for a 6-week period, making weekly visits to the program site. This was followed by a 1-week post-drug follow-up visit. All subjects concurrently received a non-intensive psychosocial intervention (Sobell, Sellers, & Sobell, 1990).

ANALYSIS

Dependent Variables

The main dependent variables were (i) daily evening drinking urge ratings, and (ii) daily alcohol consumption.

Independent Variables

Two independent variables were defined: assigned Drug Group [0.25 mg, n=23; 2.0 mg, n=25; placebo, n=23] and Drug Perception, based on the subject's belief as to whether they had received drug or placebo [drug, n=27; placebo, n=44]. Urges to drink and amount of consumption were analyzed in 2x3 analyses of covariance (ANCOVA) with baseline scores as the covariates.

---

*The views expressed in this manuscript are those of the authors and do not necessarily reflect those of the Addiction Research Foundation.

RESULTS

Alcohol Consumption

A significant ($p<.05$) Drug Perception main effect on the number of drinks consumed during treatment was obtained. Subjects who believed that they were receiving drug reported fewer drinks per day during treatment than did subjects who believed they had received placebo, regardless of whether they had actually received drug or placebo. Further analyses showed this effect occurred only during the first three weeks of the treatment period.

Urge Scores

A significant ($p<.05$) Drug Perception main effect on the urge scores reported during treatment was obtained. Subjects who believed that they had received drug during treatment reported significantly less strong urges to consume alcohol than those who believed they had received placebo, regardless of whether they had been administered drug or placebo. In addition to this main effect, a significant Drug Group X Drug Perception interaction was observed for the second three week period of treatment with subjects who believed that they had received placebo reporting more intense urges only if they also received the lower drug dose.

DISCUSSION

In this study subjects who believed they had received drug drank less and reported weaker drinking urges than did subjects who believed they had received placebo, irrespective of whether or not they had actually been administered drug or placebo. Thus, perception of which drug was administered influenced changes in alcohol consumption and urges to a greater degree than did the actual drug administered. These findings are especially interesting in the context of no significant main effects for the Drug Group condition. That is, an analysis limited to testing the central hypothesis of this study would have found that the experimental drug was not more effective than placebo in modifying alcohol consumption and would have hidden the effect that perception of drug condition produced on alcohol consumption and urges. An implication of these results is the necessity of assessing effects due to expectancy or belief, in addition to, and independent of, the effects produced by the pharmacological effects of the agent. It is possible, therefore, that drugs that produce reliable effects on behavior as a function of their pharmacology may interact with the subjects beliefs about the drug to either enhance, or equally possibly, to attenuate any behavioral effects. The recognition of such interactions raises the possibility of manipulating subjects' perceptions to facilitate the belief that the subject is actually receiving a drug. Although the data are not presented in this report, in this study subjects who reported at least one side effect tended to report less drinking than those who did not. Whether the pharmacological effects of the drug and the psychological states concerning the drug combined to synergistically maximize treatment effects must await further research. Finally, the clinical importance of the modest effects attributed to beliefs in this study remains to be evaluated.

REFERENCES

American Psychiatric Association. (1987) Diagnostic and statistical manual of mental disorders. (rev. 3rd ed.). Washington, DC: Author.

Sobell, M.B., Sellers, E.M., & Sobell, L.C. Combining pharmacological and behavioral treatments for enhancing self-control over addictive behaviors. Poster session presented at the Fifth International Conference on Treatment of Addictive Behaviors, Sydney, Australia, January 1990.

DISULFIRAM TREATMENT OF ALCOHOLISM

J. Chick

1.1 OBJECTIVE

To assess the efficacy of supervised disulfiram as an adjunct to out-patient treatment of alcoholics.

1.2 DESIGN

Randomized, partially-blind 6-month follow up study in patients receiving 200 mgs disulfiram or 100 mgs Vitamin C under supervision of a nominated informant.

1.3 SETTING

Seven alcoholism treatment centres in the United Kingdom.

1.4 SUBJECTS

One hundred and twenty six patients (64 disulfiram, 62 Vitamin C) attending clinics for alcohol dependence or abuse, who had relapsed after previous therapy or support and were now being helped towards complete abstinence.

1.5 MAIN OUTCOME MEASURES

Total abstinent days plus total and weekly average alcohol consumption as compared to the six months prior to the study.

1.6 RESULTS

In the opinion of the (blinded) independent assessor, disulfiram patients increased average total abstinent days by 100 and Vitamin C patients by 69 ($p=0.02$). Mean weekly alcohol consumption was reduced by 162 units with disulfiram, compared to 105 units with Vitamin C ($p=0.14$) and the disulfiram patients reduced their total 6-month alcohol consumption by 2572 units compared with an average reduction of 1448 units in the Vitamin C group ($p=0.04$). Serum gamma GT showed a great improvement with disulfiram than with Vitamin C ($p=0.02$).

1.6 CONCLUSIONS

In a 6 month follow-up study, supervised disulfiram plus counselling enhanced the outcome of treatment in alcoholics as compared to a control medication (Vitamin C) plus counselling.

CONTROLLED RELEASE DISULFIRAM (DS) IMPLANT.

M.D. Faiman*, K.E. Thompson+ and K.L. Smith+.
*Department of Pharmacology and Toxicology, University of Kansas, Lawrence, KS. 66045 and +Bend Research, Inc., Bend, OR 97701.

Introduction

The inhibition of liver aldehyde dehydrogenase (ALDH) and subsequent increase in acetaldehyde after ethanol ingestion, form the basis for the clinical use of disulfiram (DS) in the treatment of alcoholism. This is referred to as the disulfiram-ethanol reaction (DER). A major problem associated with DS's usefulness is patient compliance. DS implantation, however, could alleviate this concern. Unfortunately, the use of surgery required with implantation, and the apparent variability in producing a DER with implants, has limited the usefulness of this route of administration. Studies were therefore carried out to develop a cylindrical DS implant exhibiting high loading characteristics and a well-controlled range of release rates which could be implanted with a trochar. Specific objectives of these studies were to: 1) determine target doses from animal studies and to design prototype implants which meet these targets; 2) determine the *in vivo* release rates of DS from the prototype implants; 3) test the efficacy of prototype implants and correlate *in vitro* with *in vivo* release rates; and 4) determine the bioavailability of the implanted DS.

Methods

1. Implant Preparation

DS-containing cylindrical implants were prepared by mixing together DS and other core additives, heating to 50°C to melt the drug and achieve uniform mixing, drawing the liquid mixture into glass tubing (2 mm internal diameter), and cooling to solidify the implant core. The implant core, typically 3 cm long, could then be extruded manually from the glass tubing and cut to the desired length.

This drug core was then coated by submersion in a polymer solution and slowly withdrawing it, followed by drying at room temperature. This process was repeated to vary the membrane thickness.

2. Determination of Release Rates

In vitro release rates of drug from the prototype implants were determined by measuring the quantity of DS released into solution of 500 ml of tris-buffered saline at pH 7 at 37°C over a period of time. *In vivo* release rates of DS from the prototype implants were determined by measuring the amount of DS remaining in the implants following their removal from the implantation site in rats, subtracting this quantity from the initial quantity present in the implants, and dividing by the duration (time) the implant was left in the rat.

3. Implantation in Rats and Bioavailability

Male rats (275 - 300 g) were anesthetized with ether, a small incision made in the scapula region, the DS rod implanted, and the site closed with a staple. After the rats recovered from the ether, a loading dose of DS (40 mg/kg i.p.) was administered. Rats were then killed at various times after DS implantation.

Results and Discussion

Prototype implants were designed with a drug-containing core coated with a membrane through which the drug diffused. The permeability and thickness of the membrane controlled the release rate of drug until all the drug was delivered. The membrane subsequently bioeroded to obviate the need for removal. The release of DS from prototype implants is given in Figure 1. The implants performed according to theory, as a thick membrane resulted in DS release approximately five times slower than that from a membrane that was one-fifth the thickness.

In vivo release rates from implants placed in rats were determined for several different doses of implants. The dose of DS was varied by increasing the total length of the implants. As shown in Figure 2, the implants behaved in vivo as expected as the release rate was directly proportional to the dose. The efficacy of the prototype implants, as determined by liver mitochondrial low Km ALDH inhibition in rats also was found to be dependent on implant dose (Figure 3). Higher doses generally produced greater ALDH inhibition, although there was significant scatter in the data. ALDH inhibition greater than about 40% was assumed to be required for a reproducible DER.

In conclusion, a suitable DS bioerodable implant was developed. Increasing membrane thickness slowed the DS release rate. The release rate was directly proportional to the administered dose. DS inhibited ALDH continuously in vivo in a dose dependent manner. (Supported by a contract from NIAAA, contract No. ADM 281-86-0005)

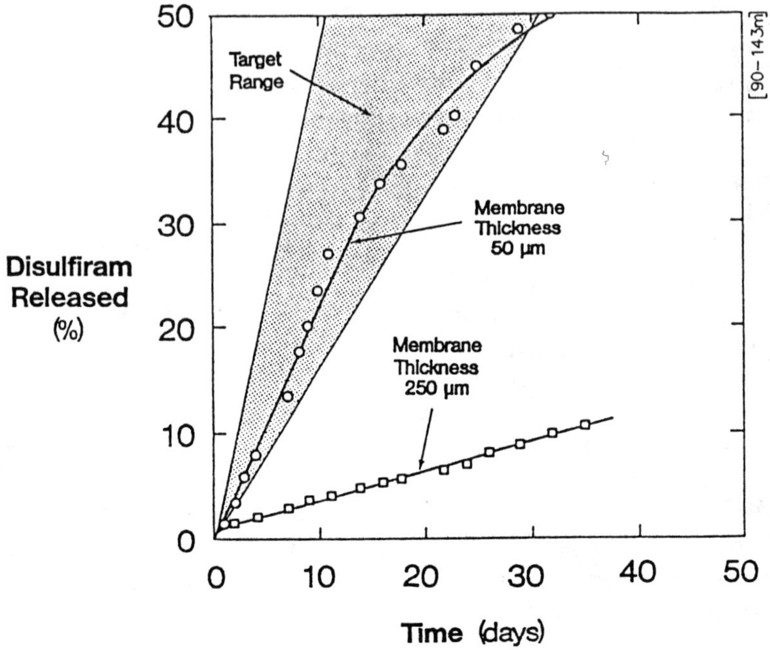

Figure 1. Disulfiram Release from Prototype Implants

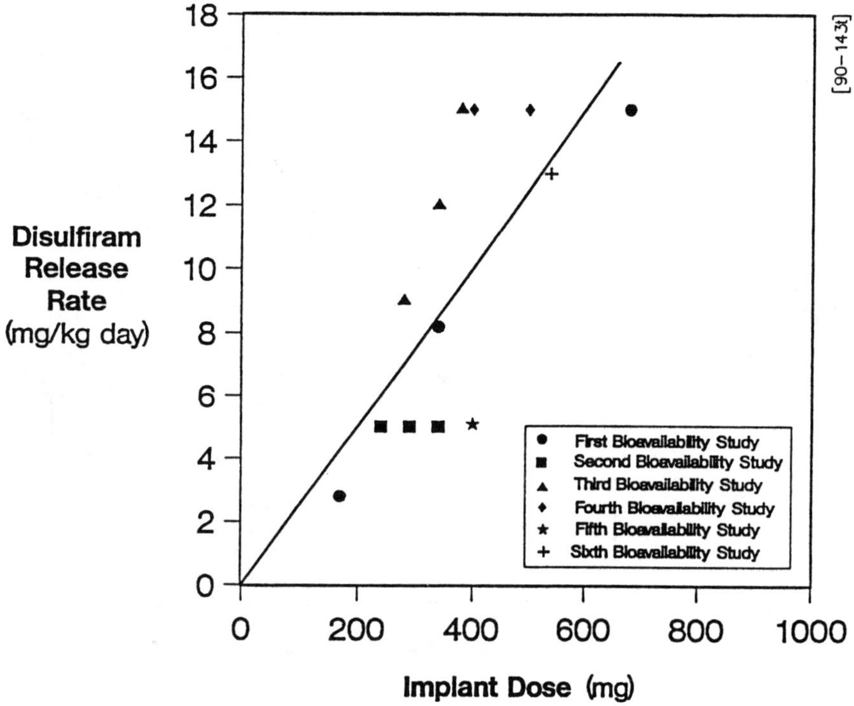

Figure 2. In Vivo Disulfiram Release Rate vs. Implant Dose

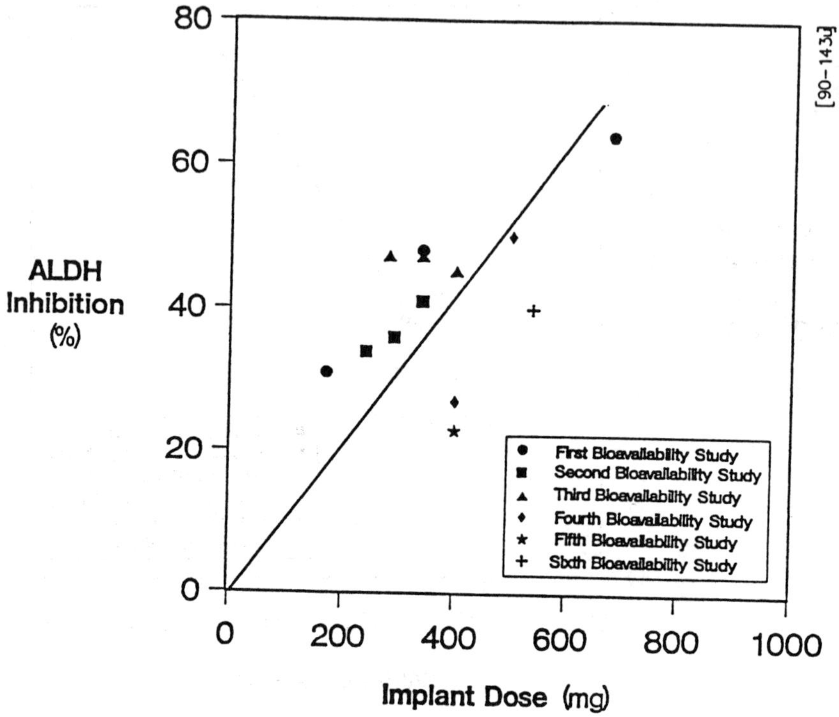

Figure 3: Implant Efficacy vs. Dose

DEPOT DISULFIRAM: PHARMACOKINETICS AND CLINICAL EFFECTS DURING 28 DAYS FOLLOWING A SINGLE SUBCUTANEOUS DOSE

Michael Phillips

1.1 OBJECTIVE

To evaluate two new sustained-release formulations of injectable depot disulfiram (DSF) for their ability to induce prolonged sensitivity to alcohol.

1.2 METHODS

Depot DSF: A single dose of depot DSF was administered in an ascending dose protocol using two different formulations:
Formulation A: Depot DSF suspended in normal saline/carboxymethylcellulose (CMC).
Formulation B: Depot DSF suspended in normal saline/polysorbate 80 (Tween 80^{R}).

1.3 HUMAN SUBJECTS

Fourteen abstinent male alcohol abusers first completed a qualifying period of four weeks of oral DSF without adverse effects. Following a one-week washout period, they each received a single treatment:
Formulation A: Five pairs of subjects received a single subcutaneous dose of 1.0, 2.0, 2.5, 3.0, or 3.5 g depot DSF.
Formulation B: Two pairs of subjects received a single subcutaneous dose of depot DSF (60 mg/kg or 75 mg/kg) accompanied by a single oral loading dose of DSF (15 mg/kg).

1.4 OUTCOME EVALUATION

Drug efficacy was monitored by the response to an alcohol challenge (0.15 kg ethanol/kg) administered prior to treatment, and repeated on days 7, 14, 21, and 28 after the injection of depot DSF. Subjective responses, skin temperature, breath ethanol and acetaldehyde levels, pulse rate and blood pressure were monitored at 5 minute intervals for 90 minutes. Pharmacokinetics of DSF were monitored by breath assays of carbon disulfide (CS_2), a metabolite of DSF, on days 0, 7, 14, 21 and 28. One hundred and twenty six patients (64 disulfiram, 62 Vitamin C) attending clinics for alcohol dependence or abuse, who had relapsed after previous therapy or support and were now being helped towards complete abstinence.

1.5 RESULTS

1.5.1 Subjective Response

Subjective responses to the alcohol challenges consistent with a DER were frequently observed. These were mild, consisting mainly of facial flushing, sweating and blurring of vision, and were usually maximal on day 7 or day 14, then declined in intensity. The reactions generally started within 10 minutes of the alcohol challenge, and were over within 35 minutes. There was no consistent relationship between the size of the dose and the intensity of the subjective responses.

1.5.2 Objective responses

Breath CS_2 levels demonstrated that the depot DSF was mobilized from the injection sites, generally peaking at day 7 or day 14. There was objective evidence of the alcohol challenges eliciting true DERs, as shown by changes in breath acetaldehyde, skin temperature, pulse rate, and systolic and diastolic blood pressure. Mean values for these variables were calculated fro the first 30 minutes following the ingestion of alcohol. The changes in several subjects achieved statistical significance when compared to baseline (pre-treatment) values, using analysis of variance (ANOVA).

1.6 FORMULATION B

Based on the finding of the low-dose study, the following changes were made in the protocol:

1. The formulation was changed. CMC was removed from the formulation, and replaced by a wetting agent, polysorbate 80 (Tween 80[R])

2. The dosage was increased. A new ascending dosage schedule was developed for an additional 10 subjects. In addition, dosage was adjusted to body weight:

Subject	Dose (mg DSF/kg)
11 & 12	60
13 & 14	75

3. An oral loading dose of DSF was administered with the depot DSF. The pharmacokinetic rationale of a loading dose is that a depot formulation, mobilized by log-linear kinetics, will be more effective over a longer period if it is administered when there is a high "baseline" level of drug in the body. For this reason, subjects were also given an oral dose of DSF on day zero (as close to 15 mg/kg as could be approximated by subdividing 250 mg tablets of DSF (Antabuse[R])

1.6.1 Subjective Responses to the Alcohol Challenges

These generally peaked on day 7 then progressively declined. The commonest complaint was flushing, which usually commenced within 10 minutes of drinking the alcohol. Flushing usually started in the face (most pronounced under the eyes), then spread to the chest, neck, and arms. Other common symptoms were blurring of vision and fatigue. There were sporadic reports of shortness of breath, chest discomfort, and numbness and tingling in the lips, fingers and toes. By testing, these symptoms caused moderate but not intense discomfort. The challenge dose of ethanol was kept low intentionally in order to elicit the typical symptoms of the DER, but not to make the patients violently ill.

1.6.2 Objective Responses

Again, there was objective evidence of the alcohol challenges eliciting true DERs, as shown by changes in breath acetaldehyde, skin temperature, pulse rate, and systolic and diastolic blood pressure. ANOVA testing of these data demonstrated a number of significant changes. In particular, it should be noted that elevations in breath acetaldehye were greater than those marked conjunctival injection was also observed but this was not quantified. The elevation in breath CS_2 varied consistently with dosage of depot DSF throughout the 28 day period, which probably reflected improved bioavailability of the drug.

1.7 CONCLUSIONS

1. Depot DSF was well tolerated by all subjects without toxicity or significant adverse effects.

2. Formulation A (DSF/CMC) exhibited erratic mobilization kinetics. Clinical effects were detectable for 28 days, but responses were mild and not consistently related to the dose.

3. Formulation B (DSF/polysorbate 80) exhibited superior mobilization kinetics. clinical responses were detectable for 28 days. Subjective and objective responses were related to the dose, and were clinically significant.

4. Formulation B combined with oral loading dose appears to offer an effective new approach to inducing and maintaining a sensitivity to alcohol for periods up to 28 days following a single treatment.

5. Further studies are needed to determine the optimal dosage of depot DSF, and to evaluate the effect of this treatment on drinking behavior in a prospective clinical trial.

MILDLY INTOXICATING LEVELS OF ALCOHOL PRODUCES DIRECT MYOCARDIAL DEPRESSION ON LEFT VENTRICULAR PERFORMANCE

Che-Ping Cheng, M.D., Ph.D.
Zak Shihabi, M.D.
William C. Little, M.D.

ABSTRACT

Previous studies of the effect of mildly intoxicating amounts of alcohol on left ventricular (LV) performance in conscious subjects have produced conflicting results. This may have resulted from the confounding influence of alcohol produced changes in loading conditions on conventional measures of LV performance. Accordingly, we recently used load-insensitive pressure (P)-volume (V) analysis of LV performance to assess the effect of alcohol (0.2 gm/kg, iv, blood level 67±14 mg/dl) in 10 conscious dogs. LV V was determined from three LV internal dimensions. Three relations that provide load-insensitive measures of LV performance were determined from variability loaded P-V loops produced by caval occlusions. Alcohol significantly decreased the slopes of the LV end-systolic P-V relation (14.7±2.2 vs 9.2±1.3 mmHg/ml, mean + SD, $p<0.05$), the dP/dt_{max}-end-diastolic volume (V_{ED}) relation (135.2±18.5 vs 99.1±15.9 mmHg/sec·ml, $p<0.05$) and the stroke work-V_{ED} relation (90.1±15.9; 85.2±9 mmHg, $p<0.05$). All three relations were shifted toward the right, indicating a depression of LV contractile performance. Similar, but more marked cardiac depression, was observed following autonomic blockade.

We conclude that mildly intoxicating levels of alcohol (blood concentration <100 mg/dl) are capable of producing myocardial depression in conscious animals, which are more marked after autonomic blockade. This suggests that patients with impaired LV function should avoid even small amounts of alcohol.

INTRODUCTION

Although the myocardial toxicity of chronic, excessive alcohol consumption is well established (1-2), the acute cardiac effects of occasional social drinking have not been clearly established. Acute, modest alcohol intake has been variably reported to improve (3), to have no direct effect (4,5), or to impair (6,7) left ventricular (LV) performance. Since conventional measures of LV performance are influenced not only by contractile state, but also loading conditions, these conflicting results may be due to the confounding influence of changes in both preload and afterload by alcohol. The influence of loading conditions can be minimized by evaluating LV performance in the pressure-volume plane (8). Thus, we recently used load-insensitive measures of LV performance derived from variably loaded pressure-volume loops, to assess the direct inotropic effects of alochol in normal conscious dogs with reflexes intact as well as after autonomic blockade (9).

MATERIALS AND METHODS

Ten healthy, adult mongrel dogs (weight 23-30 kg) were instrumented to measure LV pressure with a micromanometer and to measure three, orthogonal LV internal dimension (Figure 1) (9). All studies were performed after full recovery from instrumentation with the dogs lying on their right sides in a sling.

Data were initially recorded with the animals lying quietly on their sides without medication to obtain baseline values. Three sets of variably loaded pressure-volume loops were generated by sudden, transient occlusions of the cavae. This caused a progressive fall in LV end-systolic pressure, volume, and dP/dt_{max} over a 12-second recording period. Immediately after the recording period, the caval occlusion was released and hemodynamic parameters were allowed to restabilize. After all parameters returned to their baseline level, 0.2 gm/kg body weight alcohol was injected intravenously over 1 minute. Both new steady-state recordings and three sets of variably loaded P-V loops were generated immediately as well as 20 minutes after alcohol infusion.

To assess the interactions of alcohol with autonomic reflexes, the protocol was repeated after administering hexamethonium (5 mg/kg i.v.) and atropine (0.1 mg/kg i.v.) on the following day. The adequacy of the autonomic blockade was confirmed in each animal by a lack of an increase in heart rate after arterial pressure was reduced by >30 mmHg by caval occlusion.

Blood Ethyl Alcohol Determination

Blood samples (5 ml) were taken from a different vein than that used for alcohol infusion before, immediately after, and 20 min after alcohol infusion and analyzed by an enzymatic assay (10).

Data Processing and Analysis

The LV volume was calculated as a modified general elipsoid (9). LV stroke work (SW) was calculated by point-by-point integration of the LV pressure-volume loop for each beat as described by Glower et al (11).

From the variably loaded P-V loops produced by the transcient caval occlusions, we derived:

(1) the LV end-systolic P-V relation (P_{ES}-V_{ES}),

(2) the dP/dt_{max}-end diastolic volume (V_{ED}) relation, and

(3) the SW-V_{ED} relation (9).

Statistical Analysis

The slopes, volume intercepts, and positions of the relations for each condition were evaluated as the mean values determined from the three caval occlusions performed under each condition.

RESULTS

The blood alcohol concentration was undetectable before administering alcohol, and 125 ± 24.6 mmHg/dl immediately after alcohol. Twenty minutes after alcohol infusion, the blood level was 67 ± 14 mg/dl.

In the animals with intact autonomic nervous systems, there was no significant change in heart rate or P_{ES} in response to alcohol (9). The LV end-diastolic pressure was increased immediately after alcohol, while V_{ED} was reduced at 20 minutes after alcohol, LV end-diastoic pressure was elevated without any significant change in V_{ED}. Similar results were obtained after autonomic blockade.

With intact reflexes, dP/dt_{max} was significantly decreased immediately after infusing alcohol, but was not significantly different from control after 20 minutes. The stroke volume was significantly smaller and V_{EE} larger after alcohol. The arterial elastance was increased with alcohol. After autonomic blockade, dP/dt_{max} and SV were uniformly decreased and V_{EE} increased, but the arterial elastance was unchanged.

Representative variably loaded LV pressure-volume loops, produced by bicaval occlusion during autonomically blocked control and after alcohol infusion in a conscious dog, are shown in Figure 2. From these loops, the P_{ES}-V_{ES}, dP/dt_{max}-V_{ED}, and SW-V_{ED} relations were derived (Figures 2 -3). The slopes of all three relations, E_{ES}, dE/dt_{max}, and M_{SW}, were significantly ($p < 0.05$) decreased by alcohol. (Figures 2-3). Furthermore, all three relations were shifted toward the right. These changes were apparent both immediately after and 20 minutes after alcohol infusion. Similar changes in the relations with alcohol occurred in each animal with intact as well as after blocking the autonomic nervous systems (9).

DISCUSSION

We investigated the acute effect of alcohol on LV contractile performance in conscious animals (9). To avoid the potentially confounding effects of these changes in loading conditions on conventional measures of LV performance, we assessed LV contractile performance using variably loaded pressure-volume loops. All three measures of LV performance derived from the pressure-volume loops (the P_{ES}-V_{ES}, SW-V_{ED}, and dP/dt$_{max}$-V_{ED} relations) were shifted to the right with decrease in slopes after alcohol. The dose of alcohol used was modest, producing a steady-state blood alcohol concentration less than 100 mg/dl, below the usual legal definition of intoxication. This indicates that in conscious animals, even modest blood levels of alcohol produce a substantial depression of LV contractile performance.

The depression of LV performance was apparent with intact reflexes, but was somewhat more marked after complete autonomic blockade. In addition, alcohol's depression of LV contractile performance could be completely reversed by the infusion of a catecholamine, dobutamine (9). Thus, it appears that autonomically mediated cardiac stimulation partly offset the direct myocardial depression of alochol. This effect may be due to central sympathetic stimulation, stimulation of the adrenal medulla or other effects (12).

Our finding of a depression of LV contractile performance by alcohol in conscious animals is consistent with observations of isolated cardiac muscle (13). Although some previous studies of anesthetized animals (7), consious animals (6) and patients (5,14) have suggested that alcohol depresses LV contractile performance, other studies (3-5,15) have found little or no depression of cardiac performance with alcohol. These conflicting and inconsistent results may have resulted from the confounding influence of alcohol produced changes in loading conditions on conventional measures of LV performance, and variable effects of autonomic reflexes.

In summary, LV pressure-volume analysis indicates that even mildly intoxicating levels of alcohol are capable of producing direct myocardial depression in conscious animals (9). This myocardial depression appears to be partially offset by the automatically mediated effects. Our findings suggest that patients with impaired LV function should avoid even small amounts of alcohol.

ACKNOWLEDGEMENTS

The authors gratefully acknowledge Mary Ann Hayner and Kathy Hurdle's secretarial assistance, the technical assistance of Todd Hall and Brad Trott.

This study was supported in part by Grants-in-Aid from the North Carolina Affiliate of the American Heart Association and the NIH (R01-HL37324). Dr. Little is an Established Investigator of the American Heart Association.

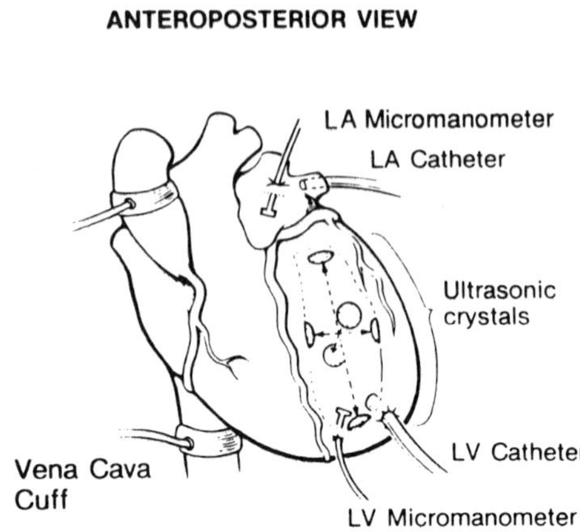

FIGURE 1. *Diagram of instrumentation.*

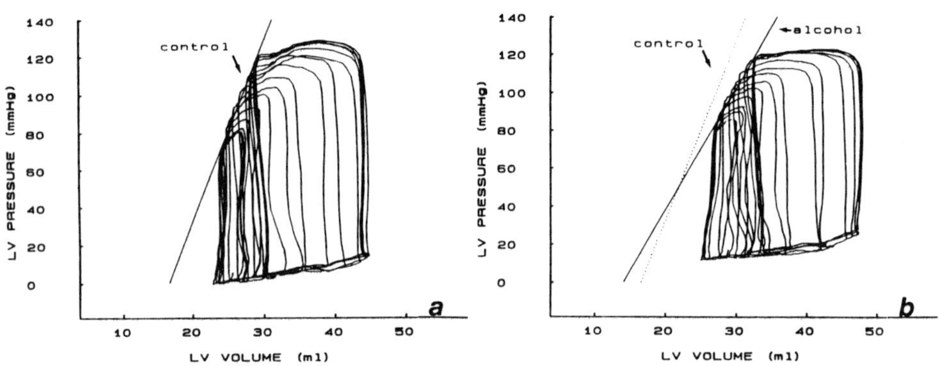

FIGURE 2. *Left ventricular pressure-volume loops produced by bicaval occlusion following autonomic blockade control (a) and after infusion of alcohol (b) in a conscious dog. End-systole occurs at the upper-left hand corner of the pressure-volume loop. The LV end-systolic pressure-volume relations are indicated by lines. Alcohol produced a rightward shift of the relation with a decreased slope. This indicates that alcohol depressed LV contractile performance.*

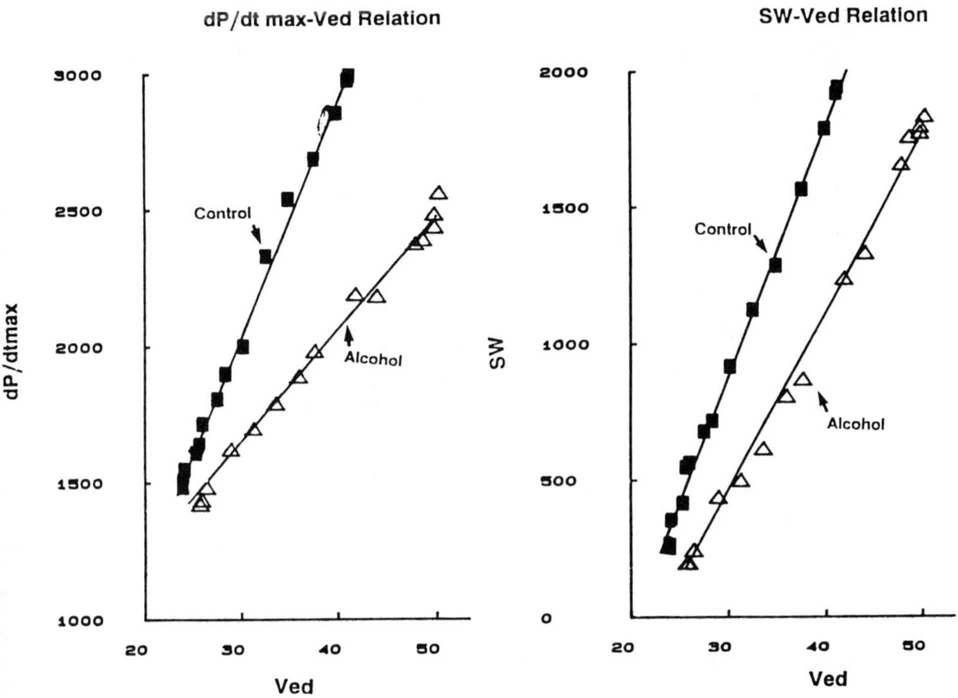

FIGURE 3. *The LV dP/dt*$_{max}$*-end-diastolic volume (*V_{ED}*) and stroke work (SW)-*V_{ED} *relations derived from the same pressure-volume shown in Figure 2. Alcohol decreases the slopes of both relations and shifts them to the right. This indicates a depression of LV contractile performance.*

REFERENCES

1. Alderman EL, Coltart DJ: Alcohol and the heart. Br Med Bull 38:77-80, 1982.
2. Gould L, Shariff M, and DiLieto M: Cardiac hemodynamics in alcoholic patients with chronic liver disease and presystolic gallop. J. Clin Invest. 48:860-868, 1969.
3. Gould L, Zahir M, DeMartino A, Gomprecht RF: Cardiac effects of a cocktail. JAMA 218:1799-1802, 1971.
4. Kupari M, Heikkila J, Ylikahri R: Acute effects of alcohol on left ventricular dynamics during isometric exercise in normal subjects. Clin Cardiol 6:103-108, 1983.
5. Riff DP, Jain AC, Doyle JT: Acute hemodynamic effects of normal human volunteers. Am Heart J 78:592-597, 1969.
6. Horwitz LD, and Atkins JM: Acute effects of ethanol on left ventricular performance. Circulation. 49:124-128, 1974.
7. Mierzwiak DS, Widenthal K, Mitchel JH: Acute effects of ethanol on the left ventricle in dogs. Arch. Int. Pharmacodyn Ther. 199:43-52, 1972.
8. Kass DA, and Maughan WL: From "E_{max}" to pressure-volume relations: a broader view. Circulation. 77:1203-1212, 1988.
9. Cheng CP, Shihabi Z, Little WC: Acute effects of mildly intoxicating levels of alcohol on left ventricular function in conscious dogs. J Clin Invest 85:1858-1865, 1990.
10. Jung G, and Ferard G: Enzyme-coupled measurement of ethanol in whole blood and plasma with a centrifugal analyzer. Clin Chem 24:873-876, 1978.
11. Glower DD, Spratt JA, Snow ND, Kabas JS, Davis JW, Olsen CO, Tyson GS, Sabiston DC Jr, Rankin JS: Linearity of the Frank-Starling relationship in the intact heart: the concept of preload recruitable stroke work. Circulation 71:994-1009, 1985.
12. Bloom FE, Siggins GR, Foote SL, Gruol D, Aston-Jones G, Rogers J, Pittman Q, Staunton D:. Noradrenergic involvement in the cellular actions of ethanol. In: Catecholamines: Neuropharmacology and Central Nervous System - Theoretical Aspects. New York: Alan R. Liss., 1984.
13. Gimeno AL, Timenom F, Webb JL: Effects of ethanol on cellular membrane potentials and contractility of isolated rat atrium. Am J Physiol 203:194-196, 1962.

14. Conway N: Hemodynamic effects of alcohol in patients with coronary heart disease. Br. Heart J. 30:638-644, 1968.

15. Regan TJ: Ethyl alcohol and the heart. Circulation 44:957-963, 1971.

A HUMAN MODEL FOR TESTING DRUG-INDUCED CONCOMITANT VARIATIONS IN ALCOHOL CONSUMPTION AND DESIRE TO DRINK*

C.A. Naranjo, K.E. Bremner, C.X. Poulos

1. ABSTRACT

A simple, economical and efficient model is needed to test new medications for alcohol consumption in humans. We compared the efficiency of two paradigms to determine the effects of a serotonin uptake inhibitor, known to decrease alcohol consumption, on alcohol intake and desire to drink. Healthy, non-depressed, alcohol-dependent subjects ($x=46$ standard drinks per week), 13 male and 3 female, aged 26 to 69 years, completed 4 one-week periods of a randomized, double-blind, crossover trial: baseline, citalopram (C) 40 mg/day, washout and placebo (P). Subjects monitored daily alcohol intake and had weekly medical and psychosocial assessments. Desire, craving, and liking for alcohol over the past week were rated on 5-point scales. C decreased total alcoholic drinks consumed to 32.2 ± 4.4 ($\bar{x} \pm$ SEM) compared with P (40.2 ± 5.4) ($p=0.01$) and increased percent of days abstinent (C: 27.7 ± 5.7; P: 15.5 ± 3.7; $p<0.01$). Subjects indicated less desire, craving, and liking for alcohol during C than P ($p<0.05$). Changes in these variables and drinks correlated ($r>0.5$, $p<0.01$). Furthermore, inpatient experimental bar sessions were conducted after C and P periods: the same subjects were offered up to 18 mini-drinks (6 standard alcoholic drinks), and rated their intoxication, mood and desire for each. There was some indication that citalopram reduced desirability for alcohol early in the experimental bar session, however, it had no significant effect when the entire session was analyzed. C had no effect on drinks consumed ($\bar{x} \pm \text{SEM} = 14.9 \pm 1.3$ after C, 16.1 ± 0.9 after P, n.s.) or intoxication. The potential sensitivity of the experimental bar sessions may have been reduced by the time of day offered for testing and restricted beverage choice. Accordingly, a more powerful experimental bar paradigm is being developed. However, a brief outpatient trial is a simple and efficient method to detect clinically important variations in desire to drink and alcohol consumption.

---

*Parts of this manuscript have been presented in abstracts and other papers by the authors.

The views expressed in this publication are those of the authors and do not necessarily reflect those of the Addiction Research Foundation.

2. INTRODUCTION

The initial testing of new medications in humans has been hampered by the lack of an adequate sensitive, simple and economical model. Such a model is crucial for the prompt and efficient identification of new pharmacological treatments for alcoholism and for testing their mechanism of action. Previous short-term (2 to 4) weeks outpatient clinical trials (Naranjo *et al*, 1984, 1989, 1990) have shown that several serotonin uptake inhibitors, including citalopram, (Naranjo *et al*, 1987) decrease alcohol consumption in subjects with mild to moderate alcohol dependence. The effect is not due to the antidepressant action of the drugs, an alcohol-sensitizing reaction, or side effects. Because of their potential therapeutic value, further research with serotonin uptake inhibitors was undertaken. This study compared the efficacy of two paradigms to test drug effects on alcohol consumption and desire to drink: 1) a short-term (4-week) outpatient trial, and 2) a drinking session in an experimental bar (Poulos and Cappell, 1987). The results have implications for the development of a standardized methodology for early studies to determine medication effects on alcohol intake and urges to drink in humans.

3. STUDY DESIGN

3.1 Outpatient Trial

The double-blind, crossover study consisted of four one-week periods: baseline, citalopram/placebo, washout and placebo/citalopram. Subjects recorded their daily intake of alcoholic drinks (one standard drink = 13.6 g absolute alcohol) and took an evening urine sample (approximately 10:00 p.m.) for measurement of ethanol (Kapur and Anderson, 1980) and riboflavin (Naranjo *et al*, 1984) concentrations. Study medication (identical appearing placebo or citalopram 40 mg capsules with a 20 mg riboflavin marker) was taken daily at 8:00 p.m. during the citalopram and placebo treatment periods. At the beginning of the study and weekly thereafter, subjects were assessed for depression, anxiety and side effects and had a physical examination including laboratory tests, as in our previous citalopram study (Naranjo *et al*, 1987). Blood samples were taken for assay of citalopram and metabolites in plasma and for uptake of serotonin by human platelets (Naranjo *et al*, 1987). Also, desire, craving, and liking for alcohol over the previous week were measured by ratings (0=not at all, 1=slight, 2=moderate, 3=a lot, 4=an awful lot), based on a scale designed by Fraser *et al* (1961). No advice or other treatment was offered to the subjects.

3.2 Experimental Drinking Sessions

Immediately after completion of the citalopram and placebo treatment periods the same subjects participated individually in an experimental bar session. In a relaxed bar setting, they were offered up to 18 alcoholic mini-drinks (equivalent to 6 standard drinks) at 5-minute intervals. For a 70 kg person, each drink was 35 ml in volume, with an ethanol concentration of 12% (approximately 4.2 g of ethanol). The volume of alcohol per drink was adjusted to each subject's body weight so that blood alcohol concentration (estimated by breathalyzer) would reach a maximum of approximately 100 mg/100 ml if every drink were consumed. Subjects indicated the desirability of each drink on a rating scale (integers between -100 and +100, where -100 = the strongest possible aversion I can imagine for the next drink in this situation, 0 = I don't care one way or another whether I have the next drink or not, and +100 = the strongest possible desire I can imagine having for this next drink) and could stop drinking before consuming all the scheduled drinks. Subjective level of intoxication (from 1.0 = not at all intoxicated to 10.0 = extremely intoxicated with intervals of 0.5) and other feelings and moods (18 items relating to present feelings (1 = not at all, 2 = slightly, 3 = moderately, 4 = quite a bit, 5 = extremely)), were indicated on self-rating scales during the experimental bar session. Once the maximum number of drinks (18) had been consumed, or the subject indicated that he/she desired no more, the experimental bar session was terminated and the subject remained under supervision until a breathalyzer reading of zero was obtained. The subject was then sent home by cab.

4. RESULTS

4.1 Subjects

The subjects, (13 male and 3 female) ranged in age from 26 to 69 years, and they drank an average of 46 standard drinks per week (6.6 per day). They were socially stable, well-educated (10 had attended college or university), and of average intelligence. They satisfied the DSM-III-R criteria for mild to moderate alcohol dependence (American Psychiatric Association, 1987), but abused no other drugs. They were not clinically depressed or anxious, and had no evidence of liver damage. All subjects were compensated for their participation.

4.2 Outpatient Trial

All measures of compliance (e.g., concentrations of citalopram and its metabolites in plasma) confirmed that subjects adhered to the study protocol.

4.2.1 Changes in Alcohol Intake

Alcohol intake was assessed in terms of mean daily drinks, percent of days abstinent and drinks per drinking day. Mean daily drinks (including drinking and abstinent days) significantly decreased during citalopram ($\bar{x} \pm SEM$ = 4.6±0.6) compared with placebo (5.7±0.8) ($F_{1,14}$ = 8.6, p = 0.01). Average alcohol intake during citalopram and placebo periods was significantly dependent upon baseline alcohol intake ($F_{1,13}$ = 25.4, p < 0.001). Order of treatment had no significant effect ($F_{1,13}$ = 1.4, n.s.) or interaction with the treatment effect ($F_{1,14}$ = 0.2, n.s.).

The average change in mean daily drinks when citalopram was compared with placebo was a 17.45% decrease with responses ranging from a 21.2% increase to a 41.7% decrease. Twelve of the 16 subjects decreased their alcohol intake during citalopram compared with placebo; the average decrease for these subjects was 28.9% with a range from 12.5% to 41.7%.

Percent of days abstinent during citalopram ($\bar{x} \pm SEM$ = 27.7±5.7) was significantly greater than during placebo (15.5±3.7) ($F_{1,14}$ = 14.4, p = 0.002). Order of treatment had no significant effect ($F_{1,13}$ = 1.9, n.s.) or interaction with the treatment effect ($F_{1,14}$ = 1.4 n.s.).

Drinks per drinking day were similar during citalopram ($\bar{x} \pm SEM$ = 7.0±1.0) and placebo (6.7±0.8), ($F_{1,14}$ = 0.4, n.s.). Therefore, subjects decreased their alcohol intake during citalopram treatment by decreasing the number of days on which they drank, rather than by decreasing the number of drinks per day.

4.2.2 Changes in Desire, Interest, Craving and Liking for Alcohol

Subjects indicated less desire and craving for alcohol during the citalopram treatment outpatient periods than during placebo (both p < 0.05), (Figure 1). This indicates an attenuation of the urge to drink. Similarly, citalopram decreased the liking for alcohol ($p<0.05$) (Figure 1), suggesting a decrease in its reinforcing effects. The variations in interest, desire, craving and liking correlated with alcohol intake (all $r>0.50$, $p<0.05$), indicating that the self-ratings may be a factor determining drinking level and that they are modifiable by citalopram.

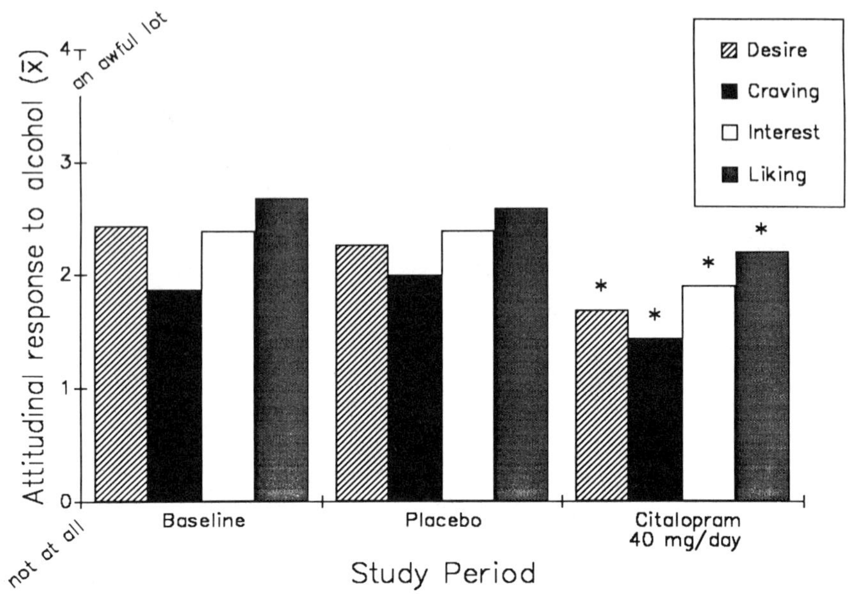

Fig. 1. Desire, craving, interest and liking for alcohol during the one-week outpatient study periods (* = $p < 0.05$ compared with placebo).

4.3 Experimental Bar Sessions

4.3.1 Desirability of Alcohol

Most subjects consumed 18 drinks during each experimental bar session. If the last drink taken was not drink 18, the last desirability rating was carried forward so that, for purposes of data analysis, each subject had 18 desirability ratings per session. Mean and maximum desire ratings during each experimental bar session were calculated for each subject. The number of drinks taken was also analyzed.

Citalopram had no significant effect on the number of drinks consumed during the experimental bar sessions ($\bar{x} \pm$SEM = 14.9 ± 1.3 after citalopram, 16.1 ± 0.9 after placebo, n.s.). Citalopram decreased the average desirability ratings for drinks 3 to 10 compared with placebo. However, in a multivariate set-up, comparing desire for drink 1 after citalopram with desire for drink 1 after placebo, etc., univariate F-tests with 1,15 degrees of freedom indicated a significant decrease in desire for alcohol after citalopram compared with placebo for only the fourth drinks ($p = 0.046$, with no adjustment made for multiple analyses). The mean desirability ratings for drinks 1 to 10 and drinks 11 to 18 did not differ between or within the two nor was the interaction (drug treatment wih drink number) significant. No effect of order of allocation to drug treatment, or interactions between order and treatment, were detected in any of the analyses.

4.3.2 Feelings of Intoxication and Changes in Mood

Subjective feelings of intoxication and blood alcohol concentrations (i.e. breathalyzer readings) increased with the number of drinks consumed but no differences in maximum or mean values between the citalopram and placebo experimental sessions were detected.

Before every third drink, subjects rated themselves on 18 items related to their mood at that moment. Maximum ratings for each item per experimental bar session were analyzed in a multivariate analysis of variance design. Citalopram decreased ratings for "my face feels warm" and "I feel depressed" ($p \leq 0.05$).

4.4 Adverse Events

All adverse events were mild to moderate and could not account for the decrease in alcohol intake or desire to drink during the citalopram periods. Symptoms included appetite loss, fatigue, headache and dry throat, but no symptom was reported more frequently during citalopram treatment than during placebo (McNemar's tests, all n.s.). However, four subjects dropped out because of adverse events while receiving citalopram 40 mg/day. One experienced fatigue and disorientation; one had headache and dry mouth; one felt tense, nervous, weak, fatigued and had insomnia; and one reported heart pounding, excess sweating, loss of appetite and insomnia. All subjects were followed until the symptoms disappeared.

5. DISCUSSION

This study compared two paradigms for assessing drug effects on alcohol consumption and their possible mechanisms of action. In the outpatient trial, citalopram 40 mg/day (one week) reduced alcohol intake in mildly to moderately dependent alcoholics, mainly by increasing the number of abstinent days per week. Citalopram also decreased desire, craving, interest and liking of alcohol, as assessed by retrospective self-report, and these changes correlated with drinking. These results confirm previous findings with citalopram (Naranjo *et al*, 1987). During the experimental bar sessions, citalopram 40 mg/day had no effect on the number of drinks consumed or intoxication from alcohol. However, there was some indication that citalopram 40 mg/day reduced the desirability of alcohol early in the experimental bar sessions but there was no significant overall effect. Therefore, while citalopram 40 mg/day effects on alcohol consumption and desire to drink alcohol are easily detected in short-term outpatient trials, drinking in an experimental bar seems to be less sensitive to citalopram effects. The potential sensitivity of the experimental bar session may have been reduced by the time of day offered for testing and restricted beverage choice. Therefore, the bar session is being developed into a more powerful experimental paradigm. In conclusion, a short-term outpatient trial is a simple, economical and efficient method to study the effects of a drug on desire to drink and the reinforcing effects of alcohol, and to test new pharmacological interventions for alcoholism.

6. REFERENCES

American Psychiatric Association (1987). DSM-III-R Diagnostic and Statistical Manual of Mental Disorders (Third Edition-Revised), Washington D.C.

Fraser, H.F., G.D. Van Horn, W.R. Martin, A.B. Wolback and H. Isbell (1961). Methods for evaluating addiction liability, a)"attitude" of opiate addicts toward opiate-like drugs, b) a short-term "direct" addiction test. *J. Pharmacol. Exp. Ther.*, 133, 371-387.

Kapur, B., and M. Anderson (1980). Enzymatic determination of ethanol in urine with the American monitor KDA. *J. Clin. Chem.*, 26, 1063.

Naranjo, C.A., E.M. Sellers, C.A. Roach, D.V. Woodley, M. Sanchez-Craig, and K. Sykora (1984). Zimelidine-induced variations in alcohol intake by non-depressed heavy drinkers. *Clin. Pharm. Ther.*, 35, 374-381.

Naranjo, C.A., E.M. Sellers, J.T. Sullivan, D.V. Woodley, K. Kadlec, and K. Sykora (1987). The serotonin uptake inhibitor citalopram attenuates ethanol intake. *Clin. Pharm. Ther.*, 41, 266-274.

Naranjo, C.A., J.T. Sullivan, K.E. Kadlec, D.V. Woodley-Remus, G. Kennedy, and E.M. Sellers (1989). Differential effects of viqualine on alcohol intake and other consummatory behaviors. *Clin. Pharmacol. Ther.*, 46, 301-309.

Naranjo, C.A., K.E. Kadlec, P. Sanhueza, D. Woodley-Remus, and E.M. Sellers (1990). Fluoxetine differentially alters alcohol intake and other consummatory behaviours in problem drinkers. *Clin. Pharmacol. Ther.*, 47, 490-498.

Poulos, C.X. and H. Cappell (1987). The self-regulation of alcohol consumption in heavy and light drinkers. 4th International Conference of Treatment of Addictive Behaviors, Bergen, Norway.

Poster Papers: Serotonin and Alcohol Consumption

MIANSERIN, A SEROTONERGIC ANTAGONIST, AND INTAKE OF AN ALCOHOLIC BEVERAGE

Edward J. Bilsky, John D. Delconte, Christopher L. Hubbell and Larry D. Reid

There is evidence showing that manipulations of serotonergic systems affect ingestion. In general, agents enhancing serotonergic activity decrease ingestion, while serotonergic antagonists block this effect and, by themselves, appear to potentiate ingestion [1,2,3,4,5,6,7,8,9]. In addition, there are a number of reports that enhanced serotonergic activity reduces intake of ethanol (E) [10, 11,12,13,14,15]. If serotonergic systems are saliently related to propensity to take E, and if increases in serotonergic activity decrease intake, then it is reasonable to predict that decreases (or antagonism) in serotonergic activity should enhance intake of alcoholic beverages. In the present study, we assessed the effects of mianserin, a general serotonergic antagonist, across a range of doses, on rats' intakes of a sweetened alcoholic beverage.

METHOD

Sixty, male, Sprague-Dawley rats (Taconic Farms, Germantown, NY) were maintained on a daily regimen of 22 hr fluid deprivation followed by a 2-hr opportunity to take water and a sweetened ethanol solution (ES). Each 100 g of ES contained 12 g of pure E, 5 g of sucrose and 83 g of tap water. Each day, rats' body weights and intakes of fluids were tabulated. The data associated with rats' intake of E are presented in terms of g/kg (g of pure E taken per kg of body weight).

Subsequent to being maintained on the daily regimen, just described, for 80 days, a dose-response assessment of mianserin's effects was made. The doses tested were 0.0 (physiological saline), 0.1, 1.0, 3.0 and 10.0 mg/kg. On one day, all rats received placebos (physiological saline). The rats were divided into 5 groups (n=12) such that their mean g/kg intakes were nearly equal. Doses of mianserin were then randomly assigned to each group. The following day, rats received their respective dose of mianserin. All injections were given subcutaneously, 1 ml/kg, 30 min prior to their drinking session.

RESULTS

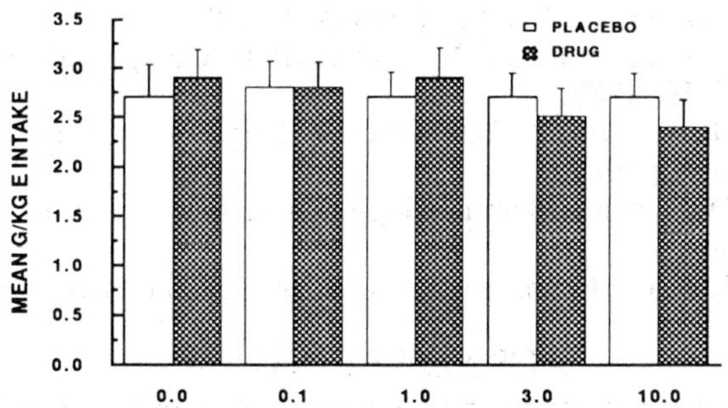

FIGURE 1. On one day, all groups received injections of physiological saline (PLACEBO). On the next day, the groups received a dose of mianserin (DRUG).

The results, in terms of mean g/kg, are depicted in Figure 1. The data conform to a 5 by 2 ANOVA, having repeated measures, with factors associated with Doses of mianserin and Days (placebo versus drug), respectively. In brief, the overall ANOVAs of the data associated with rats' intake of E and water failed to reveal reliable sources of variance associated with either factor or their interaction. For example, the interaction term of the ANOVA of the data associated with g/kg yielded an $F(4,55)=0.44$, $p=0.78$.

DISCUSSION

Since we had no independent measure of mianserin's effects, the results are difficult to interpret. It is possible that mianserin did not reach brain or a procedural error was made. On the other hand, given that mianserin was administered correctly (and there is no reason to suppose that it was not), and given that mianserin did not reliably modify intake of the sweetened alcoholic beverage, there is no support provided for the hypothesis that serotonergic systems are specifically involved in propensity to take alcoholic beverages. Mianserin, in the same doses as tested here, dose-relatedly increased 4-hr food-intake among rats that were not deprived of food or water [3]. In our study, informal observation indicated that the rats receiving the highest dose ate more food. Nevertheless, we are left with the fact that null results are difficult to interpret without another, independent measure of mianserin's effects.

REFERENCES

1. Bendotti, C., & Samanin, R. European Journal of Pharmacology 121:147-150; 1986.
2. Blundell, J.E. Neuropharmacology 23:1537-1551; 1984.
3. Dourish, C.T., et al. Psychopharmacology 97:54-58; 1989.
4. Dourish, C.T., et al. Psychopharmacology 94:58-63; 1988.
5. Dourish, C.T., et al. Psychopharmacology 86:197-204; 1985.
6. Hutson, P.H., et al. European Journal of Pharmacology 129:347-352; 1986.
7. Neill, J.C., & Cooper, S.J. Physiology & Behavior 44:453-459; 1988.
8. Neill, J.C., & Cooper, S.J. British Journal of Pharmacology 92:647; 1987.
9. Weiss, G.F., et al. Pharmacology Biochemistry & Behavior 25:1223-1230; 1986.
10. Linnoila, M., et al. International Congress of Pharmacology Abstracts:S-67A; 1987.
11. Murphy, J.M., et al. Alcohol 2:349-352; 1985.
12. Naranjo, C.A., & Sellers, E.M. International Congress of Pharmacology Abstracts:S-69; 1987.
13. Ogren, S.O., & Amit, Z. International Congress of Pharmacology Abstracts:S-70; 1987.
14. McBride, W.J., et al. Pharmacology Biochemistry & Behavior 30:1045-1050; 1988.
15. Bilsky, E.J. et al. Pharmacology, Biochemistry and Behavior 37: in press; 1990.

ACKNOWLEDGMENT

This research was supported, in part, by a grant from NIDA (DA04440).

EFFECTS OF THE 5-HT UPTAKE INHIBITOR, SERTRALINE, ON ETHANOL, WATER AND FOOD CONSUMPTION

B.Brands, H.L.Kaplan, E.M.Sellers

Introduction

Several reports in the literature (Gill et al, 1985; Lucki et al, 1988; Gill et al, 1988a, b; Wong et al, 1988) have shown that 5HT uptake inhibitors decrease ethanol and food consumption in rats.

The present study was undertaken to characterize the overall food consumption and the microdrinking patterns of ethanol and water of sertraline-treated rats using an unlimited-access, free choice paradigm.

Materials and Methods

Subjects

Male Wistar rats (Charles River, Canada) initially weighing 175-225g were housed individually in stainless steel cages in a room regulated for constant temperature (22-24 C), humidity (55%) and a 12 hour lights on (7:00 am-7:00 pm) cycle.

Procedures

Following a 2-3 day habituation period where water was the only fluid available, rats were presented with a free choice drinking schedule between water and an ethanol solution. The free choice schedule began with a 2% ethanol solution (v/v) and was slowly increased (1% every 3 days) until a final concentration of 5% (v/v) was achieved. Only rats consuming more than 2g/kg/12hr dark cycle on the 5% ethanol solution continued in the study.

The rats then entered a 7 day baseline period during which they received daily (6:00 pm) intraperitoneal injections of vehicle. Fluid intake was continuously monitored and food consumption was measured daily.

At the end of baseline, blocking of the rats was performed based on ethanol consumption. Rats then entered the first 2 day drug phase followed by two days of washout. In three subsequent treatment/washout cycles , the rats were crossed to the 3 other treatments in a Latin square design. Rats received once daily (6:00 pm) injections of Sertraline 1.0, 3.0, or 10.0 mg/kg or vehicle control. Throughout the treatment period of the study all animals continued to receive a free choice between water and 5% ethanol solution. Continuous monitoring of ethanol and water occurred. Body weight and food consumption were measured daily.

Drinkometer System

The drinkometer is a specialized testing device designed to monitor the amount of fluid consumed by a rat every minute. It consists of a microcomputer, a scanning digital voltmeter, a power supply and 60 drinking units. The drinking units track consumption by measuring the partial vacuum in the space above the fluid column of an arrangement hydraulically equivalent to a sealed-top Richter tube. Two drinking units, one filled with ethanol solution and the other with distilled water, are mounted on each individual rat's cage.

The drinkometer provides minute by minute readings of the volume of fluid remaining in the tube and stores these readings on disk. At the conclusion of the experiment, the files are transferred to a second computer where software has been written to remove noise from these data and then extract statistics of interest, typically including total volume consumed, number of individual drinks (periods of one or more consecutive minutes where the volume remaining has decreased), number of minutes of drinking activity, and the time at which the first 50% of the fluid has been consumed.

Materials

Sertraline HCL (Pfizer) was dissolved in distilled water (pH6.0) and prepared fresh daily. All doses were calculated as the HCL salt.

Analysis

Using the SAS GLM procedure, the 16 days of data for each rat were fit to a model including terms for rat, treatment cycle, dose, day (within treatment cycle), and the interactions of each cycle and dose with day. From this analysis, the residual sum of squares was used to test three specific contrasts, each contrast comparing the mean of one dose's two treatment days to the vehicle control condition, with no correction for the multiple comparisons. These contrasts were based on the fitted model, which automatically accounts for missing data in both the estimates and the error term. The same analysis was applied to each of the dependent variables.

Results

At the end of the study, only 16 rats were reliably drinking >1.5 g/kg/day on washout days, and only the data for those 16 rats are reported here. Sertraline decreased ethanol consumption in g/kg ($p=0.0009$) as well as number of drinks ($p=0.0002$); the 10 and 3 mg/kg doses of sertraline reduced ethanol consumption by 30% and 13% respectively, compared to the vehicle condition, and fewer drinks were taken in these two conditions compared to control. Water consumption was unaffected. All doses of sertraline decreased food consumption ($p=0.0001$), but only in the 10 mg/kg condition did this lead to a reduction in weight gain.

Discussion

The present study confirms the findings of Gill and her associates (1988a, b) that sertraline decreases ethanol consumption while water consumption remains unaffected. The drinkometer system has enabled us to demonstrate that this reduction in ethanol intake is due to a decrease in the number of drinks; drink size does not change. Sertraline had no effect on the volume of water consumed, number of water drinks or size of water drinks. These findings suggest a selective serotonergic regulation of ethanol drinks.

The anorexic effect of sertraline has been well documented (Gill et al, 1988b; Lucki et al, 1988). We too were able to show that sertraline decreased food consumption at all doses studied. These findings continue to implicate the 5HT system in the regulation of consummatory behaviours.

References

Gill, K., Amit, Z. and Ogren, S.O. The effects of zimeldine on voluntary ethanol consumption: studies on the mechanism of action. Alcohol 2:343-347 (1985).

Gill, K., Amit, Z. and Koe, B.K. Treatment with sertraline, a new serotonin uptake inhibitor, reduces voluntary ethanol consumption in rats. Alcohol 5:349-354 (1988a).

Gill, K., Filion, Y., and Amit, Z. A further examination of the effects of sertraline on voluntary ethanol consumption. Alcohol 5:355-358 (1988b).

Lucki, I, Kreider, M.S. and Simansky, K.J. Reduction of feeding behavior by the serotonin uptake inhibitor sertraline. Psychopharmacol. 96:289-295 (1988).

Wong, D.T., Reid, L.R. and Threlkeld, P.G. Suppression of food intake in rats by fluoxetine: Comparison of enantiomers and effects of serotonin antagonists. Pharmacol. Biochem. Behav. 31:475-479 (1988).

FLUVOXAMINE IS POORLY TOLERATED BY ALCOHOLICS

Kranzler, H., Del Boca, F., Korner, P. and Brown, J.

Fluvoxamine maleate is a monocyclic antidepressant that potently and selectively inhibits presynaptic serotonin reuptake (Claasen et al. 1977). In addition to their antidepressant effects, selective serotonin-uptake inhibitors (SUIs), have been shown to reduce ethanol consumption in both rodents and non-depressed, heavy drinking humans (Gorelick 1986, Naranjo et al. 1984, 1986, 1987, 1989, 1990). To test the utility of fluvoxamine as an adjunct to relapse prevention treatment, we conducted an open trial (OT) in 16 subjects (13 males) and then initiated a placebo-controlled, double-blind trial (CT) in 19 subjects (18 males). All subjects met DSM III-R criteria for alcohol dependence (APA 1987). Subjects were excluded if they met criteria for current drug (other than nicotine) dependence or if they had a medical or psychiatric disorder that contraindicated treatment with fluvoxamine.

Measures of alcohol consumption (Sobell et al. 1980), depressive symptoms (Hamilton 1960), and severity of alcohol dependence (Hesselbrock et al. 1983), were obtained at baseline. Side effects were monitored on a weekly basis, using a structured interview. A side effect scale was developed based on the number and intensity of symptoms reported. Prior to treatment this scale provided a general measure of symptomatology (i.e. baseline "side effects").

In both the OT and the CT, fluvoxamine treatment was begun at a dosage of 50 mg hs and was then gradually increased to a maximum of 200 mg per day over two weeks. The dosage was decreased at any time during treatment in response to adverse effects. All subjects also received weekly, individual cognitive-behavioral psychotherapy.

Results

The majority of subjects treated with fluvoxamine in both trials did not complete the 12-week treatment program. Of 16 patients who received the drug in the

OT, only six (38%) completed. Five of the subjects who left the OT prematurely attributed their dropout to intolerable side effects. Of the 10 subjects that received fluvoxamine in the CT, only two (20%) completed treatment. Six of those in the active drug group who left treatment prematurely cited intolerable side effects as the reason. Among the nine placebo-treated subjects in the CT, eight (89%) completed 12 weeks. The CT was discontinued early, given the high dropout rate in the fluvoxamine-treated subjects.

No significant diferences were found in the baseline characteristics of subjects who completed the 12-week trial, compared with those who did not (pooled across the two studies). Those who completed the trials had consistently low side effect scores. The noncompleter group had a peak mean side effect score at week two (at which time the mean score was more than double that at baseline), after which it declined (due to selective attrition) to near that of the completer group. At week two the mean ($\pm$ SD) side effect score was 1.8 ($\pm$ 1.9) for the completer group and 6.1 ($\pm$ 9.5) for the noncompleter group. While the side effect scores were not significantly different at baseline or at week 1, at week 2 the difference approached significance ($t=1.35$, $df=8$, $p=.11$). Both the small sample size and the large variability in side effect scores appear to mitigate against a significant finding. Among noncompleters, the most commonly reported side effects were gastrointestinal (e.g. nausea), followed by CNS effects (e.g. headache and sedation). Completers reported fewer and less intense treatment emergent symptoms; the symptoms reported most often were CNS effects (e.g. headache and sedation). Interestingly, all 4 females in the two studies (all of whom received fluvoxamine) completed 12 weeks of treatment.

Discussion

Fluvoxamine has been shown to be effective in the treatment of both major depression (Benfield and Ward 1986), and obsessive-compulsive disorder (Goodman et al. 1989,1990). In these trials, fluvoxamine was well tolerated. Similarly, other SUIs have been well tolerated in both heavy drinkers (Naranjo et al. 1987, 1989, 1990) and alcoholics (Gorelick 1986). In an ongoing trial of fluoxetine for alcohol dependence, which employs a design and study population similar to those used in our CT with fluvoxamine, we have also found fluoxetine to be well tolerated. To date, we have enrolled 48 subjects in the fluoxetine study. Of the 26 subjects assigned to receive fluoxetine, 4 (15%) have dropped out due to adverse effects of the medication. In comparison, 2 of 22 placebo-treated subjects (9%) have dropped out due to side effects.

In contrast, in our OT with fluvoxamine, a substantial proportion (31%) of patients treated with the drug reported adverse effects that led to study discontinuation. Despite the recruitment of less severely dependent, more socially stable subjects for the CT, fluvoxamine-induced side effects led 60% of subjects treated with the drug to drop out. Moreover, noncompleters did not differ from completers in terms of any alcohol-related variables that may have offered an alternative explanation for differential dropout. The high retention rate for placebo-treated subjects may be interpreted to reflect efficacy for the relapse prevention treatment that was provided to both groups.

Based on these results we believe that that fluvoxamine is not useful as an adjunct to relapse prevention psychotherapy for the treatment of alcoholism. An alternative application for fluvoxamine may be in a challenge paradigm, where it may serve to discriminate alcohol-dependent subjects from nonalcoholics.

Acknowledgement: This work was supported by grant AA03510 from the National Institute on Alcohol Abuse and Alcoholism.

References available on request

Poster Papers: Opioids and Alcohol Consumption

EFFECTS OF DIFFERENTIAL HANDLING ON RATS' INTAKE OF ALCOHOL

Richard C. Gilbert, John D. Delconte, Christopher L. Hubbell and Larry D. Reid

Considerations of the effects of stress on propensity to take alcoholic beverages have played a predominant role in theories of alcoholism. Generally, the idea is that stress, in one of its many manifestations, increases propensity to take alcohol. Sometimes it is explicitly stated that alcohol is anxiolytic. The mechanism by which alcohol, then, increases propensity to drink is by way of negative reinforcement, i.e., alcohol is said to provide relief from stress.

An early and persistently found effect, in the study of endogenous opioid peptides, is that stress increases some signs of increased activity of the endogenous opioids. Stress, for example, increases the release of beta endorphin as measured in samples of blood [1].

Small doses of morphine increase the intake of alcoholic beverages in rats [2]. Since these small doses might mimic the effects of endogenous opioids, and since stress increases the release of some endogenous opioids, perhaps, stress might increase propensity to take alcoholic beverages in the same circumstances that morphine does. Such a hypothesis is very compatible with the thinking of Volpicelli et al. [3] who have used naltrexone to treat alcoholics.

Bozarth [4] found that shaking rats (an activity that from the folklore of rat-laboratories is known to "calm" difficult to handle rats) produced a state that would sustain a conditioned place preference. He attributed this effect to a release of endogenous opioids. Given the line of thinking outlined above, it follows that this shaking of rats should increase rats' intake of of alcoholic beverages. Consequently, we shook rats in different ways before their daily opportunity to take sweetened, alcoholic beverage.

METHOD

Sixty, male, Sprague-Dawley rats (Taconic Farms, Germantown, NY) were maintained on a daily regimen involving 22 hr of fluid deprivation followed by a 2-hr opportunity to take water and a sweetened ethanol solution (ES). Each 100 g of ES contained 12 g of pure ethanol (E), 5 g of sucrose and 83 g of tap water. Each day, rats' body weights and intakes of fluids were tabulated to the nearest 0.1 g. The data associated with rats' intake of E are presented in terms of g/kg (g of pure E taken per kg of body weight). After 45 days of being maintained on the daily regimen, just described, the effects of differential handling on intake of E were assessed. The data obtained on the day previous to the treatment-day, was used as "placebo" data. The rats were divided into four groups (n=15) such that their mean g/kg intakes on the placebo day were nearly equal. On the day of treatment, the groups were exposed to one of four of the following types of handling, 15 min before the drinking session: (a) no handling, (b) being weighed only, (c) being weighed and swung five times at the end of an outstretched arm in a pendulum-like motion or (d) being weighed, being swung, and being shaken vigorously.

The data conform to a 4 by 2 ANOVA, having repeated measures, with factors associated with Groups (exposure to one of four types of handling) and Days (no treatment versus treatment), respectively. The body weights from the day of no treatment were used to calculate the g/kg intakes of the group that was not weighed on treatment-day.

RESULTS

The results of differential handling on rats' intake of E, in terms of mean g/kg, are presented in Figure 1. The overall ANOVAs of the data associated with rats' intake of E and water failed to reveal reliable sources of variance associated with either factor or their interaction. For example, the interaction term of the ANOVA of the data associated with rats' g/kg intakes yielded an $F(3,56)=0.21$, $p=0.89$.

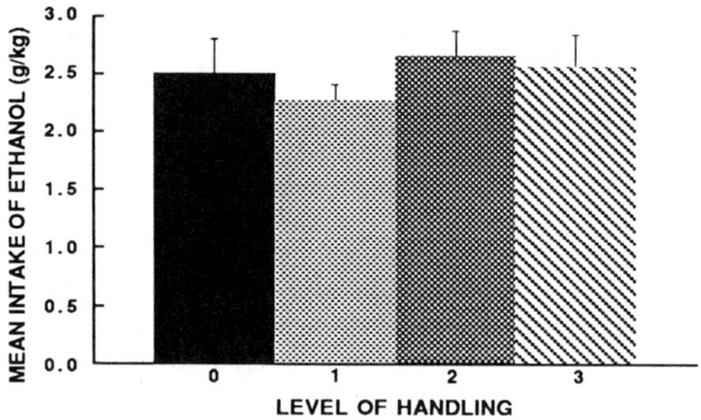

FIGURE 1. Depicted are the effects of different levels of handling on rats' intake of a sweetened alcoholic beverage. Treatments were given shortly before a 2-hr presentation of a sweetened alcoholic beverage and water, after 22 hr of deprivation of fluids. None of the levels of handling reliably modified intake of ethanol. 0 = no handling. 1 = weighing. 2 = weighing and swinging. 3 = weighing, swinging, and shaking.

DISCUSSION

Our procedures did not affect intake of E. This, of course, does not mean that stress will not contribute to a propensity to take alcoholic beverages. We did not have an independent measure of the effectiveness of our treatments in terms of producing stress or leading to a release of endogenous opioids.

Relevant to the considerations of stress and propensity to drink alcoholic beverages is a personal communication from Joseph Volpicelli. He reported that stress induces an increased propensity to take E some period of time after the stress rather than soon after stress.

The findings are comforting from one perspective. It apparently makes little difference to the outcomes of our studies, using the same general procedures that were used here, exactly how the rats are handled while they are getting injections of drugs. Our injection-procedures are surely not more gross than these procedures which have no effects.

REFERENCES

1. Millan, M.J. In: Emrich, H.M. (Ed.), Modern Problems of Pharmacopsychiatry: The Role of Endorphins in Neuropsychiatry. Basel: Karger, pp. 68-96, 1981.
2. Hubbell, C.L., & Reid, L.D. In: Reid, L.D. (Ed.), Opioids, Bulimia, and Alcohol Abuse & Alcoholism. New York: Springer-Verlag, pp. 145-174, 1990.
3. Volpicelli, J.R., et al. In: Reid, L.D. (Ed.), Opioids, Bulimia, and Alcohol Abuse & Alcoholism. New York: Springer-Verlag, pp. 195-214, 1990.
4. Bozarth, M.A. In: Bozarth, M.A. (Ed.), Methods of Assessing the Reinforcing Properties of Abused Drugs. New York: Springer-Verlag, pp. 241-273, 1987.

ACKNOWLEDGMENT

This research was supported, in part, by a grant from NIDA (DA04440).

STEREOSELECTIVITY OF OPIOIDS' EFFECTS ON INTAKE OF AN ALCOHOLIC BEVERAGE

Michael L. Nichols, Christopher L. Hubbell and Larry D. Reid

Small doses of morphine (M), the classic agonist at opioid receptors, increase rats' intake of alcoholic beverages. Naloxone (NX), the classic antagonist, decreases rats' intake. Having firmly established these basic facts (for a review see [1]), the next set of questions revolve around issues of the generality and specificity of these effects. The small-dose-M-effect is not peculiar to one or two experimental arrangements, but is observed across a variety of experimental arrangements [1]. However, small doses of M increase and NX decrease a wide array of ingesta, with effects being more pronounced when the ingesta are at the more extreme ends of preference-aversion functions. So, these opioidergic effects, although robust [1], are not specific to alcoholic beverages [2].

There are also issues of pharmacological specificity. For example, can any agent that might be self-administered by rats (or people) act similarly to M? The answer is probably no, not all agents that people take recreationally increase rats' intake of alcoholic beverages. Cocaine, MDMA, and THC, for examples, do not lead rats to take more alcoholic beverages than they would ordinarily.

There are other issues of pharmacological specificity. Are, for example, the effects of M and NX due to their effects at opioid receptors? There is clearly a possibility that the effects could be by way of other receptors or other mechanisms. The usual way of determining if an effect is opioidergic is to see if that effect is reversible by NX. If we assessed whether or not M's effects were reversed by NX and we observed a decrease in intake after a combination of M and NX, the effect could be merely a nonspecific effect of NX and not due to NX's blockade of M. There is, however, another way of asking about specificity with respect to a given receptor. The stereospecific isomers of NX should produce selective effects if the response in question is related to one kind of receptor. Consequently, to further assess the specificity of opioidergic effects on intake of alcoholic beverage, we tested the effects of the dextrorotatory (+NX) and levorotatory (-NX) stereoisomers of NX.

METHOD

Sixty, male, Sprague-Dawley rats (Taconic Farms, Germantown, NY) were maintained on a daily regimen involving 22 hr of fluid deprivation followed by a 2-hr opportunity to take water and a sweetened ethanol solution (ES). Each 100 g of ES contained 12 g of pure ethanol (E), 5 g of sucrose and 83 g of tap water. Each day, rats' body weights and intakes of fluids were tabulated to the nearest 0.1 g. The data associated with rats' intake of E are presented in terms of g/kg (g of pure E taken per kg of body weight).

After 21 days of being maintained on the daily regimen, just described, a dose-response assessment of +NX and -NX's effects on intake of E was made. The doses of each stereoisomer tested were 0.1, 1.0 and 10.0 mg/kg. Injections of drug or placebo (physiological saline) were given subcutaneously, 1.0 ml/kg, 15 min before the presentation of fluids. On one day, all rats received placebos. Subsequently, the rats were divided into 6 groups (n=10) such that their mean g/kg intakes under placebo were nearly equal. On the next day, the groups were given one of the doses of one of one of the stereoisomers. The data conform to a 2 by 3 by 2 ANOVA, having repeated measures, with factors associated with Stereoisomer, Dose and Day (placebo versus drug), respectively.

RESULTS

The results are presented in Figures 1 and 2. The overall ANOVA of the data associated with rats' intakes of E yielded a reliable main effect of Days, $F(1,54)=5.73$, $p<0.03$, and a reliable Day by Stereoisomer interaction, $F(1,54)=6.08$, $p<0.02$. Subsequently, separate 3 (Dose) by 2 (Day) ANOVAs were performed for the data obtained with each stereoisomer. No reliable sources of variance were revealed by the ANOVA of the data of g/kg for the +NX isomer. However, the ANOVA of the data of g/kg for the -NX isomer revealed a reliable main effect of Day, $F(1,27)=10.6$, $p=0.003$. Student's t-tests, for dependent measures, revealed that the 10.0 mg/kg dose of -NX reliably decreased rats' mean g/kg intakes, $t(9)=2.51$, $p<0.04$. The other two doses of -NX did not reliably modify rats' intake of E.

The overall ANOVA of the data associated with the rats' intake of water revealed reliable sources of variance associated with the Day by Stereoisomer interaction, $F(1,54)=8.26$, $p<0.006$. Again, separate 3 (Dose) by 2 (Day) ANOVAs were performed for the data obtained with each stereoisomer. No reliable sources of variance were revealed by the ANOVA of the data associated with the +NX isomer. The ANOVA of the data associated with the -NX isomer revealed a reliable main effect of Day, $F(1,27)=7.65$, $p=0.02$. Student's t-tests, for dependent measures, revealed that no individual dose of -NX reliably decreased rats' intake of water. However, the 10.0 mg/kg dose of -NX produced a marginal decrease in rats' mean intakes of water, $t(9)=2.13$, $p=0.062$.

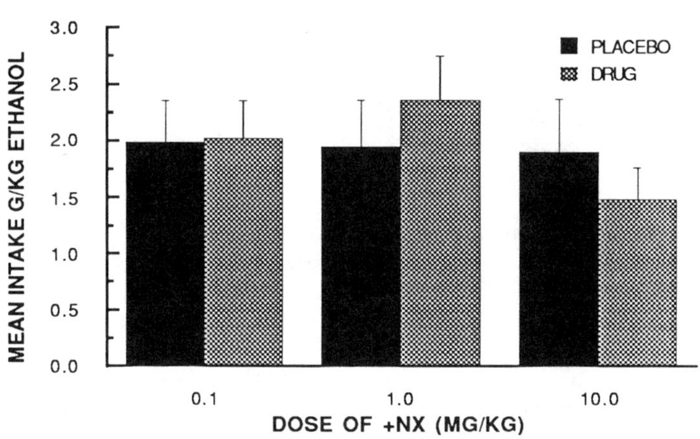

FIGURE 1. Depicted are the effects of doses of +NX on rats' intakes of ethanol. PLACEBO refers to a day when rats received an injection of saline. DRUG refers to the next day when they received one of the doses of +NX. Error bars represent standard errors of the means. In brief, none of the doses of +NX tested produced reliable shifts in rats' mean intakes of E.

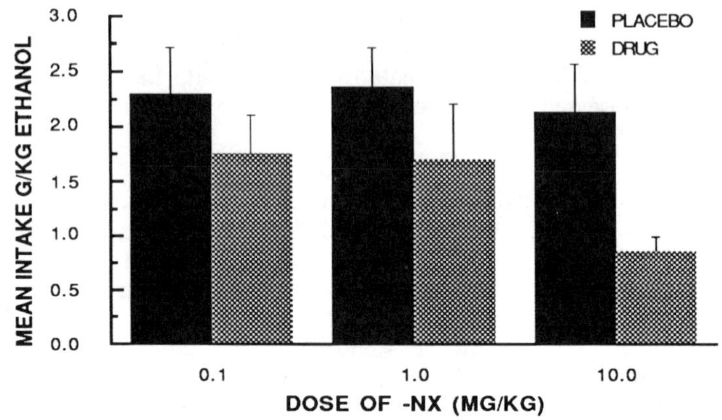

FIGURE 2. Depicted are the effects of doses of -NX on rats' intakes of ethanol. PLACEBO refers to a day when rats received an injection of saline. DRUG refers to the next day when they received a dose of -NX. The 10.0 mg/kg dose of -NX reliably decreased rats' intake of E ($p<0.04$). Error bars represent standard errors of the means.

DISCUSSION

These findings confirm that NX's effects on intake of E are due to its actions at opioid receptors and not due to an action at other kinds of receptors or by way of other nonspecific effects. It seems clear that NX's effects on intake of alcoholic beverages are related to those receptors defined as opioid, i.e., those receptors for which M is an agonist and NX is an antagonist. Both M and NX are relatively nonspecific in terms of kind of opioid receptor. Given that there are multiple kinds of opioid receptors, and that more kinds are apt to be discovered [3], there remains the possibility that only one kind of opioid receptor is, in turn, related to intake of alcoholic beverages.

REFERENCES

1. Hubbell, C.L., & Reid, L.D. In: Reid, L.D. (Ed.), Opioids, Bulimia, and Alcohol Abuse & Alcoholism. New York:Springer-Verlag, pp. 145-174, 1990.
2. Reid, L.D. American Journal of Clinical Nutrition 42:199-1132; 1985.
3. Unterwald, E.M., & Zukin, R.S. In: Reid, L.D. (Ed.), Opioids, Bulimia, and Alcohol Abuse & Alcoholism. New York: Springer-Verlag, pp. 49-72, 1990.

ACKNOWLEDGEMENTS

This research was supported, in part, by a grant from NIDA (DA04440). M.L. Nichols was supported by funds made available from the Ewing Marion Kauffman Foundation.

METABOLITES OF MORPHINE AND INTAKE OF AN ALCOHOLIC BEVERAGE

Edward J. Bilsky, Kenneth D. Wild, Michael L. Nichols,
Christopher L. Hubbell and Larry D. Reid

A number of studies have shown that small doses of morphine enhance intake of ethanol solutions among rats (for a review, see [1]). Furthermore, this effect is centrally mediated [2,3]. The two primary metabolites of morphine are morphine-6-beta-D-glucuronide (M6BG) and morphine-3-beta-D-glucuronide (M3BG) [4,5]. Among people, M6BG produces analgesia [6]. Among mice, M6BG is about 45 times more potent than morphine when given intracerebrally, but only 3 to 4 times more potent when administered subcutaneously [7]. Furthermore, it has been demonstrated that M6BG crosses the blood-brain barrier, and that its effects are not mediated by reconverting into morphine [8]. M3BG, however, is inactive with respect to analgesia.

Not all opioid agonists, with respect to analgesia, are effective at enhancing intake of ethanol solution [9]. Consequently, one approach to learning more about the specifics of how morphine increases intake of ethanol solutions is to see if a group of opioids might be isolated that produce analgesia, but not enhance intakes and another group isolated that produces enhanced intakes, but not analgesia, and then compare them. We tested, therefore, whether or not M3BG would increase rats' intake of ethanol, as well as M6BG. We assessed the effects of these two metabolites on rats' intake of a sweetened alcoholic beverage. In a pilot study, we tested the effects of M6BG on rats' intake of ethanol, in doses of 0.03, 0.1, and 0.3 mg/kg. The results of that preliminary study indicated a trend for the 0.3 mg/kg dose to increase rats' mean intake of ethanol. In the present study, we assessed the effects of a higher dose of M6BG and, in addition, the effects of a range of doses of M3BG on rats' intakes of ethanol.

METHOD

Sixty, male, Sprague-Dawley rats (Taconic Farms, Germantown, NY) were maintained on a daily regimen involving 22 hr of deprivation of fluids followed by a 2-hr opportunity to drink water and a sweetened ethanol solution (ES). The ES was 12% pure ethanol, 5% sucrose in tap water. Each day, rats' body weights and intakes of fluids were tabulated to the nearest 0.1 g. The data associated with rats' intake of ethanol are presented in terms of g/kg (g of pure ethanol taken per kg of body weight).

After 34 days of being maintained on the daily regimen just described, dose-response assessments of the effects of both M6BG and M3BG on rats' intakes of fluids were made. On one day, all rats received injections of placebo (physiological saline). Subsequently, the rats were divided into 6 groups (n=10) such that their mean g/kg intakes under placebo were nearly equal. On the next day, 5 of the groups received injections of one of the metabolites. The doses of M6BG tested were 0.3 and 1.0 mg/kg. The doses of M3BG tested were 0.3, 1.0 and 3.0 mg/kg. The sixth group received only placebo (saline) and served as the control group. Injections of drug or placebo were given subcutaneously, 1.0 ml/kg, 15 min before the presentation of fluids.

RESULTS

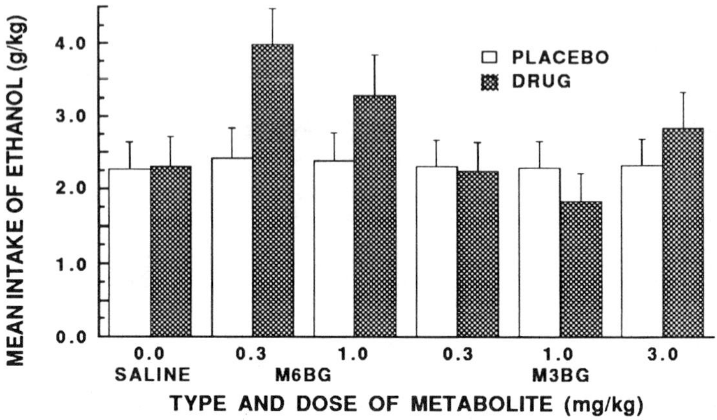

FIGURE 1. Depicted are the effects of the two major metabolites of morphine on rats' intake of ethanol. The 0.3 mg/kg dose of morphine-6-beta-D-glucuronide (M6BG) reliably increased rats' intakes. No dose of morphine-3-beta-D-glucuronide (M3BG) produced reliable shifts in rats' intakes. Error bars represent standard errors of the mean.

The results, in terms of mean g/kg, are presented in Figure 1. The data conform to a 6 by 2 ANOVA having repeated measures with factors associated with Groups (placebo or one of the doses of the metabolites) and Days (placebo versus drug), respectively. The ANOVA revealed a reliable main effect of Days and a reliable interaction term, $F(1,54)=5.98$, $p=0.018$ and $F(5,54)=3.039$, $p=0.017$, respectively. Since the groups had nearly equal mean g/kg intakes under placebo, the source of the interaction must be due to differential intakes on the day when doses of the metabolites were administered. Student's t-tests, for dependent measures, revealed that the 0.3 mg/kg dose of M6BG reliably increased rats' intake of alcoholic beverage, $t(9)=2.33$, $p=0.04$. The 1.0 mg/kg dose of M6BG also produced an increase in intake that approached standards of statistical significance, $t(9)=2.12$, $p=0.06$. No dose of M3BG produced reliable shifts in rats' intakes. Neither metabolite reliably modified rats' mean intakes of water.

DISCUSSION

The results indicate that M6BG has similar effects as morphine on intake of an alcoholic beverage, while M3BG had no discernible effect. These results are concordant with what would have been predicted from previous studies of morphine and its metabolites.

Given that morphine's analgesia and its ability to enhance intake of alcoholic beverages are separable [1], it was reasonable to ask whether or not M3BG would enhance intake of ethanol solution. It did not. M6BG is the "active" metabolite with respect to analgesia and intake of alcoholic beverage.

REFERENCES

1. Hubbell, C.L., & Reid, L.D. In: Reid, L.D. (Ed.), Opioids, Bulimia, and Alcohol Abuse & Alcoholism. New York: Springer-Verlag, pp. 145-174, 1990.
2. Linesman, M.A. Pharmacology Biochemistry & Behavior 33:407-413; 1989.
3. Wild, K.D. Is the Opioidergic Modulation of Ethanol-Intake a CNS Phenomenon? Unpublished Master's Thesis, Rensselaer Polytechnic Institute, 1989.
4. Casy, A.F., & Parfitt, R.T. Opioid Analgesics: Chemistry and Receptors. New York: Plenum Press, 1986.
5. Misra, A.L. In: Adler, M.L., Manara, L., & Samini, R. (Eds.), Factors Affecting the Action of Narcotics. New York: Raven Press, pp. 297-343, 1978.
6. Osborne, R., et al. Lancet 1(8589):828; 1988.
7. Shimomura, K., et al. Tohoku Journal of Experimental Medicine 105:45-52; 1971.
8. Yoshimura, H., et al. Biochemical Pharmacology 22:1423-1430; 1973.
9. Reid, L.D. In: Reid, L.D. (Ed.), Opioids, Bulimia, and Alcohol Abuse & Alcoholism. New York: Springer-Verlag, pp. 275-280, 1990.

ACKNOWLEDGEMENTS

This research was supported, in part, by a grant from NIDA (DA04440). M.L. Nichols was supported by funds made available from the Ewing Marion Kauffman Foundation. We thank Yizhao Hui for help with the data collection. K.D. Wild is now with the Department of Pharmacology, University of Arizona.

PERIPHERAL ADMINISTRATION OF TIQS AND INTAKE OF AN ALCOHOLIC BEVERAGE

Michael L. Nichols, Edward J. Bilsky, Christopher L. Hubbell and Larry D. Reid

In 1970, two findings indicated that a metabolite of ethanol (E) could combine with certain neurotransmitters to produce potential opioidergic products [1,2]. The idea is that acetylaldehyde (the first metabolic product of E) in the presence of either phenylethylamine, dopamine, norepinephrine or epinephrine yields a class of compounds called tetrahydroisoquinolines (TIQs). Subsequently, it was demonstrated that the central administration of a TIQ increased intake of E among rats [3,4,5]. Although a critical site of action of these putative metabolites of E must be in brain, the question remains: What effects do these agents have on intake of E when administered peripherally? Therefore, we tested the effects of 3 TIQs on rats' intake of a sweetened alcoholic beverage. The 3 TIQs tested were: (a) 1,2,3,4-tetrahydroisoquinoline (1,2,3,4-TIQ); (b) tetrahydropapaveroline (THP); and (c) l-salsolinol (SAL).

METHOD

Male, Sprague Dawley rats (Taconic Farms, Germantown, NY) were maintained on a daily regimen involving 22 hr of fluid deprivation followed by a 2-hr opportunity to take water and a sweetened E solution (ES). Each 100 g of ES contained 12 g of pure E, 5 g of sucrose and 83 g of tap water. The data associated with rats' intakes of E are presented in terms of g/kg (g of pure E taken per kg of body weight).

Various doses of each TIQ were assessed. All rats had been maintained on the regimen previously described for at least 50 days prior to any assessment. In brief, on one day all rats received placebos. Subsequently, they were divided into equally numbered groups such that their mean g/kg intakes under placebo were nearly equal. On the next day, groups received a dose of a TIQ.

1,2,3,4-TIQ was assessed in doses of 0, 1, 3, 10, 30 and 55 mg/kg among 72 rats. THP was assessed in doses of 0, 1, 3 and 10 mg/kg among 36 rats. SAL was assessed in doses of 0, 1, 3 and 10 mg/kg among 48 rats. Physiological saline served as placebo (0 mg/kg) for 1,2,3,4-TIQ and SAL, while distilled water was the placebo for THP. All injections were given subcutaneously, 1.0 ml/kg, 15 min before the session. The data of each assessment conform to a factorial ANOVA having repeated measures, with factors associated with Doses and Days (placebo versus drug), respectively.

RESULTS

The dose-response effects of 1,2,3,4-TIQ on intake of E are presented in Figure 1. The ANOVA revealed reliable main effects of Doses, $F(5,66)= 2.59$, $p<0.04$, and Days, $F(1,66)=23.2$, $p<0.0001$, and a reliable Day by Dose interaction, $F(5,66)=5.58$, $p=0.0002$. Student's t-tests, for dependent measures, revealed that the source of the interaction was due to the 10, 30 and 55 mg/kg doses reliably decreasing rats' intakes of E, $t(11)=4.19$, $p<0.002$, $t(11)=2.93$, $p<0.02$, and $t(11)=4.67$, $p=0.0007$, respectively.

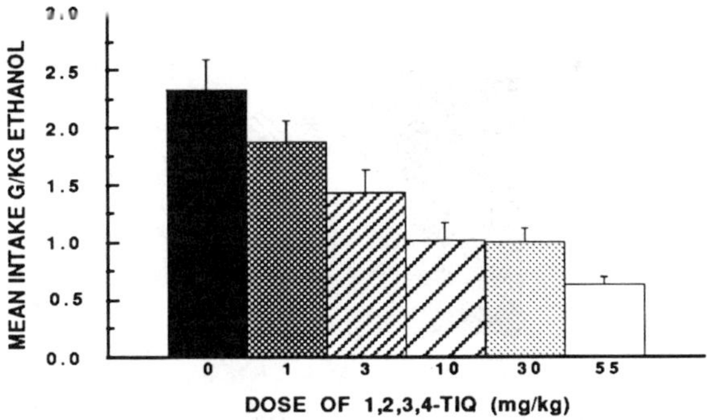

FIGURE 1. Depicted are the dose-response effects of 1,2,3,4-tetrahydro-isoquinoline (1,2,3,4-TIQ) on rats' intake of ethanol (E), in terms of g/kg, on the day of drug administration. On the previous day there were no reliable differences between groups' mean intakes of E. In brief, 1,2,3,4-TIQ dose-relatedly decreased rats' intake of E. Error bars represent standard errors of the means.

The ANOVA of the data associated with intake of water revealed a reliable main effect of Days, $F(1,66)=12.7$, $p<0.0001$. Student's *t*-tests, for dependent measures, revealed that all doses of 1,2,3,4-TIQ reliably increased intake of water, all $ps<0.05$.

The dose-response effects of THP on intake of E are presented in Figure 2. The ANOVA revealed a reliable main effect of Days, $F(1,32)=50.1$, $p<0.0001$. Student's t-tests, for dependent measures, revealed that each dose of THP reliably decreased intake of E, all $ps<0.02$. The ANOVA of the data associated with intake of water revealed a reliable main effect of Days, $F(1,32)=34.4$, $p<0.0001$. Student's t-tests, for dependent measures, revealed that 1 and 3 mg/kg doses of THP reliably increased intake of water, $t(8)=2.74$, $p<0.03$, and $t(8)=2.90$, $p<0.02$, respectively.

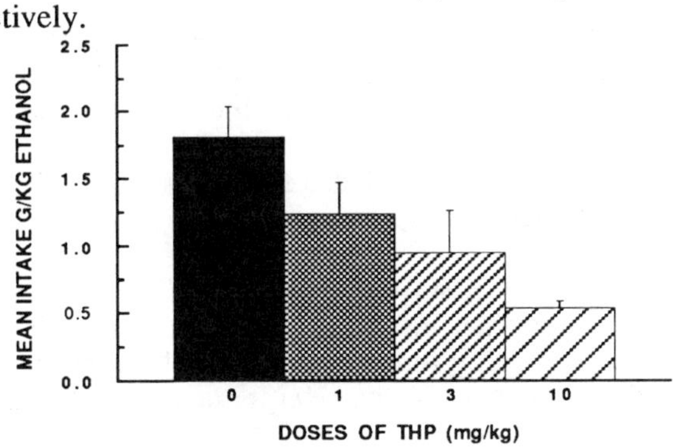

FIGURE 2. Depicted are the dose-response effects of tetrahydropapaveroline (THP) on rats' intake of ethanol (E), in terms of g/kg, on the day of drug administration. On the previous day, all rats, received placebos and there were no reliable differences between groups' mean intakes of E. In brief, all doses of THP reliably decreased rats' intake of E. Error bars represent standard errors of the means.

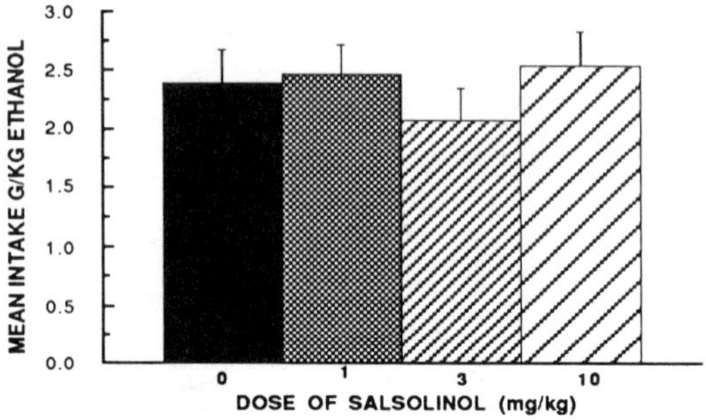

FIGURE 3. Depicted are the dose-response effects of l-salsolinol on rats' intake of ethanol (E), in terms of g/kg. In brief, l-salsolinol did not produced reliable shifts in rats' intake of E.

The dose-response effects of SAL on intake of E are presented in Figure 3. The ANOVA failed to reveal any reliable sources of variance. The ANOVA of the data associated with intake of water revealed a reliable main effect of Days, $F(1,44)=5.16$, $p<0.03$, reflecting a trend for each group to increase their mean intake of water.

DISCUSSION

THP and 1,2,3,4-TIQ produced dose-related decreases in intake of E, while SAL had no apparent effect. Given that E is primarily metabolized in liver, which is a potential site for the production of TIQs, and that injections of TIQs do not increment intakes of E, these data provide no support for the TIQ hypothesis of alcoholism. Since TIQs have been demonstrated to be produced in brain [2], further studies of TIQs' central effects are of interest.

REFERENCES

1. Cohen, C., & Collins, M. Science 167:1749-1751; 1970.
2. Davis, V.E., & Walsh, M.J. Science 167:1005-1007; 1970.
3. Melchior, C.L., & Myers, R.D. Pharmacology Biochemistry & Behavior 7:19-35; 1977.
4. Myers, R.D., & Melchior, C.L. Science 196:554-556; 1977.
5. Myers, R.D., & Oblinger, M.M. Drug and Alcohol Dependence 2:469-483; 1977.

ACKNOWLEDGEMENTS

This research was supported, in part, by a grant from NIDA (DA04440). M.L. Nichols was supported by funds made available from the Ewing Marion Kauffman Foundation. We thank Yizhao Hui for help with the data collection.

MORPHINE ENHANCES INTAKE OF AN ALCOHOLIC BEVERAGE REGARDLESS OF TYPE OF FLAVORING

John D. Delconte, Michael L. Nichols, Kenneth D. Wild, Christopher L. Hubbell and Larry D. Reid

Small doses of morphine (M) enhance intake of sweetened alcoholic beverages. Doses of naloxone (NX) reduce intakes [1]. M and NX are known to affect intake of palatable beverages [2]. This lack of specificity of opioids on intake of alcoholic beverages is obviously of some concern in terms of theorizing about the importance of endogenous opioidergic systems and alcoholism. The lack of specificity may, in fact, tell us something of importance about the nature of alcoholism (e.g., that alcoholism is more than superficially just an ingestive disorder). On the other hand, it may seriously limit the generality of the findings that opioids affect intake of alcoholic beverages in rats. Here, we provide data to indicate that M, in small doses, increments the intake of a variety of kinds of alcoholic beverages.

METHOD

Male, Sprague-Dawley rats (Taconic Farms, Germantown, NY) were maintained on a daily regimen involving 22 hr of water-deprivation followed by a 2-hr opportunity to take a sweetened ethanol solution (ES) and water. After intakes became stable, some groups were presented other kinds of ESs that varied in flavoring and concentrations of ethanol (E). All ESs were prepared by mixing weighed amounts of pure E, flavoring (in one case, no flavoring), and, most of the time, tap water. Beer solutions were made by mixing pure E into a commercially available, nonalcoholic malt beverage that had been allowed to go "flat" overnight.

Each day, rats' bodyweights and intakes of fluids were tabulated to the nearest 0.1 g. The data associated with rats' intake of E are presented in terms of g/kg (g of pure E taken per kg of body weight). The dose of M tested was 1.0 mg/kg. All injections were given subcutaneously, 15 min before the daily session, in a volume of 1.0 ml/kg.

RESULTS

The results are summarized in Figure 1. Please notice that intakes on day of placebo differed considerably, depending on the kind of alcoholic beverage. In each instance, dependent t-tests indicated that M reliably increased intake. It is, however, probably not realistic to compare degree of increase across kinds of beverage. These data were collated from a number of experiments. Placebo (also baseline rates, i.e., days before placebo and after M) were considerably different for some of the solutions than for others. There is no scaling of effects with respect to amount of intake of E. All increases, although different, may have been nearly the same in terms of some meaningful psychological scale.

DISCUSSION

Small doses of M increase intake of a variety of kinds of alcoholic beverages. For those who feel face validity of a model is important, it is probably important to note that the small dose of M increased intake of beer of the kind that people take.

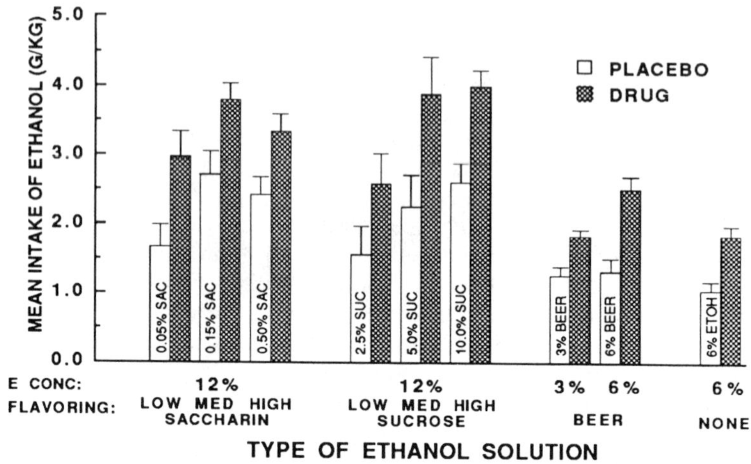

FIGURE 1. Depicted are the effects of morphine on intakes of ethanol (E) presented in a variety of concentrations and with a variety of flavorings. The data are in terms of g/kg E by different groups of rats after being presented day after day with an alcoholic beverage. The different beverages are characterized by type and concentration of E. On one day rats received PLACEBO and on the next, 1.0 mg/kg morphine (DRUG). Error bars represent standard errors of the means.

The comparison between the effects of M on intake of saccharin solutions and sucrose solutions (both containing E) indicate that the calories of sucrose is not critical to the small-dose-M-effect. Please notice that M increased intake of a solution of only E in water. Evidently, it is not necessary to have any additional flavoring in the alcoholic beverage to observe the small-dose-M-effect. The small-dose-M-effect is manifest when rats are taking substantial amounts of alcohol and when they are taking small amounts. Combined with other data [1], it is possible to conclude that small doses of M enhance intake of alcoholic beverages under a wide variety of circumstances.

The importance of the finding that M increases intake of alcoholic beverages to people's alcoholism is, of course, still subject to debate. There is no need, however, to debate the issue of whether or not M's effects in rats are limited to one kind of alcoholic beverage.

REFERENCES

1. Hubbell, C.L., & Reid, L.D. In: Reid, L.D. (Ed.), Opioids, Bulimia, and Alcohol Abuse & Alcoholism. New York: Springer-Verlag, pp. 145-174, 1990.
2. Cooper, S.J., & Kirkham, T.C. In: Reid, L.D. (Ed.), Opioids, Bulimia, and Alcohol Abuse & Alcoholism. New York: Springer-Verlag, pp. 91-110, 1990.

ACKNOWLEDGEMENTS

This research was supported, in part, by a grant from NIDA (DA04440). M.L. Nichols was supported by funds made available from the Ewing Marion Kauffman Foundation. We thank Yizhao Hui for help with the data collection. K.D. Wild is now with the Department of Pharmacology, University of Arizona.

LY78335, AN INHIBITOR OF PHENYLETHANOLAMINE N-METHYLTRANSFERASE, AND RATS' INTAKE OF AN ALCOHOLIC BEVERAGE

John D. Delconte, Christopher L. Hubbell and Larry D. Reid

Norepinephrine is converted to epinephrine by the enzyme phenylethanolamine N-methyltransferase (PNMT) [1,2,3]. Recently, it has been demonstrated that LY78335 (2,3-dichloro-alpha-methylbenzylamine), a PNMT inhibitor, antagonizes the intoxicating effects of ethanol (E) among rats [4]. This suggests that adrenergic systems in brain may mediate some of the effects of E.

We have assessed the effects of a number of agents on intake of E among rats. Mildly water-deprived rats are provided with a limited, daily opportunity to take water and a sweetened alcoholic beverage. Across days, rats steadily increase their intakes until after about 3 weeks they take, on the average, around 2 to 2.5 g of pure E per kg body weight (g/kg). Subsequently, and without further manipulation, their intakes are relatively stable across days [5]. It can be argued that intakes become stable because further intake of E leads to a level of intoxication that is aversive. So, if rats drink to experience the effects of E, but limit their intakes to avoid aversive levels of intoxication, and if LY78335 blocks the intoxicating effects of E, then would an effective dose of LY78335 lead rats to increase their intake of E? Since small doses of morphine (M) increase rats' intake of E [6], would a small dose of M in combination with a dose of LY78335 lead to even greater intake of E? To provide germane information, we performed the following study.

METHOD

Sixty, male, Sprague-Dawley rats (Taconic Farms, Germantown, NY) were maintained on a daily regimen involving 22 hr of fluid deprivation followed by a 2-hr opportunity to take water and a sweetened E solution (ES). Each 100 g of ES contained 12 g of pure E, 5 g of sucrose and 83 g of tap water. Each day, rats' body weights and intakes of fluids were tabulated to the nearest 0.1 g. The data associated with rats' intake of E are presented in terms of g/kg of pure E.

After 56 days of being maintained on the daily regimen, just described, a 2-day series of injections was begun. On the 1st day, all rats received two placebos (physiological saline). Subsequently, the rats were divided into 6 groups (n=10) such that their mean g/kg intakes of E on the placebo day were nearly equal. On the 2nd day: (a) a Control group again received two placebos, (b) three groups received saline and one of three doses of LY78335 (3.0, 10.0 or 30.0 mg/kg), (c) one group received M (1.0 mg/kg) and saline, and (d) one group received 1.0 mg/kg M and 30.0 mg/kg LY78335. All injections were given in a volume of 1.0 ml/kg, the 1st injection 15 min before the session and the 2nd 5 min before. Injections of M and its placebo were given subcutaneously, while LY78335 and its placebo were give interperitoneally. The data conform to a 6 by 2 ANOVA, having repeated measures, with factors associated with Groups and Days (placebo versus drug), respectively.

RESULTS

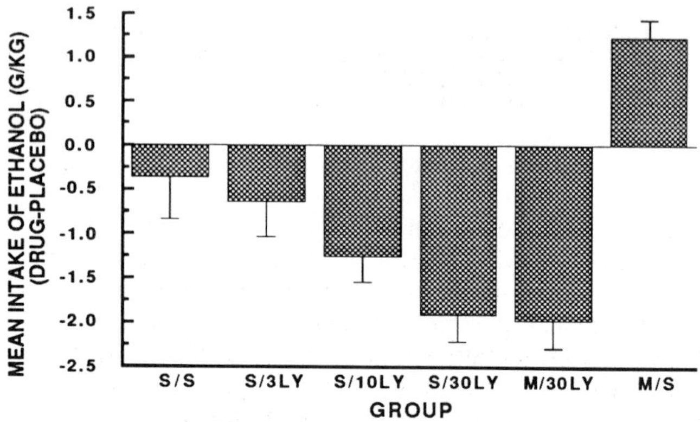

FIGURE 1. Depicted are mean difference scores, in terms of g/kg of E. In summary, LY78335 dose-relatedly decreased intake of E. Morphine increased intake of E but did not overcome the ability of the high dose of LY78335 to decrease intake of E. Error bars represent standard errors of the mean difference scores.

The results, in terms of rats' intake of E, are summarized in Figure 1. The ANOVA revealed reliable main effects of Groups, $F(5,54)=5.57$, $p=0.0005$, and Days, $F(1,54)=34.3$, $p<0.0001$, and a reliable Day by Group interaction, $F(5,54)=12.2$, $p<0.0001$. Since the groups were arranged to have nearly equal g/kg intakes of E on the day of placebo, the source of the interaction must be due to the differential treatment on the 2nd day of these procedures. Indeed, a one-way ANOVA of the scores obtained on the day of treatment revealed that there was a reliable source of variance among groups, $F(5,54)=17.7$, $p<0.0001$. Subsequently, Student's t-tests, for dependent measures, revealed that the 10.0 and 30.0 mg/kg doses of LY78335 reliably decreased intake of E, $t(9)=4.46$, $p<0.002$, and $t(9)=6.19$, $p=0.0002$, respectively. In addition, the combination of M and 30.0 mg/kg of LY78335 also decreased intake of E, $t(9)=6.12$, $p=0.0002$. The 3.0 mg/kg dose of LY78335 did not reliably modify intake of E. As expected [6], M reliably increased intake of E, $t(9)=6.27$, $p=0.0001$. Intake of E by the Control group did not reliably change across days.

The data associated with rats' intakes of water are summarized in Figure 2. The ANOVA yielded a Day by Group interaction of $F(5,54)=5.04$, $p=0.0007$. One-way ANOVAs revealed that the groups' mean intakes of water did not reliably differ on the day of placebo, but did on the day of treatment, $F(5,54)=7.90$, $p<0.0001$. Subsequently, Student's t-tests, for dependent measures, revealed that the 10.0 mg/kg dose of LY78335 reliably increased intake of water, $t(9)=3.51$, $p<0.007$. None of the other groups' mean intakes of water were reliably different across days.

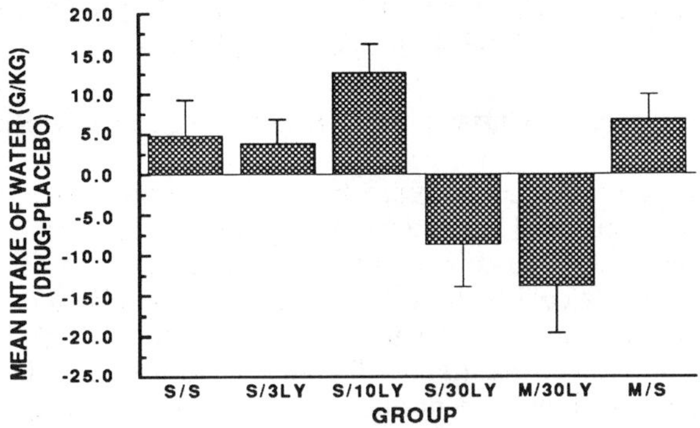

FIGURE 2. Depicted are mean difference scores, in terms of g/kg of water. Error bars represent standard errors of the mean difference scores.

DISCUSSION

Since this was only a preliminary study of the effects of manipulating adrenergic systems on intake of one alcoholic beverage, it is difficult to draw firm conclusions concerning the involvement of noradrenergic and adrenergic systems in regulating intake of alcohol. Also, decreases in intakes, as a result of giving a drug, are difficult to interpret. The drug may have had a number of nonspecific effects that are incompatible with taking alcohol, in addition to its potential specific effect on ingestion of alcohol. Nevertheless, the findings have some interesting features.

Provided that LY78335 does, indeed, block some of the intoxicating effects of E, such a blockade does not apparently "release" rats from having a "brake" on their intake. Given that LY78335 does not lead to greater intakes and given that LY78335 plus M does not lead to greater intakes, it is more difficult to conclude that M achieves its incrementing effects by somehow reducing the intoxicating effects of alcohol.

As mentioned, the fact that the compound blocked M's ability to increment intake of E could be due to a number of reasons. An interesting reason is that M may achieve its augmenting effects on intake of the alcoholic beverage by way of adrenergic systems. A less interesting explanation is that LY78335 led to a malaise for which M was not an antidote. Further research is required to distinguish these effects.

REFERENCES

1. Hokfelt, T., et al. Acta Physiologica Scandinavia 89:286-288; 1973.
2. Hokfelt, T., et al. Brain Research 66:235-251; 1975.
3. Vogt, M. Journal of Physiology 123:451-481; 1954.
4. Mefford, I.N., et al. Alcoholism: Clinical and Experimental Research 14:53-57; 1990.
5. Hubbell, C.L., et al. Alcohol 3:39-54; 1986.
6. Hubbell, C.L., & Reid, L.D. In: Reid, L.D. (Ed.), Opioids, Bulimia, and Alcohol Abuse & Alcoholism. New York: Springer-Verlag, pp. 145-174, 1990.

ACKNOWLEDGMENT

This research was supported, in part, by a grant from NIDA (DA04440).

LY255582, AN OPIOID ANTAGONIST, AND INTAKE OF AN ALCOHOLIC BEVERAGE

John D. Delconte, Christopher L. Hubbell and Larry D. Reid

Manipulations of opioidergic systems have been shown to modulate rats' consumption of ethanol (E) [1]. In general, agonists (e.g., morphine, in small doses) at opioid receptors (opioceptors) increase, and antagonists (e.g., naloxone) decrease rats' intakes of alcoholic beverages [1]. The accumulated data lead to the suggestion that prescribing an antagonist at opioceptors might be a useful pharmacological adjunct to treatments for alcohol abuse and alcoholism [2]. LY255582 [3] is a novel and potent antagonist of opioids' analgesia [4,5] that has been shown to decrease intake of food and water among obese Zucker rats [4,5,6]. Indeed, LY255582 appears to be about 40 times more potent than naltrexone (a long-lasting opioid antagonist) at reducing intake of food [6]. In the present study, we assessed the effects of LY255582, across a range of doses, on rats' intake of a sweetened alcoholic beverage.

METHOD

Twenty-four male, Sprague-Dawley rats (Taconic Farms, Germantown, NY) were maintained on a daily regimen involving 22 hr of fluid deprivation followed by a 2-hr opportunity to take water and a sweetened E solution (ES). Each 100 g of ES contained 12 g of pure E, 5 g of sucrose and 83 g of tap water. Each day, rats' body weights and intakes of fluids were tabulated. The data associated with rats' intake of E are presented in terms of g/kg (g of pure E taken per kg of body weight).

After 25 days of being maintained on the daily regimen, just described, an initial dose-response assessment of LY255582's effects was performed. The doses tested were 0.0, 0.001, 0.01 and 0.1 mg/kg. 10% DMSO in physiological saline served as placebo (0.0 mg/kg). All injections were given subcutaneously, 1.0 ml/kg, 15 min prior to the presentation of fluids. On one day, all rats received placebo. Subsequently, they were divided into 4 groups (n=6) so that the groups' mean g/kg intakes under placebo were nearly equal. On the next day, each group was injected with one of the doses of LY255582. Initial analyses of the data led to the conclusion that we had not tested an effective range of doses. Therefore, 8 days later we tested the effects of LY255582 in doses of 0.0, 0.1, 1.0 and 10.0 mg/kg in the same manner as that of the lower range of doses.

RESULTS

The results are summarized in Figures 1 and 2. As mentioned, the analyses of the data associated with the 1st assessment of LY255582's effects revealed that we did not test a wide enough range of doses, i.e., the ANOVA's of those data of intake of E and water failed to reveal reliable sources of variance associated with either factor or their interaction. Upon closer inspection of that data, it was determined that there was a trend for LY255582 to decrease intake of ES and water. This is supported by the reliable Doses by Days interaction, $F(3,20)=5.88$, $p<0.005$, associated with the data of total intake of fluids (ES plus water), which indicated that total-fluid intake was dose-relatedly decreased.

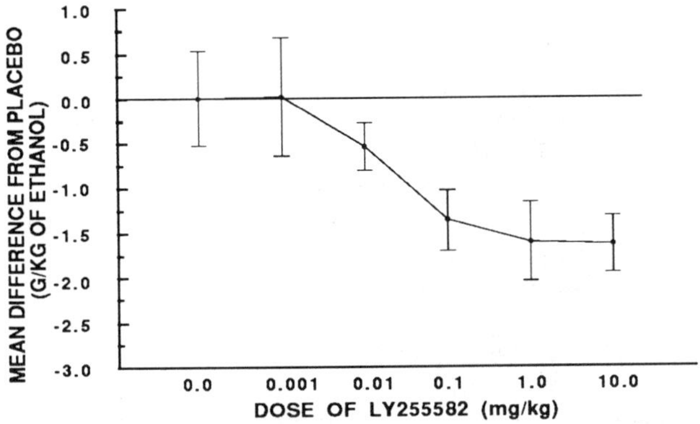

FIGURE 1. The data are presented in the form of mean difference scores (placebo minus drug). The data presented for the 0.001 and 0.01 mg/kg doses are from the 1st assessment while the rest are from the 2nd assessment (see Method). In brief, LY255582 dose-relatedly decreased rats' intake of ethanol. Bars represent standard errors of the means.

The data obtained from each assessment conform to 4 by 2 ANOVAs, having repeated measures, with factors associated with Doses of LY255582 and Days (placebo versus drug), respectively. The analyses of the data obtained from the 2nd assessment with larger doses revealed that we had tested an effective range of doses. In terms of mean g/kg intakes, the ANOVA revealed a reliable main effect associated with Days, $F(1,20)=30.3$, $p<0.0001$, and a reliable Day by Dose interaction, $F(3,20)=3.49$, $p<0.04$. One-way ANOVAs revealed that the groups' mean g/kg intakes did not differ on the day of placebo, but did on the day of LY255582, $F(3,20)=6.86$, $p<0.003$. Student's t-tests, for dependent measures, revealed that all three doses reliably decreased rats' g/kg intakes, all $ps<0.03$.

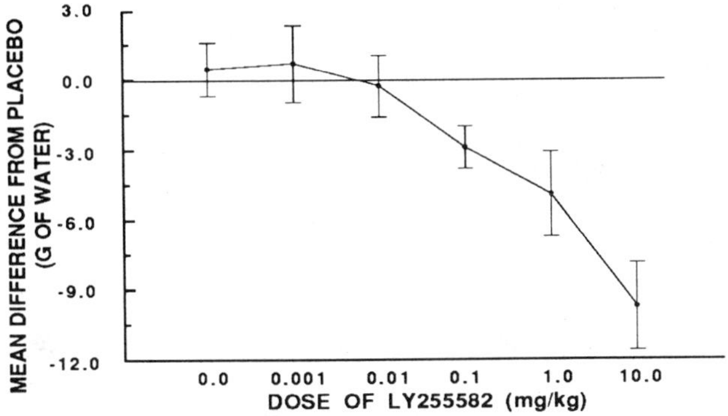

FIGURE 2. The dose-response effects of LY255582 on rats' intake of water, are summarized. The data, g of water taken, are presented in the form of mean difference scores (placebo minus drug). The data presented for the 0.001 and 0.01 mg/kg doses are from the 1st assessment while the rest are from the 2nd assessment (see Method). In brief, LY255582 dose-relatedly decreased rats' intake of water. Bars represent standard errors of the means.

DISCUSSION

LY255582, which other data clearly indicates is antagonistic to opioid analgesia, acts similarly to naloxone, the classic antagonist, with respect to intake of alcoholic beverage and intake of water. LY255582 produces no analgesia by itself, blocks other opioids' analgesia [4,5] and reduces, dose-relatedly, intake of ES and intake of water (when presented by itself [4,5,6] and when presented concurrently with the ES). These data provide, in general, confirmation of the idea that opioidergic processes are involved in ingestion of fluids, including alcoholic beverages.

When testing is done using the general procedures we typically use (22 hr of water deprivation followed by 2 hr of access to ES and water), some antagonists are more effective in reducing intake of water than others. Naloxone, for example, sometimes reliably reduces intake of water and sometimes it does not; at the same time, it reliably reduces intake of the alcoholic beverage. Furthermore, when naloxone is given before a series of daily sessions, it does not reduce intake of water beyond the 1st day of administration [7]. In these tests of LY255582, the antagonist produced marked reductions in intake of water. Agonists such as morphine increase intake of alcohol while not affecting total intake of fluids [7] (also, morphine does not reliably increase intake of water when water is the only fluid presented [7]). For an antagonist to be effective in curbing people's intake of alcoholic beverages, it should produce its effects day after day and not interfere with basic processes such as maintaining a proper balance of fluids in the body. LY255582 needs to be assessed, therefore, when given daily while continuing to monitor intake of E and water.

REFERENCES

1. Hubbell, C.L., & Reid, L.D. In: Reid, L.D. (Ed.), Opioids, Bulimia, and Alcohol Abuse & Alcoholism. New York: Springer-Verlag, pp. 145-174, 1990.
2. Reid, L.D. In: Reid, L.D. (Ed.), Opioids, Bulimia, and Alcohol Abuse & Alcoholism. New York: Springer-Verlag, pp. 275-280, 1990.
3. (3S,4R)-1-((S)-3-hydroxy-3-cyclohexylpropyl)-4-(3-hydroxyphenyl)-3,4-dimethyl-1-piperidine.
4. Leander, J.D., et al. International Narcotics Research Conference Abstracts:0.61; 1988.
5. Mitch, C.H., et al. Society for Neuroscience Abstracts 14(445.2):1106; 1988.
6. Zimmerman, D.M., et al. International Narcotics Research Conference Abstracts:P.186; 1988.
7. Akkok, F., et al. Bulletin of the Psychonomic Society 26:556-558; 1988.

ACKNOWLEDGEMENT

This research was supported, in part, by a grant from NIDA (DA04440).

EFFECTS OF NALTREXONE ON THE COGNITIVE FUNCTIONING OF RECENTLY ABSTINENT ALCOHOL DEPENDENT PATIENTS

Adam Jaffe, Stephanie S. O'Malley, Mary Hickcox, Grace Chang, Richard S. Schottenfeld, Bruce J. Rounsaville

INTRODUCTION

Past studies have suggested that the endogenous opioid system may have a modulating influence on memory storage (Reisberg, et al., 1983; Rigter, et al., 1980; Izquierdo, et al., 1980) and may play a role in the regulation of attention (Arnsten, et al., 1981; Arnsten, et al., 1983; Arnsten & Segal, 1979). Naloxone, an opiate antagonist, has shown promise in facilitating attention (Arnsten, et al., 1983) and some memory processes (Gallagher, 1982, 1983). In addition, naloxone may improve cognitive deficits associated with ischemia (Baskin & Hosobuchi, 1981), senile dementia of the Alzheimers type (Reisberg, et al., 1983) and post-concussional syndrome (Tennant, 1987). Thus, naloxone or other opioid antagonists may also be useful in other clinical populations which have associated cognitive deficits, such as alcoholics.

The purpose of the present study was to examine whether naltrexone improves attention and concentration as well as verbal and nonverbal learning and memory processes in recently abstinent alcoholics. This paper reports preliminary analyses using data from the first 20 subjects to complete the trial.

METHODS

Subjects

Twenty treatment seeking subjects who met DSM-III-R criteria for alcohol dependence were recruited. Eleven subjects received naltrexone and nine received placebo. There were no significant differences between groups on demographic variables or drinking history measures. Overall, subjects drank heavily for an average of 10.5 years and achieved an average of 9.6 days of abstinence prior to testing. The mean age of the subjects was 40.5 years, 85% had a high school education, 63% were male and 100% were Caucasian.

Acknowledgements: This research was supported in part by grant AA-P50-03-510 from the National Institute of Alcohol Abuse and Alcoholism.

The subjects consisted of a consecutive subsample of those entered into a double blind placebo controlled treatment outcome study designed to look at the effectiveness of naltrexone in combination with psychotherapy (O'Malley, Jaffe, Chang, Witte, Shottenfeld & Rounsaville, in press). Subjects received either (1) naltrexone and coping skills therapy, (2) placebo and coping skills therapy, (3) naltrexone and supportive psychotherapy, or (4) placebo and supportive psychotherapy.

Procedures

Subjects who were abstinent from alcohol for at least seven days were screened by a research assistant. Subjects who met eligibility criteria were invited to participate and informed consent was obtained. Alcohol abuse was diagnosed with the Structured Clinical Interview for DSM-III-R (Spitzer & Williams, 1985).

The study psychiatrist reviewed the patient's medical records for eligibility criteria and met with the patient to discuss the study medication and the research protocol. The patient was then randomly assigned to receive naltrexone or placebo together with one of the two psychotherapies. In order to comply with standard clinical doses of naltrexone, the dosage level for the study was either 50 mg. of naltrexone or a placebo. The patient began the medication on the day of their first session with their individual therapist. The psychiatrist, therapist, research assistant, and patient were all blind to the study medication.

Baseline neuropsychological assessment measures were administered by the research assistant on the day of the subject's first therapy session and prior to their first dose of medication. These tests were readministered prior to their second therapy session which occurred on average 7.7 days after the initial testing. Order of administration was counter balanced across testing sessions in order to control for sequence effects. At the time of the second testing, patients completed self report measures designed to assess the number of days they drank and the number of standard drinks consumed during the period between baseline and outcome neuropsychological testing.

Measures

Symbol Digit Modalities Test. This is a standard neuropsychological screening test that requires the learning of new associations between numbers and symbols (Smith, 1973) and assesses sustained attention and concentration.

Digit Vigilance Test. This is a subtest of the Lafayette Repeatable Neuropsychological Assessment Battery (Rennick, et al., 1974). The subject is instructed to find and delete all occurrences of a specific number that is embedded in a page of numbers. This test assesses sustained visual attention and concentration.

Wechsler Memory Scale (WMS). An adapted version of the Wechsler Memory Scale (Wechsler, 1945) was used to assess verbal and nonverbal learning and memory (Heaton et al., 1978). Verbal learning was evaluated with the logical memory subtest in which the subject receives up to three trials to learn a one-paragraph story to criterion (15 points) and obtains a point for each idea he or she recalls. The subject's recall of the story after a twenty minute delay is then compared with his or her performance on the last learning trial to assess memory functions (i.e., forgetting). Nonverbal learning and memory assessment involves similar learning to criterion and delayed recall using the Figure Memory subtest of the WMS.

RESULTS

The amount of alcohol consumed between testing sessions for the placebo group (Mean number of drinking days = .3; mean number of drinks = 4) and the naltrexone group (Mean number of drinking days = .65; mean number of drinks = 1) were not significantly different. [t (19) = 1.2, p = .25]

Analyses of covariance were used to compare group means on the assessment measures at time 2, after an average of 7.7 days on naltrexone. Figure 1 presents the results for verbal learning and memory. Scores on each of the neuropsychological assessment

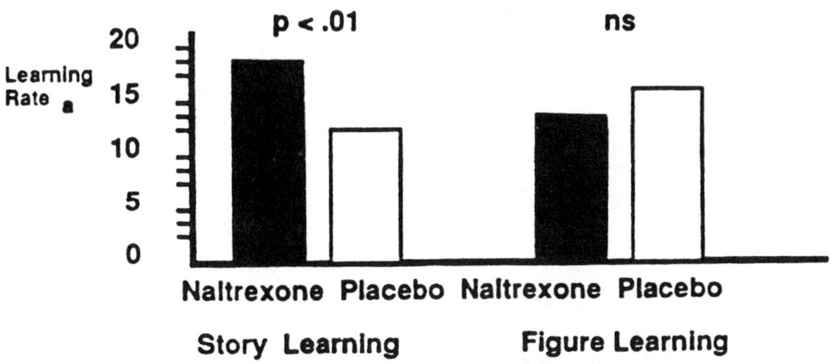

Figure 1 MEAN SCORES ON STORY LEARNING AND FIGURE LEARNING TESTS AT TIME 2

a = # of features learned on last trial ÷ # of trials

measures at baseline were used as covariates in these analyses. Significant mean differences at time 2 were evident on the story learning subtest of the Wechsler Memory Scale [$F(2,17) = 9.48$, $p < .01$]. Subjects taking naltrexone performed significantly better ($M = 16.9$, $SD = 4.1$) on this subtest than the placebo group ($M = 12.2$, $SD = 5.6$) No significant group differences were found on the verbal memory and nonverbal learning and memory subtests of the Wechsler Memory Scale, the symbol digit modalities test or digit vigilance.

DISCUSSION

Nalaxone, an opiate antagonist, has shown promise in facilitating attention and memory as well as in improving cognitive deficits associated with a variety of clinical populations. Preliminary results of the current study support this research and suggest that naltrexone may be helpful in facilitating verbal learning in recently detoxified alcoholics.

Previous research suggests that naltrexone may reduce relapse rates with alcoholics. The current results provide additional support for the use of naltrexone with a treatment seeking alcoholic population. In particular, alcohol treatment programs often require the learning of large amounts of new information. Since alcohol abuse and recent abstinence from alcohol are associated with deficits in verbal learning (see review by Grant, 1987), an agent that might facilitate the remediation of such a deficit as well as enhance treatment effects would be clearly beneficial. Given the small sample size, however, the current results should be considered preliminary. Ongoing research in our laboratory with a projected sample size of 100 subjects should provide additional validation for these findings.

REFERENCES

Arnsten AT, Segal DS: *Life Science* 1979; 25:1035-42.

Arnsten AT, Segal DS, Loughlin SE, Roberts DCS: *Brain Research* 1981; 222:351-63.

Arnsten AT, Segal DS, Neville HJ, Hillyard SA, Janowsky DS, Judd LL, Bloom FE: Naloxone augments electrophysiological signs of selective attention in man. *Nature* 1983; 304:725-27.

Baskin DS, Hosobuchi Y: Naloxone reversal of ischemic neurological deficits in man. *Lancet* 1981; ii:272-75.

Grant Igor: Alcohol and the Brain: Neuropsychological Correlates. *Journal of Consulting and Clinical Psychology* 1987; 55:310-24.

Heaton RK, Chelone GJ, Lehman RAW: Using neuropsychological and personality tests to assess the likelihood of patient employment. *Journal of Nervous and Mental Disease* 1978; 166:408-416.

Izquierdo I, Paiva ACM, Elisabetsky E: Post-training intraperitoneal administration of leu-enkephalin and ß-endorphic causes retrograde amnesia for two different tasks in rats. *Behavioral and Neural Biology* 1980; 28:246-50.

O'Malley, SS, Jaffe, AJ, Chang, GM, Witte, G, Schottenfeld, RS, Rounsaville, BJ. Naltrexone in the Treatment of Alcohol Dependence: Preliminary findings. In CA Naranjo & EM Sellers (eds.) *Novel Pharmacological Interventions for Alcoholism.* New York: Spring-Verlag, in press.

Osterreith PA: Le teste de copie d'une figure complexe. *Archives de Psychologie* 1944; 30:206-356.

Reisberg B, Ferris SH, Anand R, Mir P, deLeon MJ, Roberts E: Naloxone effects on primary degnerative dementia (PDD). *Psychopharmacology Bulletin* 1983; 19(1):44-47.

Rennick PM, Keiser T, Rodin E, Rim, Lennox K: Carbamazepine: Behavioral side effects in temporal lobe epilepsy during short-term comparison with placebo. Paper presented at the annual meeting of the American Epilepsy Society, New York, NY, December 1974.

Rigter H, Hannan TJ, Messing RB, et al: Enkephalins interfere with acquisition of an active avoidance response. *Life Science* 1980; 26:337-45.

Smith A: Symbol Digit Modalities Test. Los Angeles: Western Psychological Services, 1973.

Tennant FS, Wild J: Naltrexone Treatment for Postconcussional Syndrome. *American Journal of Psychiatry* 1987; 144:813-14.

Wechsler D: A standardized memory scale for clinical use. *Journal of Psychology* 1945; 19:87-95.

Poster Papers: The Role of Other Neurotransmitters in Regulating Alcohol Intake

CALCIUM-DIACETYL-HOMOTAURINATE WHICH PREVENTS RELAPSE IN WEANED ALCOHOLICS DECREASES THE ACTION OF EXCITATORY AMINO ACIDS IN NEOCORTICAL NEURONS OF THE RAT IN VITRO.

WALTER ZIEGLGÄNSBERGER AND MARC L. ZEISE

The behavioural disorder of compulsive drinking and the severe medical and social consequences urge research to find effective prevention and intervention strategies. The acute and chronic action of ethanol have been studied with quite a variety of techniques, but the mechanism(s) of action still remain an unresolved puzzle. Although we do not have any unifying hypothesis about the action of ethanol on synaptic transmission, there is growing evidence that in addition to biogenic amines (see Naranjo et al. this meeting), neuropeptides and steroids (2), amino acids like L-glutamate (L-GLU) (8) and y-amino butyric acid (GABA) (1) are involved in the acute and chronic action of ethanol. In particular, a subtype of the excitatory amino acid neurotransmitter (EAA), the N-methyl-D-aspartate (NMDA) receptor, has gained considerable attention in recent alcohol research. A synopsis of the available evidence suggests that NMDA receptor mediated responses may be primary targets for acute and chronic alcohol action (8). This receptor subtype appears to play important roles in learning and memory, developmental plasticity, epilepsy and various neurodegenerative disorders. L-homocysteic acid (L-HCA) is a putative endogenous ligand (besides L-GLU) for the NMDA receptor in central neurons (13; 17).

In the present study, we employed intracellular recording techniques to investigate the action of calcium-diacetyl-homotaurinate (AOTAL, LIPHA, France) on neocortical neurons (n= 35) in an in vitro preparation. This compound, which can be considered as an analogue of a sulfur-containing EAA L-HCA, has proven in a double blind study to be therapeutically useful in the prevention of relapses in weaned alcoholics (14). The present data suggest that AOTAL reduces EAA induced depolarizations in neocortical neurons without a direct effect on GABAergic neurotransmission.

In vitro preparations allow activation of synaptic connections between cells and long term stable intracellular recordings as well as the topical application of drugs in given concentrations (for technical details see: 12; 18). AOTAL is stable in biological media where it probably is readily dissociated. It remains unclear how it crosses the blood brain barrier under therapeutic conditions and whether a carrier system is used (5). AOTAL is most likely not a precursor of homotaurine in the CNS (10).

In neocortical neurons, AOTAL reduced the depolarization induced by iontophoretic application of EAA (Fig. 1) when applied locally (multibarrelled micropipette) or when added to the perfusion medium (up to 1 mM; L-GLU 52 ± 26%, n = 12; L-HCA 43 ± 20%, n = 5; NMDA 45 ± 35%, n = 5). Since, in contrast to L-GLU which elicits response mainly via non-NMDA receptors, NMDA and L-HCA very selectively activate NMDA receptors (17), these results suggest that AOTAL does not interact specifically with an EAA receptor subtype. Responses to iontophoretically applied GABA were not influenced (n = 6) by AOTAL.

The amplitude of excitatory postsynaptic potentials (EPSP) was reduced by AOTAL (average 21%). The reduction depended on the strength of synaptic stimulation. At increased stimulation intensity, AOTAL reduced the EPSP more effectively. AOTAL did not change resting membrane potential (RMP), action potential amplitude, or membrane input resistance near RMP (current voltage relation was slightly changed near spike threshold; inward rectification was attenuated).

Since the action of AOTAL was antagonized by bicuculline, it was postulated that stimulation of GABA receptors in the CNS by AOTAL reduces the voluntary intake of ethanol in rats (6; cf. 4, 3; 5). In rodents, AOTAL significantly reduced the voluntary ingestion of alcohol. In these studies, Na-homotaurine, homotaurine, Na-acetyltaurine and Ca-chloride were ineffective (4).

These authors postulated that AOTAL might be acting through various mechanisms on multiple targets hypothetically involved in alcohol dependence: through its taurine structure, its GABAmimetic action, its anti-opiate or naloxone-like effects and also as a subcellular Ca-carrier (7). AOTAL has no apparent abuse potential (9). It failed to engender drug-appropriate response at any dose or pretreatment condition in monkeys. Interestingly, specific competitive blockers for NMDA receptors (phospor-containing EEA analogues) are not discriminated from alcohol in drug discrimination tests (see 8 for refs.).

The present electrophysiological study suggests that AOTAL interacts quite selectively with EAA receptor mediated synaptic mechanisms and does not directly influence GABAergic transmission in neocortical neurons in vitro (see also 18). Since a drug which reduces the efficacy of EAAs and spike threshold is anticonvulsive, it is conceivable that this increased threshold for seizures would be therapeutically beneficial for alcoholics which, in general, have a higher incidence of seizures than the normal population. Ethanol selectively inhibits the ligand-gated inward current mediated via NMDA receptor activation without affecting GABA-activated currents (16; cf. 11; 15).

Most interestingly, chronic exposure of neurons to ethanol increases the NMDA receptor density and increases the number of Ca-channels, (see: Littleton, this meeting) thereby increasing the excitability of these neurons. NMDA antagonists for therapeutical use have not yet been developed as they all invoke serious psychotoxic side-effects. AOTAL is apparently devoid of such side-effects to a large extent and could become a lead substance in the development of clinically effective drugs to prevent relapse in alcoholics.

ACKNOWLEDGEMENT: AOTAL was kindly provided by LIPHA Arzneimittel GmbH, Essen F.R.G.

REFERENCES:

1. Bloom, F.E. and G.R. Siggins. Alcohol **4**: 331-337, 1987.
2. Bloom, F.E. J. Psychopharmacol **1** (4): 227-236, 1987.
3. Boismare, F., Daoust, M., Lhuintre J.P., Moore N., Saligaut, C. and Flipo J.L. Alcohol and Alcoholism 21: A30, 1986.

4. Boismare, F., Daoust, M., Moore, N., Salingaut, C., Lhuintre, J.P., Chretien, P. and J. Durlach. Pharmacol. Biochem. Behav. **21** (5) 787-789, 1984.
5. Chabenat, C., Chretien, P., Daoust, M., Moore, N., Andre, D., Lhuintre, J.P., Saligaut, C., Boucly, P. and F. Boismare. Methods Find. Exp. Clin. Pharmacol **10** (5): 311-317, 1988.
6. Daoust, M., Lhuintre, J.P., Saligaut, C., Chretien, P., Moore, N. and F. Boismare. J.Pharmacol **16**: 521-529 (1985).
7. Durlach, J., Rinjard, P., Sprince, H., and Smith, G.G. Methods Find. Exp. Clin. Pharmacol. **10** (7): 437-447, 1988.
8. Gonzales, R.A. Trends in Pharmacological Sciences **11**: 137-139,1990.
9. Grant, K.A., and W.L. Woolverton. Pharmacol. Biochem. Behav. **32**: 607-611, 1989.
10. Guiet-Bara, A., Bara, M., Durlach, J., and C. Pechery. Alcohol **5** (1): 63-71, 1988.
11. Hoffman, P.L., Rabe, C.S., Moses, F. and B. Tabakoff. J. Neurochem. **52**: 1937-1940, 1989.
12. Howe, J.R., Sutor, B., and W. Zieglgänsberger. J. Physiol. **384**: 539-570, 1987.
13. Knöpfel, T., Zeise, M.L., Cuenod, M., and W. Zieglgänsberger. Neurosci. Lett. **81**: 188-192, 1987.
14. Lhuintre, J.P., Daoust, M., Moore, N.D., Chretien, P., Saligaut, C., Tran, G., Boismare, F., and B. Hillemand. Lancet **1** (8436): 1014-1016, 1985.
15. Lima-Landman, M.T.R., and E.X. Albuquerque. FEBBS Lett. **247**: 61-67, 1989.
16. Lovinger, D.M., White, G., and F.F. Weight. Science **243**: 1721-1724, 1989.
17. Zeise, M.L., Knöpfel, Th., Cuenod, M., and W. Zieglgänsberger. In: E.A. Cavalheiro et al. (eds.) Frontiers in Excitatory Amino Acid Research. New York: Alan R. Liss, 1988 (pp. 187-192).
18. Zeise, M.L., Kasparow, S., Capogna, M., and W. Zieglgänsberger. In: H. Pasantes-Morales et al.(eds.) Taurine: Functional Neurochemistry, Physiology, and Cardiology. New York : Wiley-Liss Inc. 1990 (pp. 237-242).

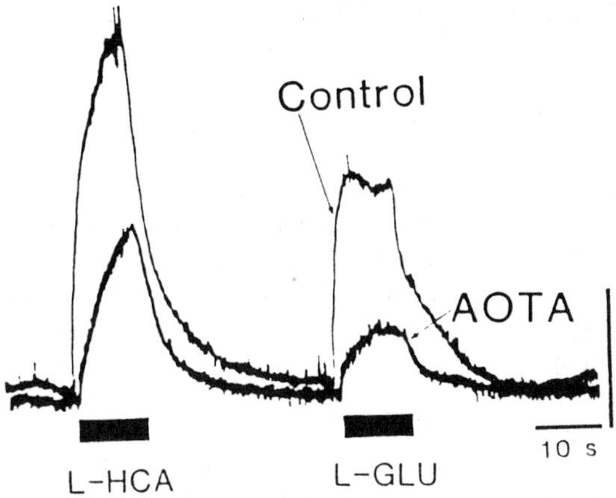

Fig 1: AOTAL depresses the depolarizing responses to iontophoretically applied EAAs (L-HCA, L-GLU, phoretic currents 90 nA and 130 nA resp.) in a neocortical neuron of the rat (RMP:-75mV). Superimposed traces of control and recording 25 min after AOTAL (1 mM) was added to the perfusion medium.

THC, AN ACTIVE INGREDIENT IN MARIJUANA, AND RATS' INTAKE OF A SWEETENED ALCOHOLIC BEVERAGE

Edward J. Bilsky, Christopher L. Hubbell and Larry D. Reid

There is substantial evidence to indicate that some drugs that are often used recreationally modify intakes of palatable ingesta [1]. For example, delta-9-tetrahydrocannabinol (THC) in small doses enhances caloric intake [1,2]. Among people, THC is also used in combination with other drugs such as ethanol (E). It is interesting to see if a drug such as THC also increases intake of a sweetened alcoholic beverage.

METHOD

Fifty, male, Sprague-Dawley rats (Taconic Farms, Germantown, NY) were maintained on a daily regimen involving 22 hr of fluid deprivation followed by a 2-hr opportunity to take water and an ethanol solution (ES). Each 100 g of ES contained 12 g of pure E, 5 g of sucrose and 83 g of tap water. Each day, rats' body weights and intakes of fluids were tabulated. The data associated with rats' intake of E are presented in terms of g/kg (g of pure E taken per kg of body weight).

After 55 days of being maintained on the regimen described, a dose-response assessment of THC's effects on intake of E was made. The doses tested were 0.0 (placebo), 0.01, 0.1, 1.0 and 3.0 mg/kg. Injections of drug or placebo were given subcutaneously, 1.0 ml/kg, 30 min before the presentation of fluids. THC's carrier, a small amount of pure E dissolved in oil, served as placebo. On one day, all rats received placebos. Subsequently, the rats were divided into 5 groups (n=10) such that their mean g/kg intakes under placebo were nearly equal. On the next day, the groups were given one of the doses of THC.

RESULTS

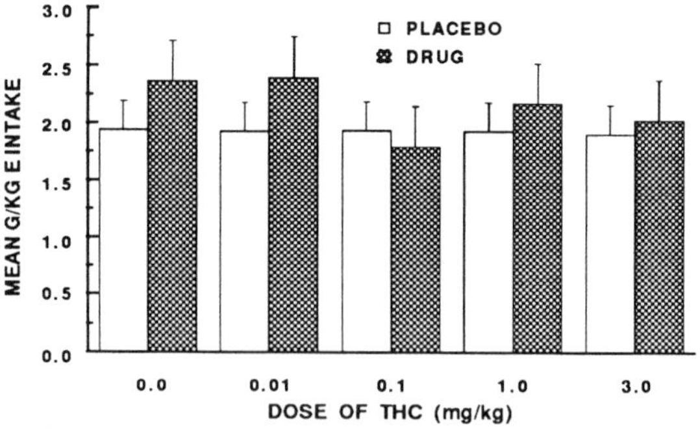

FIGURE 1. The effects of a range of doses of THC (delta-9-tetrahydrocannabinol, the active ingredient of marijuana) on rats' intake of ethanol (E), in terms of mean g/kg intakes, are depicted. PLACEBO refers to a day when rats received injections of placebo. DRUG refers to a day when they received a dose of THC. Injections were given shortly before a 2-hr presentation of a sweetened alcoholic beverage and water, after 22 hr of deprivation of fluids. None of the doses tested reliably modified intake of E.

The results are presented in Figure 1. The data conform to a 5 by 2 ANOVA, having repeated measures, with factors associated with Dose of THC and Days (placebo versus drug), respectively. In brief, the overall ANOVAs of the data associated with rats' intake of E and water failed to reveal reliable sources of variance associated with either factor or their interaction. For example, the interaction term of the ANOVA of the data associated with rats' g/kg intakes yielded an $F(4,45)=0.80$, $p=0.53$.

DISCUSSION

Since we had no independent measure of THC's effects, the results of our study should be viewed cautiously. It is possible that THC did not reach brain in the way one would expect. We may have made a procedural error. On the other hand, given that THC was administered correctly (and there is no reason to suppose that it was not), and given that THC did not reliably modify intake of the sweetened alcoholic beverage, there is no support provided for the hypothesis that THC administration leads to increased intake of alcoholic beverages.

Our findings indicate that THC reliably increases rats' intakes of sucrose solutions [2], but does not reliably increase intake of a solution of E and sucrose. We have shown time and time again that morphine, and related opioids, increase intake of sweetened and unsweetened alcoholic beverages (for a review see [3]). Morphine will also increase intake of sucrose solutions [4]. There are questions, however, about morphine's specificity with respect to its effects on intake of E. These data indicate that a psychotropic drug could increase intake of sucrose without increasing intake of an alcoholic beverage. Drugs which produce signs of incrementing positive affect, such as cocaine and MDMA, do not reliably increase intake of alcoholic beverages [5]. So morphine's effects are different than other drugs, in terms of increasing ingestion. It is one of the few we have tested that reliably increases intake of alcoholic beverages.

REFERENCES

1. Foltin, R.W., et al. Pharmacology Biochemistry & Behavior 25:577-582; 1986.
2. Milano, W.C., et al. Pharmacology Biochemistry & Behavior 31:893-897; 1989.
3. Hubbell, C.L., & Reid, L.D. In: Reid, L.D. (Ed.), Opioids, Bulimia, and Alcohol Abuse & Alcoholism. New York: Springer-Verlag, pp. 145-174, 1990.
4. Czirr, S.A., & Reid, L.D. Brain Research Bulletin 17:639-642; 1986.
5. Bilsky, E.J., et al. Pharmacology Biochemistry & Behavior 37:in press; 1990.

ACKNOWLEDGEMENT

This research was supported, in part, by a grant from NIDA (DA04440).

COCAINE AND RATS' INTAKE OF AN ALCOHOLIC BEVERAGE

Edward J. Bilsky, John D. Delconte, Christopher L. Hubbell and Larry D. Reid

There are a number of reasons to observe cocaine's effects on intake of ethanol (E). Among those reasons are: (a) There is a continuing assessment of the specificity of morphine's effects and results from tests using cocaine can be used as part of that assessment [1]. Morphine increases intake of E [2]. Perhaps, any agent that induces positive affect would also increment such intake. Since cocaine is an agent that induces positive affect, it can be used as part of the assessment of morphine's specificity. (b) Dopamine (DA) is a neurotransmitter that seems to be critical to a number of motivated behaviors [3]. Consequently, it is of interest to see how agents that modulate endogenous DA levels might affect intake of E. Cocaine increases DA levels by blocking its reuptake [4,5]. If increased DA levels is a setting condition potentiating intake of E, then injections of cocaine should also increase intake of E. (c) A recent report indicated that the gene for the DA D2 receptor was a possible marker for alcoholism among people [6]. This possibility also suggests that manipulation of DA levels should produce systematic shifts in propensity to take E. An additional indication that dopaminergic systems might be critically involved in propensity to take E is the finding that alcohol preferring rats have about a 25% lower content of DA and its metabolites in the nucleus accumbens [7]. McBride et al. suggested that this "abnormality in the dopaminergic system projecting from the ventral tegmental area to the nucleus accumbens" ([7], p. 202) promotes high levels of drinking of E. (d) There has been some controversy concerning whether or not dopaminergic systems are saliently involved in rats' intake of E from studies using the DA antagonist pimozide [8,9,10,11,12]. And (e), Joseph Volpicelli (personal communication) related that alcoholics who relapse into taking alcohol frequently relapse into taking cocaine. This observation might lead to the suggestion that cocaine augments E's reinforcing capability (or that E might augment cocaine's).

Toward getting information about how cocaine might affect rats' intake of E, we tested a number of doses of cocaine on rats' intake of a sweetened alcoholic beverage after the rats had established stable levels of intake of E. We also tested the after-effects of cocaine on intakes. Presumably, as cocaine's effects wane, there is a period when DA levels are less than ordinary.

METHOD

Male, Sprague-Dawley rats (Taconic Farms, Germantown, NY) were maintained on a daily regimen involving 22 hr of fluid deprivation followed by a 2-hr opportunity to take water and a sweetened E solution (ES). Each 100 g of ES contained 12 g of pure E, 5 g of sucrose and 83 g of tap water. Each day, rats' body weights and intakes of fluids were tabulated. The data associated with rats' intake of E are presented in terms of g/kg (g of pure E taken per kg of body weight). After 67 days of being maintained on this daily regimen, a dose-response assessment of cocaine's effects on intake of E was made among 60 rats. The doses tested were 0.0 (physiological saline), 0.1, 1.0, 3.0 and 10.0 mg/kg.

Injections of drug or placebo (physiological saline) were given subcutaneously (SC), 1.0 ml/kg, 15 min before the presentation of fluids. On one day, all rats received placebos. Subsequently, the rats were divided into 5 groups (n=12) such that their mean g/kg intakes under placebo were nearly equal. On the next day, the groups were given one of the doses of cocaine. The data conform to a 5 by 2 ANOVA, having repeated measures, with factors associated with Dose of cocaine and Days (placebo versus drug), respectively.

In a 2nd set of procedures, 48 rats that had been maintained on the daily regimen for 32 days were used. Across the next 2 days, the rats received an injection (SC, 1.0 ml/kg) at 6, 4 and 2 hr prior to the drinking session. On the 1st day, all rats received three placebos. Subsequently, the rats were divided into 4 groups (n=12) such that their mean g/kg intakes under placebo were nearly equal. On the next day, one group again received three placebos. The 3 remaining groups received a 10.0 mg/kg dose of cocaine at one of the injection-times and placebos at the other times. The data conform to a 4 by 2 ANOVA, having repeated measures, with factors associated with Groups and Days, respectively.

RESULTS

The results of the dose-response assessment of cocaine's effects on intake of E are presented in Figure 1. The ANOVA of the data associated with rats' mean g/kg intakes revealed a reliable Day by Dose interaction, $F(4,55)=3.77$, $p<0.009$. Subsequently, Student's t-tests, for dependent measures, revealed that 10.0 mg/kg of cocaine reliably decreased rats' mean g/kg intakes, $t(11)=2.72$, $p<0.03$. No other dose tested produced a reliable shift in E-intake. The ANOVA of the data associated with rats' intakes of water failed to reveal any reliable sources of variance associated with either main effect or their interaction. In summary, the 10.0 mg/kg dose of cocaine reduced intake of the E, while none of the doses tested modified intake of water.

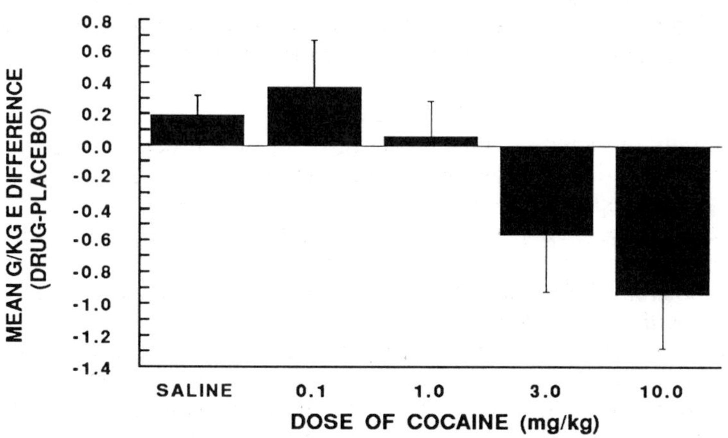

FIGURE 1. Depicted are the dose-response effects of cocaine on rats' intakes of ethanol (E). The data are presented as mean difference scores, in terms of g/kg. On the day of placebos, all groups took equivalent amounts of E, i.e. 2.7 g/kg across the 2-hr session. On the next day, the groups received one of the doses of cocaine. Error bars represent standard errors of the mean difference scores.

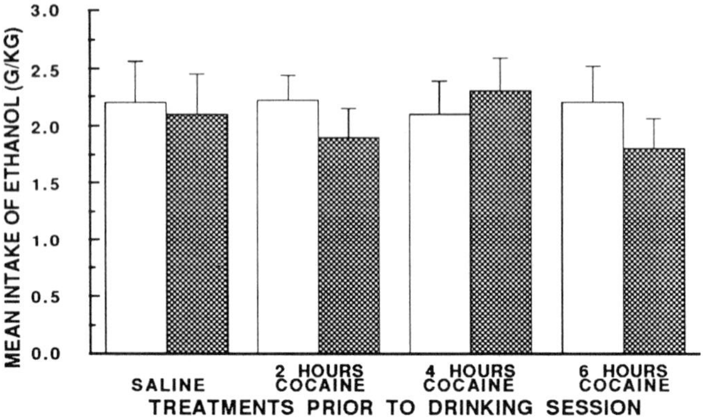

FIGURE 2. Depicted are the after effects of 10 mg/kg of cocaine on rats' intake of ethanol (E), in terms of g/kg, given at either 2, 4, or 6 hr before the opportunity to drink. On the day of placebo (open bars), all groups received injections of saline at at 2, 4, and 6 hr before the session. Under placebos all groups took equivalent amounts of E. On the next day, one group again received 3 injections of saline while the other groups received cocaine at one of the times of injections and saline at the other two (shaded bars).

The results of the 2nd procedure, in terms of mean g/kg, are depicted in Figure 2. In brief, the overall ANOVA of that data failed to reveal reliable sources of variance associated with either factor or their interaction. The ANOVA associated with rats' intake of water revealed a main effect of Days, $F(1,44)=7.02$, $p<0.02$. Subsequent analyses revealed that there was a general trend for all groups to increase their mean intakes of water on the day of treatment. In brief, although there was a trend for all groups to increase their mean intakes of water across the 2-day period of injections, cocaine (10.0 mg/kg), given at 2, 4, or 6 hr before the opportunity to drink, did not reliably modify rats' intake of E.

DISCUSSION

Cocaine did not augment rats' intake of E. In fact, it decreased intake. This result is similar to that of another report showing that an agonist at the post synaptic DA receptor, bromocriptine, decreases rats' pressing for E [13]. It seems that increases in dopaminergic activity tend to decrease intake of alcoholic beverages. This occurs, however, at a dose that might interfere with any ordinary motivated behavior with the exception of those that are manifest by, and synergistic with, increased propensity to be active.

Pimozide, a dopaminergic antagonist, also decreases rats' intakes of alcoholic beverages [10,12]. Both increases and decreases in dopaminergic activity lead to decreases in intake of E. This lack of bipolar effects with agents that produce opposite effects on DA systems does not support the idea that DA systems are salient to propensity to take E. Of course, a more specific dopaminergic manipulation, e.g., in terms of an action at a particular receptor might augment rats' propensity to drink E.

Not all agents that can elicit positive affect among rats will, in turn, increment rats' intake of E. MDMA is another agent that produces positivity, but does not increment intake of E [14]. Consequently, it is inappropriate to conclude that any agent incrementing positive affect will increment intake of E. Opioids eliciting positivity are unique in their ability to increment intake of alcoholic beverages.

REFERENCES

1. Reid, L.D. In: Reid, L.D. (Ed.), Opioids, Bulimia, and Alcohol Abuse & Alcoholism. New York: Springer-Verlag, pp. 275-280, 1990.
2. Hubbell, C.L., & Reid, L.D. In: Reid, L.D. (Ed.), Opioids, Bulimia, and Alcohol Abuse & Alcoholism. New York: Springer-Verlag, pp. 145-174, 1990.
3. Wise, R.A., & Bozarth, M.A. Psychological Review 94:469-492; 1987.
4. Galloway, M.P. Trends in Pharmacological Sciences 9:451-454; 1988.
5. Ritz, M.C., et al. Science 237:1219-1223; 1987.
6. Blum, K., et al. Journal of the American Medical Association 362:2055-2060; 1990.
7. McBride, W.J., et al. Alcohol 7:199-205; 1990.
8. Amit, Z., & Brown, Z.W. Pharmacology Biochemistry & Behavior 17:233-238; 1982.
9. Brown, Z.W., et al. Behavioral Neurological Biology 36:291-294; 1982.
10. Hubbell C.L., et al. Alcohol: In editorial review.
11. Mudar, P.J., et al. Alcohol 3:303-308; 1986.
12. Pfeffer, A.O., & Samson, H.H. Alcohol 2:693-697; 1984.
13. Weiss, F., et al. Psychopharmacology 101:178-186; 1990.
14. Bilsky, E.J., et al. Pharmacology, Biochemistry & Behavior 37:In press; 1990.

ACKNOWLEDGEMENTS

This research was supported, in part, by a grant from NIDA (DA04440). We thank Yizhao Hui for help with the data collection.

CALCIUM-ACETYLHOMOTAURINATE FOR MAINTAINING ABSTINENCE IN WEANED ALCOHOLIC PATIENTS: A PLACEBO-CONTROLLED DOUBLE-BLIND MULTICENTER STUDY

I. Pelc[1], O. Le Bon[1], P. Verbanck[1], Ph. Lehert[2] and L. Opsomer[3]

1 : Department of Psychiatry and Medical Psychology. Free University of Brussels - Brugmann Campus. Place Van Gehuchten,4 - 1020 Brussels . BELGIUM
2 : Department of Informatics and Statistics. University of Mons . BELGIUM
3 : Lipha Pharmaceuticals, Lyon. FRANCE

INTRODUCTION

Drugs used for attenuating alcohol intake consist of two types:

1. Agents postulated to attenuate drinking by causing aversive consequences if alcohol is consumed after they are ingested, including disulfiram.

2. Agents postulated to attenuate directly the desire to drink, including such drugs as lithium, fenfluramine, zimelidine and bromocriptine.

Recently, a new drug , Calcium acetyl homotaurinate (Ca AOTA) , has been shown to be of interest in reducing craving for ethanol in the animal[1] and in the human[2 3]. The pharmacological properties of this agent are quite unknown, but interactions with GABA[4] and excitatory amino acids[5] transmission have been suggested.

We present here the results of a multicentric double-blind study, comparing Ca AOTA and placebo for the prevention of relapse in recently detoxified alcoholics.

MATERIAL AND METHODS

A multicentric double-blind parallel placebo-controlled study was performed, in order to test the efficacy of Ca AOTA (1999 mg/day) on the maintain of abstinence in recently detoxified alcoholics.
102 patients were included in the assay; all of them met the DSM III-R criteria for alcohol dependence and were free of other mental or physical illness.
They were followed and assessed during 180 days.

RESULTS

At the inclusion time, no clinical or biological differences between the placebo and the Ca-AOTA groups were observed.
The compliance to treatment was better in the Ca-AOTA group, as presented in Figure 1: at the end of the follow-up, a significant excess of drop-outs was present in the placebo group ($p < 0.05$) .

The efficacy of the treatment was estimated by the abstinence survival curves (Figure 2) in the two groups and by the mean number of days without alcohol. For both the parameters, Ca-AOTA was superior to placebo ($p < 0.01$) after 180 days. This was confirmed by a better score at the clinical global impression scale in the Ca-AOTA group ($p < 0.05$) at the end of the study.
The analysis of the adverse events did not show any serious side effects; however, gastralgia, diarrhea, headache, paresthesia, diaphoresia and palpitations are significantly more frequent in the Ca-AOTA group.

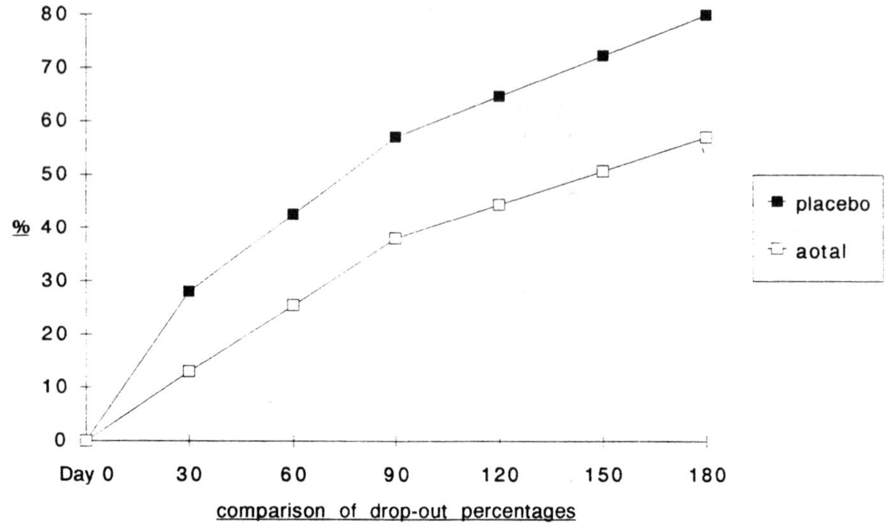

Figure 1: Evolution of the drop-outs during the follow-up period. Since the first evaluation, there are significantly more drop-outs in the placebo group.

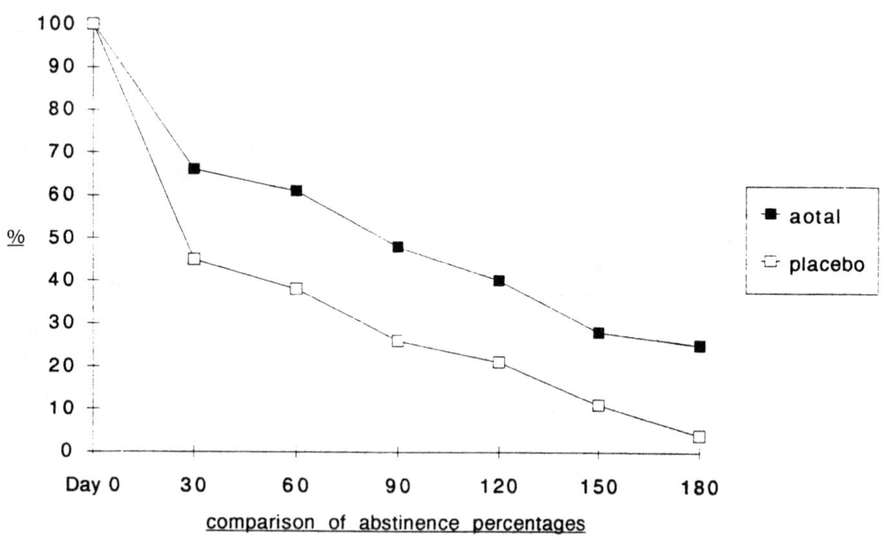

Figure 2: Evolution of the proportions of abstinent patients during the follow-up period. Since the first evaluation, there are significantly more abstinent patients in the AOTAL group.

DISCUSSION AND CONCLUSIONS

This study underlined two main points:
- such a double-blind follow-up study is difficult to carry out in ambulatory alcoholic patients, because most of the relapsing patients are lost for assessment. However, the compliance to follow-up was significantly better in the Ca-AOTA group.

- furthermore, abstinence was significantly longer in the Ca-AOTA group, and the global clinical assessment of these patients was better.

Thus, a better clinical outcome was present in patients receiving Ca-AOTA, suggesting that this drug could be of value in the treatment of detoxified alcoholics. These observations confirm previous reports on Ca-AOTA. However, for the moment, there is no indication that this drug is able to reduce the desire to drink in the human; its efficacy in reducing relapses after alcohol detoxification could also be due to indirect effects, for example on depression, anxiety, sleep disturbances or memory troubles.
Further investigations are needed in order to clarify this point.

REFERENCES

[1]LE MAGNEN J, TRAN G, DURLACH J and MARTIN C. Dose-dependent suppression of the high alcohol intake of chronically intoxicated rats by Ca-acetylhomotaurinate. Alcohol, 4: 103-8, 1987

[2]LHUINTRE JP, DAOUST M, TRAN G, MOORE N, CHRETIEN P, HILLEMAND B and BOISMARE F. Calcium acetyl-homotaurinate Ca-AOTA reduces alcohol consumption by ethylics. Alcohol Clin Exp Res 8: 103, 1984

[3]LHUINTRE JP, MOORE N, SAUGAUT C, BOISMARE M, DAOUST M, CHRETIEN P, TRAN G and HILLEMAND B. Efficacy of calcium bis acetyl homotaurine, a gaba agonist to prevent relapse in weaned alcoholics. Lancet i: 1014-16, 1985

[4]DAOUST M, SAUGAUT C, MOORE N, CHRETIEN P and BOISMARE F. The effect of calcium acetylhomotaurinate on the constants of accumulation kinetics of tritiated gamma aminobutyric acid in the striatal synaptosomes of which prefer alcohol. J Pharmacol 15: 458-9, 1984

[5]BOUCHENAFA O, CWYNARSKI K and LITTLETON JM. Interactions between excitatory amino-acids and AOTAL in a cell culture model of ethanol dependence. 5th Congress of The International Society for Biomedical Research on Alcoholism. Abstract book: abstract 30, 1990

EFFECTS OF ANGIOTENSIN CONVERTING ENZYME INHIBITORS ON FREE CHOICE ETHANOL CONSUMPTION BY RATS

B.Brands, C.A.Naranjo, J.W.Tighe, R.S.Collis, and E.M.Sellers

Introduction

Recent reports in the literature (Lingham et al, 1990; Spinosa et al, 1988) have shown that angiotensin converting enzyme (ACE) inhibitors decrease ethanol consumption in rats. A clinical trial by Naranjo and his colleagues (see these proceedings) was conducted to determine whether enalapril was effective in decreasing ethanol consumption in normotensive moderately dependent drinkers. We concurrently tested three ACE inhibitors, enalapril, benazepril and abutapril in rats using a 24 hour unlimited access free choice drinking model.

Materials and Methods

Subjects

Male Wistar rats (Charles River, Canada) initially weighing 175-225g were housed individually in stainless steel cages equipped with two 100 mL Richter tubes in a room maintained at 22-24 C, 55% humidity, and a 12 hour day-night cycle (7:00pm-7:00am darkness).

Procedures

After a two day acclimitization period during which water was the sole fluid available in both tubes, the fluid in one of the tubes was replaced by 2% ethanol (v/v). The ethanol concentration was increased by 1% every three days until a final concentration of 6% was achieved.

Rats then entered a 7 day baseline period during which the animals received daily (6:00pm) i.p. injections of Ringer's solution. Fluid consumption (including both water and ethanol) and body weights were measured daily.

Following baseline rats (n=93) were randomized to one of ten treatment groups: benazepril 1, 5 or 10 mg/kg, enalapril 1, 5 and 10 mg/kg abutapril 1, 5 and 10 mg/kg and vehicle control. All drugs were injected once daily at 6:00pm for 14 consecutive days. Fluid consumption and body weights were recorded daily.

Materials

Benazepril (Ciba-Geigy), enalapril (Merck) and abutapril (CGS 16617, Ciba-Geigy) were dissolved in Ringer's solution and prepared fresh daily. All doses were calculated as the HCL salt.

Statistical Analyses

For each rat, daily ethanol (g/kg) and water (mL) consumption levels were averaged by period (baseline, week1, week2). For each drug, a one within (period) and one between (dose level) analysis of variance (ANOVA) was performed. Pairwise differences among treatments were determined using the Student-Neuman Keuls test.

Results

Analysis of variance showed that ethanol (g/kg) and water (mL) consumption did not differ significantly among the doses of the three ACE inhibitors studied. A significant period effect was seen for ethanol consumption (g/kg) in the abutapril-treated rats ($p<.001$). The Student-Newman Keuls test showed that Week 2 was significantly lower than Baseline and Week 1 ($p<.05$) (see table 1). A period effect was also seen in water consumption in the abutapril-treated rats ($p<0.001$). The Student-Newman Keuls test showed that all three periods were significantly different ($p<.05$) (see table 1). Similar trends in ethanol consumption were noted in the benazepril and enalapril groups. However, these differences were not significant.

Table 1: Mean 14 Hour Ethanol and Water Consumption in Abutapril-Treated Rats

	ETOH (g/kg)	Water (mL)
Baseline	5.2 (1.43)	7.4 (10.79)
Week 1	5.5 (1.96)	12.0 (15.73)
Week 2	4.7 (1.94)	18.0 (19.58)

Note: Standard Deviations are in brackets

Discussion

Under the experimental conditions defined, abutapril decreased ethanol consumption during week two of treatment. Water consumption increased during both weeks of treatment. A dose effect was not seen. These findings are in agreement with those reported in the literature (Lingham et al, 1990).

Although the ACE inhibitors studied here did decrease ethanol or showed a tendency towards decreasing ethanol consumption, the decrements were small and perhaps not clinically relevant. Indeed, the results of the clinical study conducted by Naranjo and his colleagues showed that enalapril failed to decrease ethanol consumption in normotensive, moderately dependent drinkers.

References

Lingham, T., Perlanski, E. and Grupp, L.A. Angiotensin converting enzyme inhibitors reduce alcohol consumption: Some possible mechanisms and important conditions for its therapeutic use. *Alcoholism: Clin. Exp. Res.* **14** (1): 92-99 (1990).

Spinosa, G., Perlanski, E., Leenan, F.H.H., Stewart, R.B. and Grupp, L.A. Angiotensin converting enzyme inhibitors: Animal experiments suggest a new pharmacological treatment for alcohol use in humans. *Alcoholism: Clin. Exp. Res.* **12**(1): 65-70 (1988).

CALCIUM CHANNEL ANTAGONISTS ATTENUATE THE ALCOHOL DEPENDENCE SYNDROME

C.A Naranjo, T. Fan

1. ABSTRACT

Dihydropryridine calcium entry blockers (e.g., nifedipine) delay the acquisition of tolerance to ethanol, attenuate the symptoms of alcohol withdrawal and decrease alcohol consumption and preference, in rodents. These effects should be tested in humans to determine their potential therapeutic application.

2. INTRODUCTION

The alcohol dependence syndrome has various clinical manifestations such as acute intoxication, tolerance to ethanol, alcohol withdrawal and excessive alcohol consumption. In this review we will briefly discuss the effects of calcium channel antagonists on the clinical manifestations of the alcohol dependence syndrome. Calcium is essential for neurotransmitter release (Blaustein et al 1981). Neuronal calcium channels maintain intracellular calcium homeostasis and control the influx of extracellular calcium into nerve terminals. Calcium uptake into synaptosomes occurs in two phases. In the initial fast-phase calcium enters through calcium channels and inactivates within the first few seconds after depolarization (Leslie et al 1983, Leslie et al 1985). The slow phase that follows does not involve calcium channels, and calcium is transported through sodium/calcium exchange. It seems that calcium entry is mainly though voltage-sensitive calcium channels (Miller 1987).

Ethanol inhibits neurotransmitter release by altering calcium entry into the nerve terminal (Lynch et al 1983). Low concentrations of ethanol (25 mM) have been reported to inhibit the fast-phase component of calcium uptake into cerebrocortical synaptosomes (Leslie et al 1983), but much larger concentrations were required to inhibit the slow-phase calcium entry (Leslie et al 1983, Skattebol et al 1987). It is evident that calcium channels are important sites of action of ethanol on calcium uptake. Chronic ethanol treatment to animals caused an elevation of synaptosomal calcium content (Ross 1977). It is possible that ethanol inhibits calcium entry directly or indirectly through elevation of intracellular calcium which in turn inactivate calcium channels. The increased sensitivity to calcium entry and adaptive response in calcium channels may underlie alcohol tolerance, dependence and withdrawal syndrome (Dolin et al 1987). The existence of voltage-dependent calcium channels and high affinity dihydropyridine (DHP) binding sites in the brain has been demonstrated and evidence suggests a physiological role for the sites (Ramkumar et al 1986). This manuscript will review the effects of calcium channel antagonists on the various manifestations of the alcohol dependence syndrome.

3. ALCOHOL INTOXICATION

The dihydropyridine calcium channel blockers bind to the periphery and in the brain with few overt action on the central nervous system. They produce very little behavioral changes of their own in normal animals, but exaggerate the intoxicating effects of ethanol. Isaacson et al (1985) reported that administration of 5 mg/kg i.p. of nimodipine alone to Binghamton Heterogeneous adult mice did not alter rectal temperature or motor-coordination after 20 and 60 minutes. However, it potentiated hypothermia induced by 2.0 g/kg of ethanol and reduced the amount of time the animals could maintain themselves on the motorod after 0.5, 1.0, 2.0 g/kg ethanol i.p., by an unexplained mechanism. Little et al (1986) also confirmed that nitrendipine (100 mg/kg) and nimodipine (200 mg/kg) did not change the locomotor activity counts 1 and 3 hours after their administration. Flunarizine 80 mg/kg caused no change in activity 3 to 5 hours after injection and verapamil 20 mg/kg 2 hours after administration. Ethanol's effect on locomotor activity is biphasic (Engel 1977 & Engel et al 1983). Low doses, 2.5 g/kg, caused locomotor stimulation whereas high doses, 4.5 g/kg, caused sedation. Engel et al (1988) further investigated the effects of calcium channel antagonists on the stimulatory effect of ethanol. Oral administration of 1.0, 5.0, 10 mg/kg nifedipine to female NMRI mice completely antagonized the locomotor stimulatory effect of low doses of ethanol, and slightly potentiated the sedative effect of higher doses of ethanol. Although nifedipine alone (less than 5 mg/kg p.o.) has very little effect on locomotor activity, 5.0 mg/kg caused a slight statistically significant decrease in locomotor activity, whereas 10 mg/kg actually produced a slight but significant stimulation. The effect of nifedipine appeared to be more pronounced during the first 30 minutes of administration. The observation that dihydropyridine calcium channel blockers antagonized the stimulatory effects of ethanol suggested that an enhancement of calcium-mediated mechanisms may be involved. The dihydropyridines may act by changing the gating properties of voltage-sensitive calcium channels. In summary, the calcium channel antagonist potentiated the sedative effects of alcohol and antagonized the stimulatory effects of ethanol. The mechanism of these effects is unclear.

4. TOLERANCE TO ETHANOL

Calcium channel antagonists (e.g., nifedipine) delayed the acquisition of tolerance to ethanol in rats (Wu et al 1987). Trained Wistar male rats were tested for motor impairment after a challenge dose of ethanol 2.0 g/kg i.p. on the test days. When rats were chronically treated with ethanol 2.0 g/kg, tolerance to test-doses of ethanol developed 23 days after treatment (demonstrated by 50% reduction in ethanol-induced impairment). The development of tolerance to ethanol was significantly prolonged (>35 days) in rats that received both chronic nifedipine (75 mg/kg, twice daily) and ethanol. Similar observations were reported with nitrendipine (Dolin et al 1989). Concurrent administration of nitrendipine 50 mg/kg during chronic ethanol treatment (1.5 and 2.0 g/kg i.p. once daily for 10 days) prevented the development of tolerance to ethanol.

5. ALCOHOL WITHDRAWAL SYNDROME

The effects of calcium channel antagonists were studied in rats dependent on alcohol which developed symptoms of withdrawal. Discontinuation of chronic ethanol intake results in tremor and hyperexcitability, which can progress to seizures and death. The effects of four calcium channel antagonists were tested on the ethanol withdrawal syndrome (Little et al 1986). The most marked effects were obtained with nitrendipine 100 mg/kg which completely prevented spontaneous and audiogenic seizures and mortality during withdrawal. Nitrendipine 50 mg/kg and 100-200 mg/kg of nimodipine abolished all spontaneous seizures and prevented or reduced audiogenic seizures and mortality. Verapamil 10-20 mg/kg significantly decreased seizures incidence, and both it and flunarizine 40-80 mg/kg lower mortality. These findings were confirmed by Little et al (1988). They reported that concurrent injection of nitrendipine 50 mg/kg, twice daily to TO strain male mice while they were exposed to ethanol in an inhalation chamber for two weeks showed no sign of handling-induced seizures. Whereas mice given ethanol alone displayed convulsive behavior upon handling, representing a withdrawal reaction to ethanol. However, when nitrendipine was administered only during the last two days of ethanol treatment, convulsive behavior was seen on withdrawal. The opposing effect of nitrendipine and ethanol may be responsible for the prevention of ethanol withdrawal symptoms. In summary, calcium entry blockers attenuate the manifestations of alcohol withdrawal syndrome in rats.

6. ALCOHOL CONSUMPTION

Calcium channel antagonists attenuate the consumption of ethanol in rats. Engel et al (1988) demonstrated that nifedipine 5 mg/kg p.o twice daily significantly decreased ethanol preference in a free choice paradigm (6% ethanol solution), and significantly decreased the amount of ethanol consumed without affecting the amount of total fluid intake. Reduction in consumption (22%) and preference (33%) are of a similar magnitude to those reported with other drugs.

7. NEUROPHARMACOLOGICAL STUDIES

Calcium channel blockers modify the binding sites of brain synaptosomal membranes in rats when co-administered with chronic ethanol treatment. Chronic administration of ethanol in doses sufficient to induce tolerance and dependence (2 to 3 g/kg) for 10 days modify the binding sites for the dihydropyridines calcium channel blockers in cerebral cortex (Littleton et al 1988, Dolin et al 1987). They reported a 50% increase in B_{max} for ^{3}H-nimodipine binding in the cortical membrane of ethanol dependent rats. However, Little et al 1988 reported that concurrent treatment of chronic ethanol and nitrendipine 50 mg/kg decreased B_{max} for nimodipine binding significantly, whereas chronic nitrendipine treatment alone did not change the binding. K_d was not affected. We extended the investigation further by looking at nitrendipine binding sites after acute and chronic ethanol treatment and alcohol withdrawal. As shown in Figure 1, and Table 1, B_{max} increased by 25% after 4 days of ethanol treatment (3 g/kg p.o. twice daily, at 12 hours apart) and 42% after 10 days, and returned to control levels when alcohol was withdrawn for 17 hours after 10 days of treatment. No noticeable change was observed 40 minutes after an acute dose of ethanol. K_d showed no significant increase except after 4 days of ethanol treatment. It seemed that the increase in B_{max} after chronic ethanol treatment followed a similar time course to the development of tolerance to ethanol and was reversible after alcohol withdrawal. This finding strongly suggested that an upregulation in dihydropyridine calcium channels may be associated with the development of tolerance to ethanol. Co-administration of nitrendipine and ethanol prevented the increase in B_{max}. These results support the notion that dihydropyridine sites are involved in the development of tolerance to ethanol.

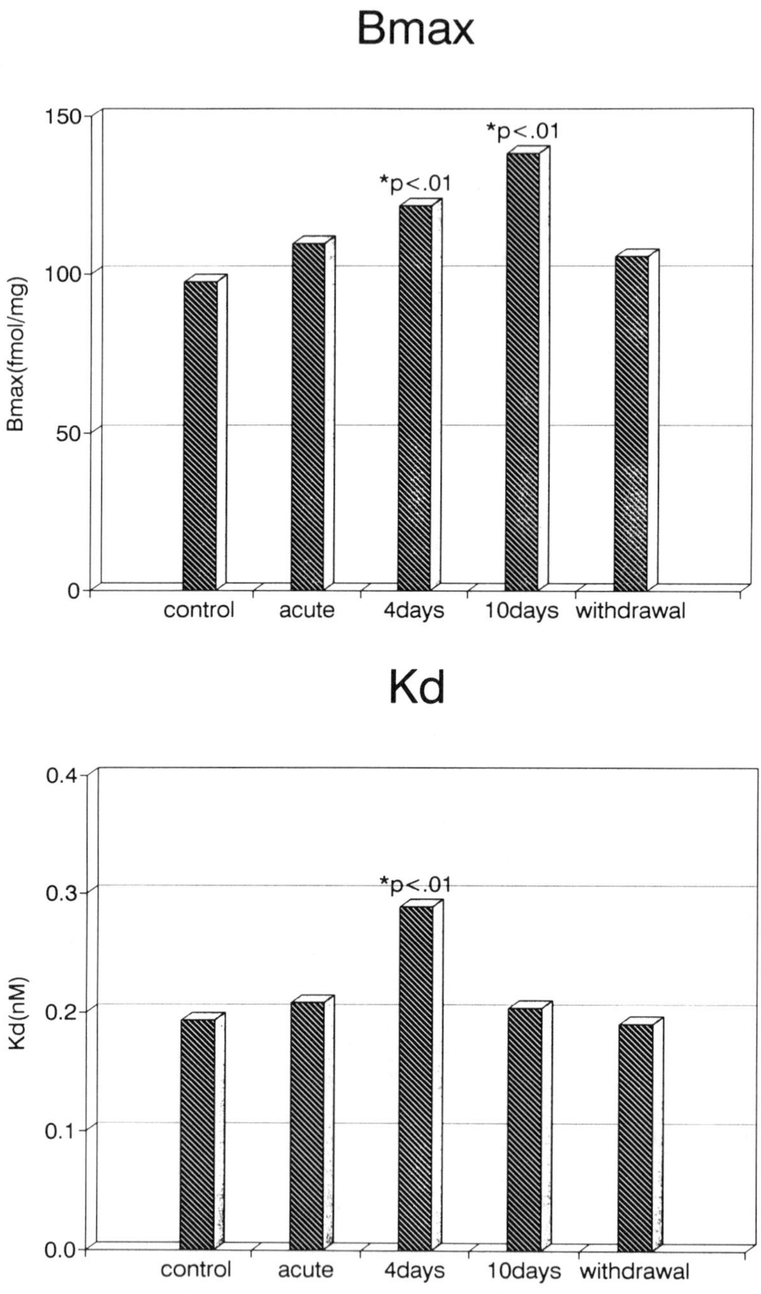

Figure 1. Effects on acute ethanol , chronic ethanol and ethanol withdrawal on nitrendipine binding (B_{max} upper panel; Kd, lower panel), to cortical membranes.

Table 1: Effects of acute ethanol, chronic ethanol and ethanol withdrawal on nitrendipine binding to cortical membranes.

	**1 control	**2 acute	**3 4 days	**4 10 days	**5 withdrawal
mean Bmax (fmol/mg)	97.50	109.73	121.83	138.18	105.70
S.D.	8	7.79	6.83	5.32	5.66
n	4	4	4	4	3
significant level			*p<.01	*p<.01	
%increase			25 %	42 %	
mean Kd (nM)	0.1932	0.2078	0.2892	0.2034	0.1902
S.D.	0.01	0.024	0.017	0.01	0.042
n	4	4	4	4	3
significant level			*p<.01		
%increase			49.7 %		

**1; control: rats received Ringers solution by intubation twice daily at 12 hours apart.

**2; acute: rats received a single ETOH dose 3 g/kg p.o., and were sacrificed 40 minutes later.

**3; 4 days: rats received ETOH 3 g/kg p.o., twice daily at 12 hours apart, sacrificed 3 hours later after the last dose on the fourth day.

**4; 10 days: rats received ETOH 3 g/kg p.o., twice daily at 12 hours apart, and were sacrificed 3 hours later after the last dose on the tenth day.

**5; withdrawal: rats received ETOH 3 g/kg p.o., twice daliy for 10 days, and were sacrificed 16½ to 18 hours after the last dose.

8. NMDA RECEPTOR COMPLEX

Ethanol has a potent and selective inhibitory effect on biochemical and electrophysiological responses to NMDA-receptors in certain brain areas (Hoffman et al 1990). Recent electrophysiological and biochemical studies by Hoffman et al (1989), Lovinger et al (1989) and Dildy et al (1989) suggested that ethanol concentrations as low as 5-10 mM, is a potent and selective inhibitor of N-methyl-D-aspartate (NMDA)-receptor complex, whereas high concentrations of ETOH (45 to 150 mM) inhibit synaptosomal depolarization-induced calcium uptake (Leslie 1986; Leslie et al 1983). Thus, the NMDA-receptor may also play a key role in mediating some of the in vivo behavioral actions of ethanol. Grant et al (1990) showed that ethanol dependent C57 BL mice treated with MK-801, a non-competitive NMDA-receptor antagonist, in doses of 0.3,1.0, 3.0 mg/kg i.p. at 0,3,7, hours after ethanol withdrawal decreased the occurrence and severity of handling-induced withdrawal seizures in a dose dependent manner. However, administration of 30 mg/kg NMDA, an agonist, at 8 hours after alcohol withdrawal enhanced handling-induced withdrawal seizures. These findings are in agreement with Morrisett et al (1990) who demonstrated that 0.33 mg/kg MK-801, i.p. suppressed audiogenic-induced seizures in Sprague-Dawley rats 12 hours after ethanol consumption of 8 g/kg daily for 10 days was withdrawn. The increase in B_{max} of MK-801 binding in hippocampus (Grant et al 1990) indicated an increase in NMDA-receptor/ionophore complex. The mechanisms of ethanol withdrawal may also be associated with sensitization and upregulation of NMDA receptor function. However, the number of ^{3}H-MK-801-binding sites did not increase in cerebral cortex of ethanol withdrawn mice. The heterogeneity of NMDA receptors may explain this finding (Hoffman et al 1990). Since the hippocampus has been regarded as an important site for ethanol withdrawal seizures, this increase in the number of NMDA-receptor complex in certain brain areas may be related to hyperexcitability and seizure activity associated with ethanol withdrawal in dependent mice. Thus, it becomes apparent that compensatory upregulation by both voltage-sensitive calcium channels and NMDA-receptor operated calcium channels is a very important process of neuroadaptation to the effects of ethanol dependence. Like the dihydropyridines, MK-801 has the ability to compensate hyperexcitability and seizure activities associated with ethanol dependence.

9. CONCLUSIONS

Although calcium channel antagonists produce very little behavioral changes of their own, they potentiate the sedative-hypnotic properties of ethanol, delay the development of tolerance, attenuate the alcohol withdrawal syndrome and decrease alcohol consumption in rats. The increase in the number of binding sites (a neuronal adaptive process to oppose the inhibitory effect of alcohol) seen after chronic ethanol treatment was also prevented. These findings clearly indicate that calcium channel antagonists can alter various aspects of the alcohol dependence syndrome. These effects are unique and have not been previously reported with any other class of agents that do not have cross-dependence/tolerance with ethanol. The dihydropyridine calcium channel blockers may be valuable as an effective, non-addictive treatment for alcohol dependence and withdrawal. The clinical effects of calcium channel blockers should be tested once agents with enhanced penetration to the CNS are found and the chances of peripheral cardiovascular side effects are diminished.

The views expressed in this publication are those of the authors and do not necessarily reflect those of the Addiction Research Foundation.

10. REFERENCES

Blaustein M.P., D.A. Nachshen, P. Drapeau (1981). Excitation-secretion coupling: The role of calcium. In: *Chemical Neurotransmission*, L. Stjarne, P. Hedqvist, H. Lagercrantz, A. Wennmalm eds.) Academic Press, London, 125-138.

Dildy, J.E. and S.W. Leslie (1989). Ethanol inhibits NMDA-induced increases in free intracellular calcium in dissociated brain cells. *Br. Res.*, 499, 383-387.

Dolin, S.J. and H.J Little (1986). Augmentation by calcium channel antagonists of general anesthetic potency in mice. *Br. J. Pharmacol.*, 88, 909-914.

Dolin, S.J. and H.J. Little (1989). Are changes in neuronal calcium channels involved in ethanol tolerance. *J. Pharm. & Exp. Ther.*, 250(3), 985-991.

Dolin, S.J., H.J. Little, M, Hudspith, C. Pagonis and J.M. Littleton (1987). Increased dihydropyridine calcium channels in rat brain may underline ethanol physical dependence. *Neuropharmacology*, 26, 275-279.

Engel, J. (1977). Neurochemical aspects of the euphoria induced by dependence - producing drugs. In: *Recent advances in the study of alcoholism*, (C-M. Idestrom ed.), Excerpta Medica, Amsterdam (International Congress Series No. 407), 16-22.

Engel, J. and S. Liljequist (1983). The involvement of different central neurotransmitters in mediating stimulatory and sedative effects of ethanol. In: *Stress and alcohol use*, (L. Pohorecky, J. Brick eds.), Elsevier, New York, 153-169.

Engel, J.A., C. Fahlke, P. Hulthe, E. Hard, K. Johannessen, B. Snape and L. Svensson (1988). Biochemical and behavioral evidence for an interaction between ethanol and calcium channel antagonists. *J. Neural. Transm.*, 74, 181-193.

Grant, K.A., P. Valverius, M. Hudspith and B. Tabakoff (1990): Ethanol withdrawal seizures and NMDA receptor complex. *Eur. J. Pharmacol.*, 176: 289-296.

Hoffman, P.L., C.S. Rabe, F. Moses and B. Tabakoff (1989). NMDA-receptors and ethanol: inhibition of calcium flux and cyclic GMP production. *J. Neurochem.*, 52, 1937-1940.

Hoffman, P.L., C.S. Rabe, K.A. Grant, P. Valverius, M. Hudspith and B. Tabakoff (1990). Ethanol and the NMDA receptor. *Alcohol*, 7, 229-231.

Isaacson, R.L., J.C. Molina, L.J. Draski and J.E. Johnston (1985). Nimodipine's interactions with other drugs: I. Ethanol. *Life Science*, 36, 2195-2199.

Leslie S.W., L.M. Brown, J.E. Dildy and J.S. Sims (1990). Ethanol & neuronal calcium channels. *Alcohol*, 7, 233-236.

Leslie, S.W., E. Barr, J. Chandler and R.P. Farrar (1983). Inhibition of fast- slow-phase depolarization dependent synaptosomal calcium uptake by ethanol. *J. Pharmacol. Exp. Ther.*, 225, 571-575.

Leslie, S.W., J.J. Woodward, R.E. Wilcox (1985). Correlation of rats of calcium entry and endogenous dopamine release in mouse striated synaptosomes. *Brain Research*, 325, 99-105.

Little, H.J., S.J. Dolin and M.A. Whittington (1988). Possible role of calcium channels in ethanol tolerance and dependence. *Annals of New York Academy of Sciences*, *560*, Calcium Channels - Structure & Function, 465-466.

Little, H.J., S.J. Dolin and M.J. Halsey (1986). Calcium channel antagonists decrease the ethanol withdrawal syndrome. *Life Sci.*, 39, 2059-2065.

Littleton, J.M. and M.A. Lynch (1983). Possible association of alcohol tolerance with increased synaptic calcium sensitivity. *Nature*, 303, 175-176.

Littleton, J.M., J.H. Harper, M. Hudspith, C. Pagonis, S.J. Dolin and H.J. Little (1988). Adaptation in neuronal calcium channels may cause alcohol physical dependence. In: *The Psychopharmacology of Addiction*, (M. Lader ed.), British association for psychopharmacology monograph, Oxford University Press, Oxford, Great Britain, 60-72.

Lovinger, D.M., G. White, F.F. Weight (1989). Ethanool inhibits NMDA-activated ion current in hippocampal neurons. *Sci.*, 243: 1721-1724.

Miller, R.J. (1987). Multiple Ca++ channels and neuronal functions. *Science*, 235, 46-52.

Morrisett, R.A., A.H. Rezvani, D. Overstreet, D.S. Janowsky, W.A. Wilson and H.S. Swartzwelder (1990). MK-801 potently inhibits alcohol withdrawal seizures in rats. *Eur. J. Pharmacol.*, 176, 103-105.

Ramkumar, V. and E.E. El-& Fakahany (1986). The current status of the dihydropyridine calcium channel antagoinist binding sites in the brain. *Trends Pharmacol. Sci.*, 7, 171-172.

Ross, D.H. (1977). Adaptive changes in Ca^{2+} membrane interactions following chronic ethanol exposure. In: *Alcohol intoxication and withdrawal - IIIa*, (M.M. Gross ed.), Plenum Press, New York, 459.

Skattebol, A and R.A. Rabin (1987). Effects of ethanol in $^{45}CA^{++}$ uptake in synaptosomes and in PC12 cells. *Biochem. Pharmacol.*, 36, 2227-2229.

Wu, P.H., T. Pham and C.A. Naranjo (1987). Nifedipine delays the acquisition of tolerance to ethanol. *Eur. J. Pharmacol.*, 139, 233-236.

PHARMACOLOGICAL ANTAGONISM OF ETHANOL BY *dl*-α-TOCOPHEROL

D.V. Gauvin, D.J. Brackett, J.R. Criado, M.R. Lerner, M.F. Wilson, and F.A. Holloway
University of Oklahoma Health Sciences Center and Veteran Affairs Medical Center, Oklahoma City, OK 73190

1.1 Abstract

There is an evergrowing data base which links ETOH with perturbations of polyunsaturated fatty acids (PUFAs), lipids, prostaglandins, and serum α-tocopherol levels (cf. Gordis, Tabakoff, Linnoila, & Stimmell, 1989). However, there is a paucity of information regarding the reverse relationship. Our laboratories have collaborated on an investigation of ETOH's deleterious effects on a composite of physiological and behavioral indices in intact conscious animals. As an experimental precursor of future protocol designs, we investigated the interaction between *dl*-α-tocopherol (VIT E) preloads and blood ETOH (alcohol) concentrations (BACs) in rats. VIT E has been linked to the conjugation of arachidonic acid with PUFAs, and the production of prostaglandins within lipid cell membranes *in vivo*. Using an isothermal gas chromatograph head-space sampling procedure to quantify BACs, we measured blood ETOH from different groups of rats treated chronically (3-5 days) with either VIT E or soybean oil (control), during inhalation chamber, intragastric, and intraperitoneal ETOH administration. Significant reductions in group BACs ($p<.01$) were found in all VIT E treated groups when compared to control cohorts. Behavioral indices of intoxication were used to assess ETOH levels. ETOH's effects on locomotor activity, drug discriminative performance, and response rates (FR10) were antagonized by prior treatment of VIT E.

1.2 Introduction

Our two laboratories have collaborated on a set of studies designed to analyze the deleterious effects of ethanol (ETOH) on the structural and ultrastructural components of a number of organ tissues, and correlating these perturbations with behavioral indices of intoxication, tolerance development, an dependence. There is a rich and vast literature linking ETOH's effects on membrane lipid, lipid peroxidation and its associated by-products, and the production of free-radical-induced tissue damage (Nordman, Ribiere, & Rouach, 1988).

Our original focus of these experiments was directed toward the effects of both acute and chronic ETOH exposure and the interaction between ETOH and *dl*-α-tocopherol (Vitamin E). Vitamin E (VIT E) has a number of physiological effects, is a naturally occurring substance found in a number of plants, and is a potent biologically active antioxidant (Porter & Whelan, 1983). VIT E's unique molecular structure enables specific physico-chemical interactions to take place between its phytyl side-chain and some of the arachidonyl chains of membrane phospholipids (Diplock, 1983; Diplock & Lucy, 1973) and also increases the uptake of cholesterol into the membrane layer (*ibid;* Patel & Edwards, 1988). Although there is a vast literature linking ETOH with perturbations of these same physiological effects (Sun *et al.*, 1989) there is a paucity of information regarding the effects of VIT E supplementation on ETOH and its behavioral or physiological effects.

As a precursor of future research protocols we wanted to investigate the interactive effects between VIT E and ETOH using acute and chronic exposure regimens using a number of routes of administration: inhalation, intragastric, and intraperitoneal. A gas-chromatographic head space sampling technique was used to assess the blood alcohol levels of rats exposed to VIT E or vegetable oil (Veg. oil) supplemental administration.

1.3 Methods

An isothermal head space sampling method adapted from Pohorecky and Brick (1982) was used to quantify blood alcohol levels using a Hewlett-Packard 5890 Gas Chromatograph (GC). The GC was equipped with an H_2-fueled flame-ionization detector, N_2 carrier gas, pressurized air purge, and a 6'x 1/8" stainless steel column (5% Carbowax, 20M, 60/80 mesh, Carbopack B). The temperature parameters were set at the following $^{\circ}$C: oven, 135; injection port, 200; detector, 300. A 20 μl tail blood sample was drawn and deposited in a 1-ml solution of .02% v/v 1-Propanol in distilled water (internal standard) and sealed in a 20-ml serum bottle.

General activity was measured using an automated photobeam activity chamber (King, Bouton, & Musty, 1987) connected to a Commodore 64C microcomputer system.

A two-choice drug discrimination task described in detail elsewhere (Gauvin *et al.*, 1989) was also used to assess the relative antagonism of the discriminative effects of ETOH by VIT E.

1.4 Results and Discussion

Two groups of rats (n=8/group) were placed in ETOH inhalation chambers after a short chronic (5 days) treatment period with either VIT E (100 mg/day) or vegetable (soybean) oil (.1 ml) gavaged to the back of the throat. Twenty microliter tail blood samples were drawn daily and treatments continued during ETOH exposure. Rats from both treatment groups were integrated within the same chambers. On Day 10, when the Veg. oil control group blood levels had reached an average of 300 mg/dl, the flow directed through the ETOH flasks was slowly reduced until Day 14 to prevent the expression of ETOH withdrawal. The resulting BAC demonstrated significant differences between the VIT E and Veg. oil control groups from Days 8 through 13 (Figure 1). On Day 10 of exposure, each animal was temporarily removed from the ETOH chamber and tested for general ambulatory and nonambulatory activity in a computerized activity monitoring device (5 mins). The VIT E group was significantly more active ($p<.01$, T=3.393 and 2.94, for ambulatory and nonambulatory movements, respectively) than the Veg. oil control group for ambulatory (407.6 $\pm$ 64 *vs.* 152.2 $\pm$ 16) and nonambulatory (141.8 $\pm$ 31 *vs.* 93.3 $\pm$ 16) movements.

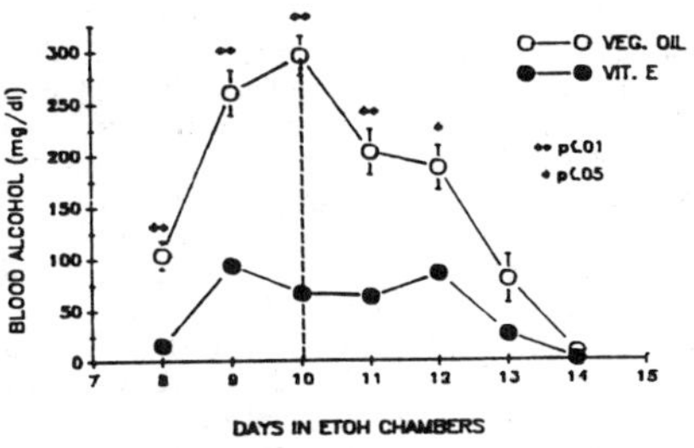

Fig. 1. ETOH chamber BAC.

Since there were significant differences between treatment groups in the ETOH inhalation chambers, we were interested in demonstrating that the efficacy of other volatile anesthetics were unaffected. Induction and recovery time for halothane anesthesia was assessed in two separate groups of rats (n=6/group) treated for 3 days prior to the test session with either VIT E or Veg. oil. Induction time was measured as the time difference between anesthetic administration and a demonstrated lack of reflexive response to tail pinch (using 8-inch locking forcep on second locking latch). Recovery time was assessed as the recovery of righting reflex after anesthetic removal. No group differences were found for either induction (120.3 $\pm$ 3.7 *vs* 105.17 $\pm$ 5.3 secs) or recovery (52.5 $\pm$ 1.9 *vs* 58.3 $\pm$ 4.1 secs) from halothane anesthesia between the VIT E and Veg. oil groups, respectively (T=1.13, 10 df, n.s.).

ETOH was administered intragastrically (i.g.) in a dose of 2 g/kg (20% w/v ETOH in distilled water) to two separate groups of rats (n=5/group) pretreated for 5 days with either VIT E or Veg. oil. Tail blood samples were drawn at the following time points after intubation: 5, 15, 30, 45, 60, 90, 120, 240 minutes. The peak of the resulting BAC occurred 30 mins post-intubation and resulted in significant differences between the VIT E (80.52 $\pm$ 4.3 mg/dl) and Veg. oil (127.14 $\pm$ 1.4 mg/dl) control groups ($p<.01$, T= 5.14, 8 df). Note that both i.g. and inhalation chamber administration of ETOH failed to increase blood levels above 100 mg/dl.

Figure 2 shows the resulting BACs for two similarly treated groups of rats (n= 10/group). After 5 daily pretreatments with VIT E or Veg. oil, animals were injected *intraperitoneally* (i.p.) with 2 g/kg (10% w/v). The time course of the BAC revealed significant group differences in blood ETOH at 5 out of 7 time points. Although statistically significant, the group differences in blood ETOH levels appear smaller in magnitude than with other routes of administration.

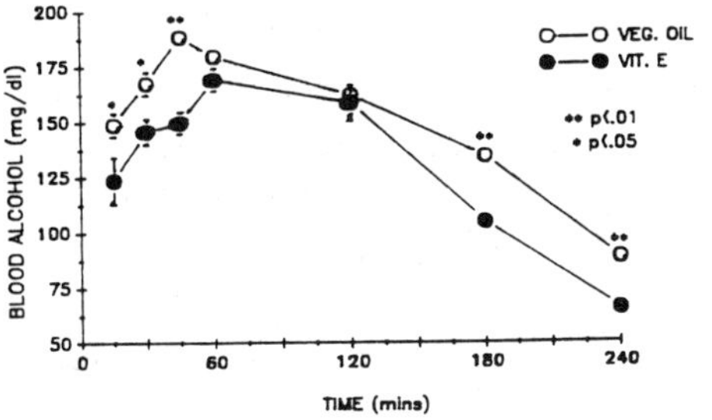

Fig. 2. ETOH i.p. injection BAC.

These results may be due to the limited pretreatment interval or VIT E dose administered compared to the total surface area available for ETOH absorption. It is possible that a longer pretreatment period, or larger doses of VIT E may have resulted in larger group differences. In order to further investigate the interactive effects between VIT E and ETOH we decided to treat rats that had been previously trained to discriminate ETOH (1.5 g/kg, i.p.) and saline in a two-lever operant task under a fixed ratio 10 schedule of food reinforcement. The drug discrimination task taps into the subjective properties of the drug in order to solve the discriminative task. A complete dose-effect function was generated after i.g. administration of a wide range of ETOH doses. On the training day prior to tests with VIT E and ETOH, each rat was pretreated with a total of 1.5 g/kg of VIT E (500 mg t.i.d.). Figure 3 shows the results of testing 2 and 4 g/kg ETOH in combination with VIT E pretreatments. Shifts to the right in the dose-effect functions of discriminative and rate-reducing properties of ETOH were demonstrated. This data clearly indicates a significant interaction between VIT E and ETOH when compared to a Veg. oil (control) pretreatment. The mechanism of action of this interaction is not known at present, but we believe these data are convincing evidence to support future research. The data more firmly supports the hypothesis that VIT E blocks (antagonizes) the absorption of ETOH into the vascular system (regardless of route of administration) rather than alterations in metabolism, for at least two reasons: 1) regardless of whether or not ETOH was administered via i.g. or inhalation routes, we could never quantify blood levels in the VIT E groups >100 mg/dl. If we could not record significant ETOH levels in the vascular system, we do not believe a metabolic mechanism could be hypothesized; 2) when significant elevations in blood levels (i.e. > 100 mg/dl, via i.p. administration) were achieved in the VIT E group, the slope of the declining limb of the BAC was not different from the Veg. oil control group, these lines were also parallel (Parallel Line Test) suggesting similar mechanisms of metabolism.

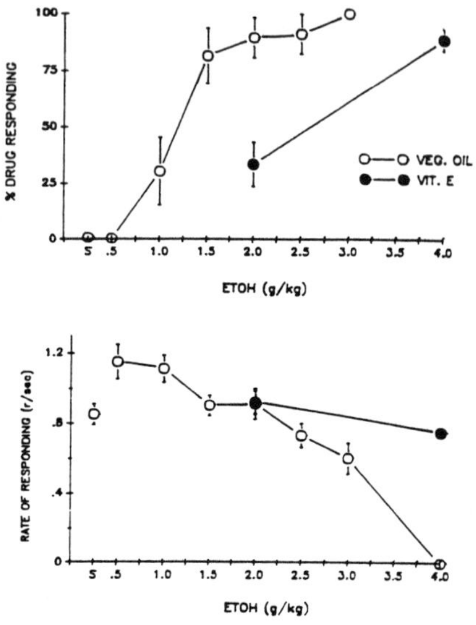

Fig. 3. ETOH's subjective and rate effects.

It is interesting to note the linkage between VIT E, membranes, and ETOH. VIT E interacts with arachidonic acid (AA) and increases cholesterol uptake into the lipid bilayer of membranes. AA increases lipid peroxidation, membrane permeability, and "order" of cell membranes (cultured cerebrovascular endothelium, Villacara *et al.,* 1989). AA is also the precursor for a number of biologically active substrates, the eicosonoids (prostaglandins). These links are important since they have been previously suggested to link ETOH with a wide range of behavioral, toxicological, and teratological events.

1.5 Acknowledgements

Supported in part by NIAAA 5T32 AA07222, 1R01 AA08338, and RO1 AA06351 to F.A. Holloway.

1.6 References

Diplock, A.T. (1983). In: *Biology of Vitamin E.* Pittman Books, London, pp. 45-56.

Diplock, A.T., & Lucy, J.A. (1973). *FEBS Lett.,* 79, 205-210.

Gauvin, D.V., Harland, R.D., Criado, J.R., Michaelis, R.C., & Holloway, F.A. (1989). *Drug and Alcohol Dependence,* 24, 103-113.

Gordis, E., Tabakoff, B., Linnoila, M, & Stimmell, B. (1989). *Alcohol Research from Bench to Bedside.* The Haworth Press, London.

King, D.A., Bouton, M.E., & Musty, R.E. (1987). *Behavioral Neuroscience,* 101(1), 104-114.

Nordman, R., Ribiere, C., & Rouach, H. (1988). *Alcohol Toxicity and Free Radical Mechanisms. Advances in the Biosciences,* Volume 71. Pergamon Press, Oxford, England.

Patel, J.M., & Edwards, D.A. (1988). *Toxicology & Applied Pharmacology,* 96, 101-114.

Pohorecky, L.A., & Brick, J. (1982). *Pharmacology, Biochemistry & Behavior,* 16, 693-696.

Porter, R., & Whelan, J. (1983). *Biology of Vitamin E.* Pittman Books, London.

Sun, G.Y., Rudeen, P.K., Wood, W.G., Wei, Y.H., & Sun, A.Y. (1989). In: *Molecular Mechanisms of Alcohol: Neurobiology and Metabolism.* Humana Press, Clifton, NJ.

Villacara, A., Spatz, M., Dodson, R.F., Corn, C., & Bembry, J. (1989). *Acta Neuropathol.,* 78, 310-316.

CHARACTERIZATION OF DSM-IIIr CRITERIA FOR UNCOMPLICATED ALCOHOL WITHDRAWAL: PROPOSAL FOR A DIAGNOSTIC INVENTORY AND REVISED WITHDRAWAL SCALE

E.M. SELLERS, J.T. SULLIVAN, G. SOMER, K. SYKORA*

Systematic studies to determine validity, reliability and limitations of the DSM-IIIr items to improve their clinical utility are needed (Knott et al, 1981; Shaw et al, 1981; Knott et al, 1981; Adinoff et al, 1988). We have studied the severity and frequency of the DSM-IIIr alcohol withdrawal items in a well characterized group of patients in alcohol withdrawal and from this analysis can propose both a simplication of the criteria and several approaches to their operationalization and clinical use (Sellers et al, 1990).

INTRODUCTION

The DSM-IIIr criteria for uncomplicated alcohol withdrawal (291.80) include the cessation of prolonged heavy ingestion of alcohol followed by coarse tremor of hands, tongue or eyelids plus at least one of nausea or vomiting, malaise or weakness, autonomic hyperactivity (elevated blood pressure, pulse or sweating), anxiety, depressed mood or irritability, transient hallucinations or illusions, headache, insomnia (APA, 1987).

METHODS AND RESULTS

The alcohol withdrawal syndrome was characterized in 137 patients using the 15-item Clinical Institute Withdrawal Assessment for Alcohol (CIWA-A), a scale of known reliability and validity (Shaw et al, 1981). The correlation of each DSM-IIIr item with CIWA-A total score and frequency distribution of scores were determined. Hand tremor, nausea or vomiting, headache, transient hallucinations, autonomic hyperactivity (pulse or sweating) and anxiety correlated with total score and distinguished among clinical severity ($r = 0.54$-0.27, $p < 0.001$). These items regressed on the original CIWA-A total scores (adjusted $R^2 = 0.84$, $p < 0.001$). Addition of "agitation" improves the correlation. The presence of two or more items diagnoses AW in 95% of patients. The number of positive items grades clinical severity "very mild" = 2, "mild" = 3, "moderate" = 4, "severe" = 5.

---

*The views expressed in this manuscript are those of the authors and do not necessarily reflect those of the Addiction Research Foundation.

DISCUSSION

Our study shows that increased hand tremor amplitude is very common in alcohol withdrawal of all severity and is typically present in moderate and severe withdrawal. Even though tremor amplitude varies considerably and hence some criterion variability will exist based on the ability to detect tremor size, of all the clinical features of withdrawal it is the most robust. However, the 95% confidence interval indicates that up to 9% of patients in moderate to severe withdrawal may score below 2 on tremor, and so tremor is best included as one of a number of criteria, rather than as a "gateway" criterion the way DSM-IIIr currently does.

Of the other clinical features anxiety and perceptual disturbances have quite high discriminant value. Only 5.1% and 19% of patients failed to have anxiety and perceptual disturbances respectively. A number of other DSM-IIIr items correlated with total CIWA-A score (pulse rate, sweating, nausea/vomiting, headache). However, no single item taken alone had a particularly high item total correlation. The original CIWA-A contains items which do not correlate with total score or contribute usefully, e.g. seizures, quality of contact, flushing of face, thought disturbances, and systolic or diastolic pressure (Sullivan et al, 1989).

Multiple regression of the DSM-IIIr items yielded an adjusted R^2 of 0.84 suggesting these items reasonably predict withdrawal severity. Addition of the agitation item from the CIWA-A further increased this to 95.6% inclusion rate and in R^2 of 0.89.

We would therefore suggest amended DSM-IIIr diagnostic criteria for uncomplicated alcohol withdrawal as follows: recent cessation of heavy drinking; two or more of the following clinical features not due to any other disorder: anxiety; increased hand tremor; transient auditory, visual or tactical disturbances; nausea or vomiting; headache; autonomic hyperactivity (sweating or pulse rate elevation > 100). In addition, the agitation item from the CIWA-A could be added since it correlated with total CIWA score and has measurement characteristics similar to nausea and transient perceptual disturbances. Agitation is also amenable to objective clinical observation. We have formalized these items into an Alcohol Withdrawal Diagnostic Inventory (AWDI) (Sellers et al, 1990) and an 8-item clinically useful instrument that converts the DSM-IIIr items into scores for tracking clinical severity over time based on experience with the CIWA (CIWA-AD). In our experience, such an instrument improves staff awareness of the elements of the clinical syndrome, helps structure clinical treatment decisions and is an essential component of clinical research.

REFERENCES

Adinoff B, Bone GHA, Linnoila M. Acute ethanol poisoning and the ethanol withdrawal syndrome. Med Toxicol 1988; 3: 172-196.

American Psychiatric Association. Diagnostic and Statistical Manual of Mental Disorders, Third Edition, Revised. Washington, American Psychiatric Association, 1987.

Knott DH, Lerner WD, Davis-Knott T, Fink RD. Decision for alcohol detoxication. A method to standardize patient evaluation. Postgrad Med 1981; 69(5): 65-78.

Sellers EM, Sullivan JT, Somer G, Sykora K. Characterization of DSM-IIIr criteria for uncomplicated alcohol withdrawal. Arch Gen Psychiatry, 1990 (in press).

Shaw JM, Kolesar GS, Sellers EM, Kaplan HL, Sandor P. Development of optimal treatment tactics for alcohol withdrawal. I. Assessment and effectiveness of supportive care. J Clin Psychopharmacol 1981; 1: 382-388.

Sullivan JT, Sykora K, Schneiderman J, Naranjo CA, Sellers EM. Assessment of alcohol withdrawal: The revised Clinical Institute Withdrawal Assessment for Alcohol Scale (CIWA-Ar). Br J Addict 1989; 84: 1353-1357.

ETHANOL EFFECTS ON CNS DOPAMINE RECEPTORS: IN VIVO BINDING FOLLOWING VOLUNTARY ETHANOL (ETOH) INTAKE IN RATS.

E. Vavrousek-Jakuba, C.A. Cohen, and Wm. J. Shoemaker

Activation of dopaminergic neurons in the nucleus accumbens (NAC) has been observed to occur after the administration of various drugs of abuse, including ETOH (1-4). It is unclear if dopamine is released during the anticipation (5) of the ETOH stimulus, after the drink is presented, actually consumed, or in any combination of the above. We have employed the in vivo D2-dopamine receptor binding technique (6) to investigate this question.

Results of Study 1: In vivo D2-dopamine receptor binding in NAC was decreased in rats given a single subcutaneous dose of amphetamine (AMPH).

To validate the use of the in vivo binding protocol as a way to assess activation of dopaminergic pathways in awake animals, NIH male rats were given a single subcutaneous injection of amphetamine (1 mg/kg as was used by DiChiara and Imperato, ref. 3) followed by an injection of 3H-raclopride (i.v., lateral tail vein, 10 uCi/rat) at three different time points. Based on the premise that endogenously released dopamine is available at the receptor site, we expected a decrease in the in vivo binding of 3H-raclopride in AMPH-treated animals. This decrease was presumed to be a result of the competition between the exogenous ligand and the endogenously released dopamine for the available receptor sites.

As illustrated in Figure 1, the specific binding was indeed lower in the NAC ($p < 0.05$) in the AMPH-treated animals, when AMPH was administered at the same time as the radioligand (0'-A group) or 20 minutes prior to the injection of the radioligand (20'-A group). The specific binding in the NAC in rats pretreated with AMPH 40 minutes prior to the injection of the radioligand (40'-A group) was not different from that of controls (0'-S). A similar trend in the effect of amphetamine on the binding of the exogenous radioligand was also observed in the CP region, but these changes did not reach statistical significance.

Results of Study II: Anticipation, as well as actual consumption of the expected ETOH drink (5% sucrose, 10% ETOH) resulted in the activation of dopaminergic neurotransmission in the NAC and CP.

Twenty Wistar male rats were trained to drink ETOH solutions during a single daily 30 min. session (5 days per week) utilizing a modification (7) of a sucrose fading procedure (8). Control rats (10 rats) received water in a similar bottle. For the rest of the day, all rats had an unlimited access to food and water.

Starting one week prior to the binding experiment, one wall of every animal cage was briefly swabbed, three minutes prior to the presentation of the drink, with a cotton swab saturated in 95% ETOH. This stimulus was introduced to provide an additional cue that the drink will be presented. On the day of the binding experiment, the ETOH drinking animals were divided into two groups. One group (E/E) received ethanol as expected, the other group (E/W) received water instead. The control group (W/W) received water as usual. All animals were injected with the radioligand 10 minutes after the presentation of the drink and were sacrificed 35 minutes later.

The data from the binding experiment are presented in Figure 2. Compared to the control group (W/W), a 25% decrease in the NAC and CP region specific binding was observed in both ETOH groups (E/E and E/W). This suggests that the anticipation of the ETOH containing drink may be as potent on dopamine activation as is the fulfilled expectation and/or actual consumption of the ETOH containing solution. It is of interest to note that while the experimental drink also contained 5% sucrose (in addition to 10% ETOH), 19 out of 20 rats trained to drink ETOH clearly preferred the ETOH containg drink over the one containing only 5% sucrose (Table 1).

FIGURE 1: The effect of a single subcutaneous dose of amphetamine on the in vivo D2-Dopamine receptor binding in the nucleus accumbens and caudate putamen

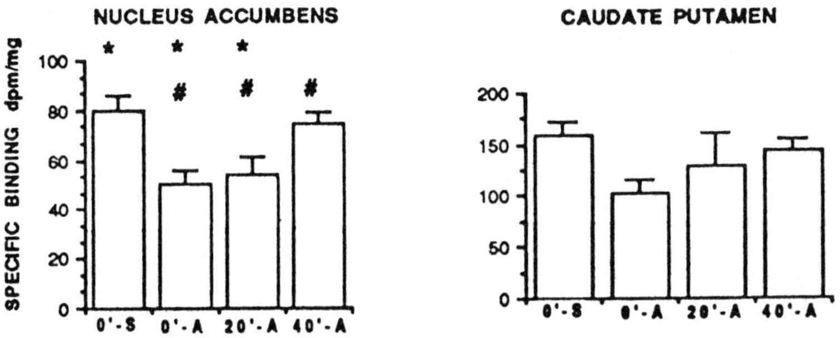

N:NIH male rats, about 200g, were used in this experiment. Amphetamine was administered subcutaneously in a dose of 1mg/kg body weight. Control rats received similar volumes of saline. All rats were sacrificed 20 minutes after the intravenous injection of ^{3}H-raclopride. Specific binding was calculated as the difference between the total radioactivity in the region/mg and that determined in cerebellum/mg. Results were analyzed by ANOVA followed by a post hoc range (SNK) test.

* Significantly different from control values and # signifcantly different from 40' amphetemine ($P < 0.05$). The nonspecific binding (cerebellum dpm/mg) was the same in all treatment groups. The four treatment groups compared in this experiments were: 0'-S= Controls given ^{3}H-raclopride immediately prior to saline injection (N=4), 0'-A= Given ^{3}H-raclopride immediately prior to amphetamine injection (N=5), 20'-A= Given ^{3}H-raclopride 20 minutes after amphetamine injection (N=5), 40'-A= Given ^{3}H-raclopride 40 minutes after amphetamine injection (N=4).

FIGURE 2: In vivo D2-Dopamine receptor binding in rats engaged or expecting to engage in drinking.

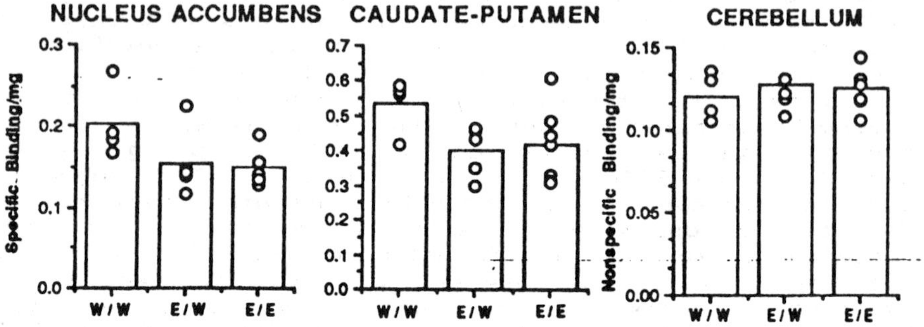

Wistar male rats, about 600g, were used in this experiment. The fluid consumption data (in g of fluid) on the experimental day were as follows: W/W: 0.3 g±0.1, range 0-0.9 g; E/W: 0.6 g±0.2, range 0-1.8 g; E/E: 5.0 g±0.6 range 2.6-7.9 g. Before statistical analysis, the complete data set were screened for technical errors and compliance with behavioral criteria. The behavioral criterion for the exclusion in the W/W group was inadvertant arousal (4 rats excluded). In the E/W group rats were excluded if they slept through, or showed an indifference after the presentation of the drink (4 rats). In the E/E group, the criteria for exclusion were either no consumption of ethanol drink, or a preference for sucrose in the prior choice test (1 rat). In addition two rats in each W/W and E/E group, and one rat in E/W group were excluded because of a technical error. This decreased the final number of rats from the original 10 to N=4 in the W/W group, N=5 in the E/W group, and N=7 in the E/E group. The binding data are expressed as % of dose x 10^{-3}

TABLE 1: Choice Test

Solution	Avg. Amt Consumed (g)	No. rats prefering each solution out of 20
Water	0.00	0/20
5% Sucrose and Water	0.84±0.29	1/20
5% Sucrose and 10% Ethanol	5.74±0.47	19/20

References
(1) Koob, G. and Bloom, F.E.: Science, 242: 715-723, 1988.
(2) DiChiara, G. and Imperato, A.: Eur. J. Pharmacol., 115: 131-132, 1985.
(3) DiChiara, G. and Imperato, A.: Proc. Natl Acad.Sci., 85: 5247-5278, 1988.
(4) Imperato, A. and DiChiara, G.: J. Pharmacol. Exp. Thera., 239: 219-228, 1986.
(5) Blackburn, J.R., et.al: Behav. Neurosci., 103: 15-23, 1989.
(6) Kohler, C., et.al: Biochem. Pharmacol., 34: 2251-2259, 1985.
(7) Gauvin, D.V., et.al.: Soc. Neurosci. Abs., 15: 28.9, 1989.
(8) Grant, K.A. and Samson, H.H.: Psychopharmacology, 86: 475-479, 1985.

Closing Remarks

Claudio A. Naranjo[1], *Edward M. Sellers*[2]

(1)Clinical Pharmacology Program, Addiction Research Foundation Clinical Institute, 33 Russell Street, Departments of Pharmacology and Medicine, University of Toronto, Toronto, Ontario, M5S 2S1, Canada.
(2)Psychopharmacology Research, Addiction Research Foundation Clinical Institute, 33 Russell Street, Departments of Pharmacology, Medicine and Psychiatry, University of Toronto, Toronto, Ontario, M5S 2S1, Canada.

Our intention in organizing this symposium was to provide a forum where researchers interested in discovering and developing new pharmacological treatments for alcoholism had an opportunity for exchanging ideas in order to identify priorities for focusing their research efforts during the coming years.

We have the impression that to a large extent we succeeded in achieving such goals. A number of important issues concerning methodology, mechanisms, clinical evaluation, and pharmaceutical and regulatory aspects were discussed. Some issues such as how the new knowledge on possible mechanisms regulating alcohol intake could be incorporated in the development and testing of a new drug were intensely debated. The need to standardize animal models and to test their predictive validity was emphasized. Of particular interest was the plea for a greater degree of collaboration among academics, pharmaceutical physicians/scientists and drug regulators. These efforts could be focused on a number of important projects in which there is a sufficient number of groups working in various aspects. With sustained efforts, progress is possible within the foreseeable future.

We hope that in a few more years this group and perhaps other new researchers will gather again to reassess progress. Only intense dialogue, collaborations and support from all the interested groups, will accelerate progress and innovation in this currently neglected therapeutic area.

Author Index